Everything
You Need to
Know about
Medical
Emergencies

Everything You Need to Know about Medical Emergencies

Springhouse Corporation
Springhouse, Pennsylvania

STAFF

Executive Director
Matthew Cahill

Editorial Director
Patricia Dwyer Schull, RN, MSN

Art Director
John Hubbard

Clinical Manager
Judith Schilling McCann, RN, MSN

Senior Project Editor
Kathy E. Goldberg

Clinical Project Manager
Helene K. Nawrocki, RN, MSN

Editors
Catherine E. Harold, Peter H. Johnson, Judith A. Lewis, Elizabeth Mauro, Andrew McPhee

Clinical Editors
Joanne Bartelmo, RN, MSN, CCRN; Stanley Nawrocki, RN, CEN; Beverly Ann Tscheschlog, RN

Copy Editors
Cynthia C. Breuninger (manager), Mary T. Durkin, Barbara Hodgson, Christina P. Ponczek, Brenna H. Mayer, Pamela Wingrod

Designers
Lesley Weissman-Cook (series designer), Joseph Clark, Amy Litz (book designer), Cindy Marczuk

Illustrators
Jacalyn Bove Facciolo, Robert Jackson, Judy Newhouse, Robert Neumann, Leonard Epstein, Eileen Rudnick, Frank Rubello

Production Coordinator
Margaret A. Rastiello

Editorial Assistants
Carol Caputo, Beverly Lane, Mary Madden, Jeanne Napier

Typography
Diane Paluba (manager), Joyce Rossi Biletz, Phyllis Marron, Valerie Rosenberger

Manufacturing
Deborah Meiris (director), T.A. Landis

This medical reference book shouldn't be used for self-treatment. It is not intended to be a substitute for emergency treatment by health care professionals. If you think you or someone you are with is having a medical emergency, call 911 or the telephone number for the local emergency medical service. However, be aware that some health insurance providers do not cover the cost of emergency care for certain medical conditions unless the person's primary care physician approves such care beforehand. To avoid problems with coverage, make sure you understand and follow your insurance company's policy regarding emergency care.

Printed in the United States of America

EYNKME-010896

Ⓡ A member of the Reed Elsevier plc group

Library of Congress Cataloging-in-Publication Data
Everything you need to know about medical emergencies.
    p. cm.
    Includes index.
    1. Medicine, Popular. I. Springhouse Corporation.
1997   96-69836
ISBN 0-87434-873-0   CIP

CONTENTS

ADVISORY BOARD

CONTRIBUTORS & CONSULTANTS

Diane Badsteubner, RN, Staff Nurse, Ambulatory and Recovery, Windham Hospital, Willimantic, Conn.

Charold L. Baer, RN, PhD, FCCM, CCRN, Professor, Clinical Knowledge Development Cluster, Oregon Health Sciences University, School of Nursing, Portland

Laura P. Barnes, RN, MSN, CNAA, Nursing Director of Critical Care Services, East Tennessee Children's Hospital, Knoxville

Ann Barrow, RN, MSN, CCRN, Clinical Editor, Springhouse Corporation, Springhouse, Pa.

Roxanne Aubol Batterden, RN, MS, CCRN, Nurse Educator, Critical Care and Medicine, Johns Hopkins Hospital, Baltimore

Jack M. Becker, MD, Chief, Allergy Services, St. Christopher's Hospital for Children, Assistant Professor of Pediatrics, Temple University School of Medicine, Philadelphia

John M. Bertoni, MD, PhD, Chairman, Department of Neurology, Creighton University, Omaha

Heather Boyd-Monk, RN, SRN, BSN, Assistant Director of Nursing for Education Programs, Wills Eye Hospital, Philadelphia

Thomas A. Brabson, DO, Emergency Physician, Emergency Department, Albert Einstein Medical Center, Philadelphia

Barbara Gross Braverman, RN, MSN, CS, Geropsychiatric Clinical Nurse Specialist, Abington (Pa.) Memorial Hospital

Lillian S. Brunner, MSN, ScD, LittD, FAAN, Nurse and Author, Brunner Associates, Inc., Berwyn, Pa.

Barry J. Burton, DO, Program Director, EMS Fellowship, Attending Physician and Faculty, Department of Emergency Medicine, Albert Einstein Medical Center, Philadelphia

Paul L. Carmichael, MD, Msc(Med), FAAO, FACS, Private practice, Ophthalmology, Lansdale, Pa.

JoAnn Coleman, RN, MS, CS, OCN, CRNP, Clinical Nurse Specialist, Gastrointestinal Surgery, Johns Hopkins Hospital, Baltimore

Robert B. Cooper, MD, Clinical Assistant Professor of Medicine, Assistant Attending Physician, New York Hospital-Cornell University, Medical Center, New York

Jerome M. Cotler, MD, The Everett J. and Marian Gordon Professor of Orthopaedic Surgery, Jefferson Medical College of Thomas Jefferson University, Philadelphia

Mary Helen Davis, MD, Associate Professor, Department of Psychiatry, University of Louisville, School of Medicine

Nancy B. Davis, RN, BSN, NP, CNOR, CRNFA, Nurse Practitioner-RN First Assistant, Cardiovascular and Chest Surgical Associates, P.A., Boise, Idaho

Brian B. Doyle, MD, Co-Director, Psychopharmacology Research Division, Director, Anxiety Disorder Program, Department of Psychiatry, Georgetown University School of Medicine, Washington, D.C.

Stephen C. Duck, MD, Associate Professor of Pediatrics, Northwestern University Medical School, Evanston (Ill.) Hospital

Nancy A. Dunbar, RN, Staff Nurse, Critical Care, Windham Hospital, Willimantic, Conn.

Maryann Foley, RN, BSN, Independent Consultant, Flourtown, Pa.

Terry Matthew Foster, RN, CEN, CCRN, Coordinator, Education Department, Clermont Mercy Hospital, Batavia, Ohio, Staff Nurse, Emergency Department, Saint Elizabeth Medical Center, Covington, Ky.

Susan Gauthier, RN, PhD, Associate Professor, College of Allied Health Professions, Department of Nursing, Temple University, Philadelphia

Roslyn M. Gleeson, RN,C, MSN, CS, APN, CRNP, Clinical Nurse Specialist, Pediatric-Spinal Dysfunction Program, Alfred I. duPont Institute, Wilmington, Del.

Kelly J. Henrickson, MD, Associate Professor of Pediatrics, Department of Pediatrics, Medical College of Wisconsin, Milwaukee

Marcia J. Hill, RN, MSN, Director of Nursing, Polly Ryon Memorial Hospital, Richmond, Tex.

Nancy M. Holloway, RN, MSN, Critical Care Educator, Nancy Holloway & Associates, Orinda, Calif.

Esther Holzbauer, RN,C, BS, MSN, Assistant Professor, Nursing, Mount Marty College, Yankton, S.Dak.

Kathleen Keenan, RN, MS, CCRN, NREMT-P, Clinical Nurse Specialist, R. Adams Cowley Shock Trauma Center, University of Maryland Medical Center, Baltimore

Lee Ann Kelly, RN, MS, PNP, Head Nurse, Antepartum-Postpartum, Hermann Hospital, Houston

Karen A. Landis, RN, MS, CCRN, Pulmonary Clinical Nurse Specialist, Lehigh Valley Hospital, Allentown, Pa.

Herbert A. Luscombe, MD, Professor Emeritus of Dermatology, Jefferson Medical College of Thomas Jefferson University, Philadelphia

Margaret E. Miller, RN, MSN, Oncology Head and Neck, Lung Clinical Specialist, Northwestern Medical Faculty Foundation, Chicago

Chris Platt Moldovanyi, MSN, RN, Nurse Consultant, Phillips and Mille Co., L.P.A., Middleburg Heights, Ohio

Roger M. Morrell, MD, PhD, FACP, Private practice, Neurology, Lathrup Village, Mich.

Helene K. Nawrocki, RN, MSN, Clinical Project Manager, Roslyn, Pa.

Stanley W. Nawrocki, RN, CEN, Staff Nurse, Emergency Department, Veterans Administration Hospital, Philadelphia

Steven J. Parrillo, DO, FACOEP, FACEP, Senior Faculty, Emergency Medicine Residency Program, Albert Einstein Medical Center, Philadelphia

Ara G. Paul, PhD, Dean Emeritus, Professor of Pharmacognosy, College of Pharmacy, University of Michigan, Ann Arbor

Rose Pinneo, RN, MS, Professor Emeritus, School of Nursing, University of Rochester (N.Y.)

Amy Perrin Ross, RN, MSN, CNRN, Neuroscience Program Coordinator, Loyola University Medical Center, Maywood, Ill.

Kristine A. Scordo, RN, Phd, Assistant Professor, College of Nursing and Health, Wright State University, Dayton, Ohio

Brenda K. Shelton, RN, MS, CCRN, OCN, Critical Care Clinical Nurse Specialist, Johns Hopkins Hospital Oncology Center, Baltimore

Harrison J. Shull, Jr., MD, Gastroenterologist, Vanderbilt University Medical Center, Nashville, Tenn.

Johanna K. Stiesmeyer, RN, MS, CCRN, Pediatric Asthma Educator, Loveless Health System, Albuquerque, Nursing Educational Consultant, Placidos, N.M.

Beverly Tscheschlog, RN, Independent Consultant, Ottsville, Pa.

Richard W. Tureck, MD, Professor of Obstetrics and Gynecology, University of Pennsylvania, Philadelphia

Naomi Walpert, RN, MS, CDE, Endocrine Clinical Nurse Specialist, Sinai Hospital, Baltimore

Fred G. Wenger, Jr., DO, FACOEP, Coordinator of Undergraduate Medical Education, Department of Emergency, Albert Einstein Medical Center, Philadelphia

Janette R. Yanko, RN, MN, CNRN, Neuroscience Clinical Nurse Specialist, Allegheny General Hospital, Pittsburgh

FOREWORD

You're driving along a country road. Suddenly, the car ahead of you swerves to avoid hitting a dog and crashes into a ditch. When you stop, you realize several people in the wrecked car have been injured. Do you know what to do?

You're wading in the surf, watching a group of children romp in the water. Suddenly one child's head disappears under the water and doesn't come up. As the adult nearest the drowning child, you pluck her from the water and carry her to shore. What should you do next?

You're at a wedding reception, watching couples dance to fast-paced music. Suddenly one of the people dancing, the bride's uncle, grabs his chest and collapses into a nearby chair. The bride rushes to his side, then calls to you, "Please, can you help?" Do you know how to respond?

Perhaps you've never encountered situations like these — but someday you might. Will you be prepared? Will you know how to prevent a bad situation from getting worse?

How this book can help you

Sooner or later, all of us experience — or see others around us experience — injuries or sudden illnesses. *Everything You Need to Know about Medical Emergencies* can help prepare you for just about any medical emergency you might encounter — at home, on the job, on the street, or anywhere else. The information it contains can help save a life, prevent permanent disability, or eliminate the need for a long hospital stay.

The latest helpful reference book from Springhouse Corporation, *Everything You Need to Know about Medical Emergencies* explains how to handle more than 200 medical emergencies. Writ-

ten for the general public, this comprehensive book offers information and advice you won't find in any other emergency book for consumers. It's written clearly and simply in everyday language you won't need a medical degree to understand. If you follow the instructions it provides, you won't feel helpless if you're ever confronted with a medical emergency.

The book has two main sections. The first tells you everything you need to know to cope with a vast range of medical emergencies — from allergic reactions and burns to head injuries, shock, and seizures. To help you find the appropriate information quickly, the emergencies are listed alphabetically. For each emergency, you'll find clear answers to these essential questions:

- What is this condition?
- What are the symptoms?
- What should I do?
- How is it treated?
- What else should I know?

You'll also find out how to set priorities. For some emergency conditions, a feature called "When seconds count," marked by a small picture, tells you which actions to take first to save the person's life.

But that's not all. Besides finding out what you should do, you'll learn what you *shouldn't* do in an emergency. This will help you avoid taking actions that could cause further injury — for example, moving a person who's suffered a spinal cord injury or giving the wrong antidote to someone who's been poisoned.

Besides this core information, you'll find many special features, each marked by a small picture. For instance, you'll find:

- *Prevention tips:* practical advice for preventing the emergency or its complications
- *How your body works:* easy-to-understand expla-

nations and illustrations of the parts of the body affected by the medical emergency

■ *Insight into emergencies:* why the emergency occurs and how it develops — clearly explained and often illustrated

■ *Especially for parents:* useful tips that will help parents prevent a child's emergency or cope with one that's already occurred

■ *Stories of survival:* inspiring accounts of rescues, told by family members, friends, and other witnesses.

The second section of the book explains how to perform a wide variety of emergency procedures, such as how to administer CPR, how to approach an injured person, and how to splint a broken limb. It also tells how you can prevent injuries at home, at work, and on the road.

Of course, this book can't replace the expertise of trained emergency-response personnel or the ad-vice of your doctor, nurse, or nurse practitioner. No book could. And even if someone receives the best emergency care available — even if you and other first responders do everything right — tragic things can still happen. But with the aid of *Everything You Need to Know about Medical Emergencies,* you can take comfort in those situations in knowing you did everything you could to help.

Injuries and sudden illnesses can strike at any time. That's why you can't afford to be without *Everything You Need to Know about Medical Emergencies.* An essential addition to any home library, this book provides useful, thorough information that isn't equalled by any other book for the general public.

Dr. Joseph A. Zeccardi
Director, Emergency Medicine
Thomas Jefferson University Hospital
Philadelphia

A

ABDOMINAL INJURIES

Abdominal injuries come from a blow to the stomach, back, or chest. These are called *blunt* injuries. The abdomen can also be injured by a penetrating object; when this occurs, the wound is called a *penetrating injury*. (See "Gunshot wounds" on page 265 and "Stabbing" on page 487.)

Even a blow fairly high in the chest can injure abdominal organs. (See *How a broken rib can injure the abdomen*, page 2.) Typically, blunt abdominal injuries occur during falls from heights, assaults, sports injuries, and car accidents. (See *Avoiding seat belt injuries*, page 3.)

Blunt abdominal injuries can be lethal if they damage major blood vessels or internal organs. Hemorrhage and shock are immediate life-threatening problems. Later, infection poses a risk.

How the damage occurs

A strike from a blunt object increases pressure within the abdomen. The blow can tear the liver and spleen, rupture the stomach, bruise the duodenum (the shortest portion of the small intestine), and damage the kidneys.

Damage to solid abdominal organs like the liver, spleen, and kidneys typically causes heavy internal bleeding. Damage to a hollow organ — the stomach, intestine, bladder, or gallbladder — causes the organ to rupture. Its contents then spill into the abdomen, where bacteria can cause infection.

What are the symptoms?

A person with a blunt abdominal injury may experience:
- severe pain
- nausea
- vomiting
- pale or bluish skin
- shortness of breath

Blunt abdominal injuries can be lethal if they damage major blood vessels or internal organs. Heavy bleeding and shock are immediate life-threatening problems.

How a broken rib can injure the abdomen

The abdomen includes more than just the stomach and intestines. It also contains organs that sit fairly high up in the chest, behind the ribs.

Chain of injuries

An abdominal injury can come from a blow to the back or chest as well as a blow to the stomach through a chain reaction. For example, a hard blow from behind can break a rib. The broken rib in turn can tear a kidney.

A dangerous weapon

A blow to the front of the ribs can break one or more ribs. The broken rib becomes a dangerous weapon within the body. It may slice into the liver or spleen.

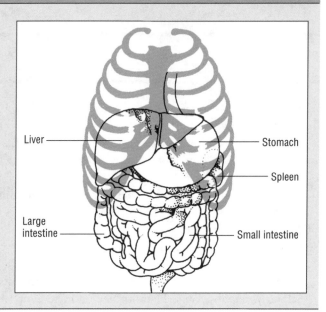

- rapid pulse
- rigid abdomen.

Sometimes the person goes into shock, with a fast pulse, light-headedness or dizziness, rapid breathing, pale skin, and sweating.

Other symptoms of a blunt abdominal injury vary with the organ that has been damaged.

Rib fracture can cause:
- sharp, severe chest pain, which gets worse when the person inhales or coughs
- shallow breathing
- shortness of breath
- cough
- tenderness and slight swelling at the fracture site.

Spleen injury can cause:
- pain in the left upper part of the abdomen
- spastic, rigid muscles
- left shoulder pain.

Liver damage can lead to:
- pain in the right upper part of the abdomen

- tender, rigid abdomen
- right shoulder pain.
   Stomach injury can cause:
- rapidly developing pain
- tenderness.
   Injury to the small intestine can result in brief pain and tenderness. *Pancreas injury* can cause a bloated abdomen.

What should you do?

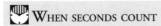 WHEN SECONDS COUNT

- Get immediate medical attention for someone who has suffered a blunt abdominal injury. Because the internal organs are hidden, you may not see outward symptoms. Even so, the person's life may be in danger from a ruptured organ or massive internal bleeding.
- While waiting for help to arrive, place the person in a comfortable position on his or her side. That way, if vomiting occurs, the person won't choke on the vomit.

⊗ Never move the person if you suspect an injury to the back, neck, or pelvis (hip area).

- Apply a clean or sterile dressing, if available, to any open wounds. If part of the intestine is exposed, apply a moist sterile or clean dressing over it.

⊗ Don't try to force a protruding part of the intestine back into the abdomen.

- If the pelvis seems to be injured, place a pillow or similar object between the person's legs and then tie the legs together. This will keep the pelvis still and help prevent further injury. Try not to move the person while tying the legs.

⊗ Be sure not to give the person anything to eat or drink.

How are abdominal injuries treated?

- The emergency rescue team makes sure the person is breathing, has a pulse, and has a clear airway. To help evaluate the person's condition, they try to find out how the injury occurred.
- In the hospital, the person receives emergency treatments like oxygen, intravenous fluids, and possibly a blood transfusion. If there's a

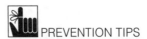 PREVENTION TIPS

Avoiding seat belt injuries

The simple act of fastening your seat belt correctly can improve your chance of escaping an abdominal injury if you are ever in a motor vehicle accident.

Fasten all restraints
If the vehicle has a shoulder harness as well as a lap restraint, be sure to fasten both. *Wearing only the lap restraint can actually cause abdominal injuries.*
   But make certain you've fastened the lap restraint the correct way. It should fall across your lap, *over your hip bones* — not across your stomach.

Watch for a seat belt bruise
If you have been in a motor vehicle accident and weren't wearing the shoulder harness, check for bruises across your abdomen. They may mean that you have hidden abdominal injuries. Get medical help at once — an internal injury may be life-threatening.

chance the abdomen was contaminated with bacteria from organ rupture, the person will receive antibiotics, too.

Assessing and repairing the damage

■ To determine which organs have been damaged, the doctor may order diagnostic tests, such as computed tomography (commonly called a CAT scan) to detect injury within the abdomen. The abdominal cavity may be washed out to detect free fluid or blood in the abdomen.

■ Sometimes a person needs immediate surgery to detect and repair the abdominal injuries. The person must also be monitored for symptoms of inflammation of the abdominal wall membranes, which can come from bacterial infection.

■ Even someone with few or no symptoms will be admitted to the hospital for observation because of the high risk of internal injury. Some abdominal injuries, such as delayed rupture of the spleen, may not become apparent for several hours or even days.

What else should you know?

A person who doesn't need surgery may be discharged after being observed in the hospital for several hours. To detect delayed symptoms of abdominal injuries, the person (and family members) should watch for and immediately report these symptoms:

■ fever
■ abdominal pain
■ loss of appetite
■ weakness
■ fatigue.

> *After the person is discharged, watch for and immediately report fever, abdominal pain, loss of appetite, weakness, or fatigue.*

ABDOMINAL PAIN

Abdominal pain can result from many conditions. Some are temporary and minor. Others demand emergency medical treatment. How can you tell when an abdominal problem needs attention — and what kind of attention it warrants?

Problems relating to abdominal organs can run the gamut from

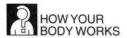

HOW YOUR
BODY WORKS

Looking at the abdominal organs

Your abdominal cavity contains much more than just your stomach. Abdominal organs and their locations are shown in this illustration. A problem with any of these organs can cause abdominal pain.

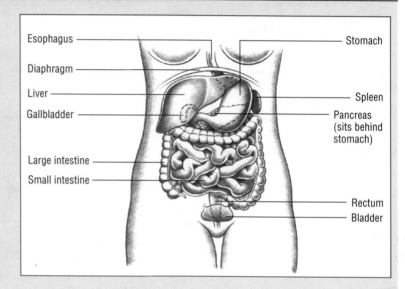

simple gas and indigestion to a long-term problem like stomach ulcer or gallbladder disease or a possible emergency like appendicitis, intestinal blockage, or poisoning. But you should suspect a medical emergency if:

- abdominal pain lasts 3 hours or longer
- the person has a fever
- the person vomits
- the pain is abnormal or unusually sharp or intense.

Where does the pain come from?
Most of us say we have a stomachache any time we have abdominal pain. But abdominal pain may have nothing to do with the stomach. Instead, it may originate in one of the many other organs in the abdominal cavity. (See *Looking at the abdominal organs.*)

What are the symptoms?
The person's symptoms may suggest the cause of the abdominal problem.

Symptoms of appendicitis

In this condition, the pain may start anywhere in the abdomen. Then it moves to the lower right side and may become constant. The person may feel sick, vomit, or have a slight fever. Eventually, the abdomen becomes rigid and increasingly tender.

Symptoms of ectopic pregnancy

This type of pregnancy occurs when a fetus grows in one of the tubes that carries the egg to the uterus (a fallopian tube) instead of in the uterus itself. The woman typically has pain in the lower abdomen. The pain may be constant or intermittent, and it may feel sharp, dull, or cramping. The woman may bleed from the vagina and experience nausea and vomiting. If the growing fetus ruptures the fallopian tube, she'll have severe lower abdominal pain that may spread to the shoulders and neck. She may become pale and sweaty and have a rapid pulse.

Symptoms of gallbladder disease

In this disease, a gallstone gets stuck in the tube leading from the gallbladder to the small intestine. The person has intense pain in the upper right part of the abdomen. The pain may begin suddenly or start out mild and steadily increase over several hours. Typically, it starts 1 to 3 hours after the person eats a fatty food like cheese or bacon. The pain may spread to the right shoulder, chest, or back. The person usually is pale and sweaty, feels sick, vomits, and has a fever and a tight, tender abdomen.

Symptoms of an abdominal aortic aneurysm

This rare condition is a life-threatening defect in the abdominal portion of a very large blood vessel called the aorta. One spot in the wall of the aorta becomes too thin, and the pressure of blood in the vessel pushes the weak spot out like a balloon. The vessel may rupture or bleeding may occur between the aorta's layers. This usually causes constant upper abdominal pain, which may worsen when the person lies down and improve when the person leans forward or sits up. An abdominal aortic aneurysm may also cause:

- dull pain in the abdomen
- low back pain
- severe chest pain.

Symptoms of a perforated ulcer

A perforated stomach ulcer typically causes sudden pain in the middle

of the upper abdomen, which may spread through the abdomen to the back. The abdomen may become as hard as a board. Usually, the person lies face down, protects the painful area, and breathes shallowly. Other symptoms may include:
- fever
- a rapid pulse
- grunting while breathing.

Other symptoms to watch for
In a *ruptured aortic aneurysm,* the person's skin below the waist may become mottled and cool because it's deprived of its usual blood supply. This condition requires immediate medical attention.

In an infant, a fever, cough, vomiting, diarrhea, or unusual or loud crying can mean a stomachache caused by a serious medical condition. (See *Is it just a harmless stomachache?* page 8.)

What should you do?

Get prompt medical attention for a person who has abdominal pain coupled with persistent nausea, vomiting, and diarrhea. Get *immediate* medical attention any time a person develops sudden, severe abdominal pain — especially if one of these additional symptoms is present:
- fever
- vomiting
- diarrhea
- vaginal bleeding
- pain lasting longer than 24 hours
- changes in pulse, breathing, or skin temperature
- rapid heartbeat
- light-headedness or faintness
- sweaty or clammy skin
- tense, rigid abdomen
- change in the pain's location or intensity
- relief from pain right after consuming a bland food like milk
- increased pain after eating fatty foods.

Make the person comfortable
Until emergency assistance arrives, help the person into the most comfortable position possible and encourage him or her to relax. Watch closely for changes in the person's condition.

Be sure to give the doctor or rescue personnel an accurate description of the pain and any other symptoms. Describe:
- the type of pain

A perforated ulcer typically causes sudden pain in the middle of the upper abdomen. The abdomen may become as hard as a board.

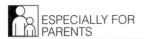

Is it just a harmless stomachache?

Like an adult's stomachache, an infant's stomachache usually isn't serious. But you *should* be concerned if your infant has a stomachache that lasts longer than 1 hour — especially if it's coupled with a fever, cough, headache, vomiting, or diarrhea.

Observe your infant
In an infant, abdominal pain can come from a serious underlying condition that requires prompt medical attention. Of course, an infant can't describe abdominal pain. So how do you know when it's there?

Observing closely is the key. Suspect abdominal pain if your infant points to the navel, bends the legs, draws the knees to the chest, or has any of these symptoms:
- unusual crying — especially if it's loud
- increased or odd-looking vomit or stools
- a hard or swollen abdomen.

When a stomachache means something serious
Infants can get several serious abdominal conditions that rarely affect older children or adults. Read on to learn about these conditions.

Intestinal problems
- *A twisted intestine.* This problem most often affects infants ages 1 to 12 months. Symptoms may include vomiting (look for greenish brown vomit), a hard and swollen abdomen, and bloody stools.
- *Sinking of a segment of the intestine into the cavity of another segment.* This condition usually arises in infants ages 8 to 18 months. The abdominal pain may come on suddenly, go away, and then suddenly recur. The infant's stools may be red and jellylike.

Other conditions
- *A strangulated hernia.* In this condition, part of the intestine or another abdominal organ pokes through an abnormal opening in the abdominal cavity, then becomes twisted or swollen. The infant with a strangulated hernia may vomit and seem irritable. You may be able to feel a lump in the scrotum, groin, or lower abdomen.
- *Narrowing of the stomach's lower opening.* Infants with this condition — usually boys ages 3 to 6 weeks — tend to vomit forcefully just after eating (called *projectile vomiting*).

Take immediate action
If you think your infant has any of these problems — or some other problem that's causing serious abdominal pain — get medical attention immediately. Don't give laxatives, enemas, drugs, food, or liquids (including water) until you talk to the doctor.

- when the pain started
- whether the pain occurs in other areas besides the abdomen
- whether the person has had the pain before.

Be as specific as possible. If the pain is intermittent, mention how long a typical episode lasts and whether it occurs after certain activities, such as eating or exercising.

Never give food or water to a person with severe abdominal pain.

Don't give a laxative or an enema.

 Be sure not to apply heat to the person's abdomen.

How is abdominal pain treated?

Treatment depends on the cause of the abdominal pain. The medical staff will probably need to identify the cause before trying specific treatments. Surgery will probably be done if the person has a disorder like:

- ectopic pregnancy
- appendicitis
- gallbladder disease.

What else should you know?

Many drugs can cause abdominal pain. Tell the doctor about any drugs the person is taking. Especially mention any antibiotics and laxatives because they can cause abdominal cramps and diarrhea.

ABUSE OF A CHILD

Child abuse is the physical, sexual, or emotional abuse or neglect of a child. A child can be abused by anyone he or she comes into contact with — a parent, other relative, teacher, family friend, babysitter, neighbor, or stranger.

Child abuse occurs among all socioeconomic and ethnic groups. It happens as often to boys as to girls, but girls are more likely to be victims of sexual abuse.

Types of child abuse

Physical abuse is an assault that involves bodily contact or injury. *Sexual abuse* occurs when an adult uses a child for his or her own or another adult's sexual stimulation. Sexual abuse can also happen when a child under age 18 sexually uses a considerably younger child or any child that he or she holds power over. An estimated 25% to 35% of women and 16% of men were sexually abused as children.

Child abuse occurs among all socioeconomic and ethnic groups. It happens as often to boys as to girls, but girls are more likely to be victims of sexual abuse.

Emotional abuse ranges from indifference to verbal threats that erode the child's self-esteem and security, causing fear or uncertainty. Such abuse can be as psychologically harmful as physical or sexual abuse. In fact, emotional abuse usually accompanies other forms of abuse.

Neglect is the failure to provide for a dependent child's basic needs — food, clothing, shelter, hygiene, medical care, and supervision.

What are the symptoms?

Child abuse can be hard to detect. The injuries that result from abuse can also occur by accident.

However, the child's physical condition, behavior, and family situation can hint at child abuse. (See *When a child's behavior suggests abuse.*)

Symptoms of physical abuse

If you suspect abuse, stay alert for:

- cigarette burns
- burns from being immersed in hot water
- broken bones
- head injuries
- injuries to the face
- adult-sized bite marks
- bald spots
- cuts
- abrasions
- welts
- genital injuries
- multiple bruises in various stages of healing. (See *How old is the bruise?* page 12.)

Be especially suspicious if the child's injuries are symmetrical, showing the same pattern on both sides of the body. Such a pattern seldom occurs naturally. Also, keep in mind that a child is most likely to be physically abused in the following sites in this order of frequency: buttocks, hips, face, arms, back, and thighs.

Check the bruising pattern

If the child has multiple bruises, the bruising pattern may suggest abuse. Here's why: When children fall, they usually get bruised on the knees, shins, forehead, nose, or other bony areas that stick out.

> *Child abuse can be hard to detect. However, the child's physical condition, behavior, and family situation can hint at child abuse.*

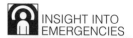
INSIGHT INTO
EMERGENCIES

When a child's behavior suggests abuse

If you think a child has been abused but you're not certain, observe the child's behavior carefully. Often, each type of abuse causes specific patterns of behavior in a child.

Physical abuse

Physical abuse includes hitting, kicking, punching, burning, tying up, or threatening with a weapon, such as a fist, knife, or gun.

Behavior clues

The child who has suffered physical abuse may:
- complain of pain
- refuse to let a doctor or nurse examine him or her
- move as if physically injured
- wear concealing clothing, even in hot weather
- avoid physical contact
- act either hostile and aggressive or timid and withdrawn
- try to cause self-injury
- stay away from home as much as possible
- run away from home.

Sexual abuse

Child sexual abuse may be committed by a family member, friend, or stranger. Rape is a violent form of sexual abuse.

Behavior clues

The sexually abused child may:
- sit or move gingerly
- show an obsession with his or her genitals
- have few, if any, friends
- seem afraid of physical contact
- know much more about sex than other children the same age
- seem introverted or depressed
- behave seductively

- have trouble falling asleep
- wet the bed
- have recently lost or gained a great deal of weight
- suddenly start doing poorly in school
- fear being alone
- show self-destructive or suicidal behavior
- seem unwilling to take part in sports, take a shower, or perform any activity that calls for changing clothes
- seem unusually concerned about siblings' safety
- try to avoid a certain person or certain people.

Emotional abuse

This type of abuse may take the form of excessive yelling, scolding, belittling, teasing, or criticizing. The child may be small for his or her age.

Behavior clues

The child who has been emotionally abused may:
- rock back and forth
- suck the thumb
- behave in a disruptive or destructive manner
- have nightmares, bedwetting, or other sleep problems
- abuse drugs or alcohol.

Neglect

A neglected child doesn't receive the basic love and nurturing necessary to develop into a productive member of society.

Behavior clues

The neglected child may:
- frequently miss school
- seem tired or fall asleep in class
- be accident-prone
- seldom smile or show emotion
- sleep poorly.

INSIGHT INTO EMERGENCIES

How old is the bruise?

A bruise isn't always a sign of abuse. But *multiple* bruises do suggest child abuse — especially if the bruises are in different stages of healing. The chart below can help you estimate the age of a child's bruises.

AGE OF BRUISE	APPEARANCE
0 to 2 days	Red and puffy
2 to 5 days	Blue to purple
5 to 7 days	Green
7 to 10 days	Yellow
10 to 14 days	Yellow to brown
14 days or older	Unblemished

Paddling, in contrast, can cause bruising on the buttocks, lower back, and lower thighs.

Some other injuries that suggest abuse include:
- bruising of the earlobes. This injury suggests the earlobes were pulled or pinched.
- upper arm bruises. These can come from being held tightly or grabbed forcefully.
- bizarre markings. These can result when a child is struck with such objects as a hot iron, a rope, or a belt buckle.
- round burns. These may come from cigarettes.

Symptoms of sexual abuse

The child who has been sexually abused may complain of pain or itching in the genital area or may have difficulty walking or sitting. Other symptoms include:
- tears or cuts in the genital or rectal area
- vaginal discharge or recurrent urinary tract or yeast infections in girls
- blood in stools
- torn, stained, or bloody underclothes.

The sexually abused child may have pain or itching in the genital area, difficulty walking or sitting, and tears or cuts in the genital or rectal area.

Symptoms of emotional abuse

If you think a child is being emotionally abused, be on the lookout for:

- speech problems
- slow physical development
- stomach pain, which could come from stress-related stomach ulcers
- asthma
- severe allergies
- substance abuse.

Symptoms of neglect

A child who has been neglected may have a swollen belly, teeth in poor condition, and rashes or other skin problems. Like an emotionally abused child, a neglected child may be small for his or her age. The child also may be:

- unusually dirty or smelly
- inappropriately dressed for the weather
- underfed or often hungry
- left alone without supervision for long periods.

What should you do?

If you suspect a child is being abused, call your local police, child protective services agency, or child abuse hot line. You can reach the National Child Abuse Hotline by calling 1-800-422-4453. To find the telephone numbers of local or state hot lines or the local child protective services agency, look in the telephone book. In many localities, you can find these numbers in the "Guide to Human Services" section (often called the "Blue Pages").

Those who come in contact with children in the course of their work are *required by law* to report child abuse. For instance, if you're a teacher, doctor, nurse, social worker, counselor, or police officer, you *must* report confirmed child abuse cases to state authorities. In some states, you must also report *suspected* child abuse.

If *you* are a child abuser, you can get help by contacting Parents Anonymous or a similar organization. (See *Help for the abused and the abuser*.)

How is child abuse treated?

Once child abuse is reported, your local or state child protective services agency will evaluate the situation. Then the agency may remove the child from the abusive household or take other action.

Help for the abused and the abuser

No matter how helpless an abused child or a child abuser may feel, various organizations exist to provide help. Read on for details.

Help for the abused child

If you're an abused child — or know of one — you can get help by contacting one of the organizations listed below. Or check the "Community Services" or "Guide to Human Services" section of your local telephone book.

- National Child Abuse Hotline: (800) 422-4453 (toll-free)
- National Committee for the Prevention of Child Abuse: (213) 663-3520

Help for the child abuser

If you're a child abuser, you can get help by contacting the groups listed below. Or check the "Community Services" or "Guide to Human Services" section of your local telephone book.

- Parents Anonymous: (800) 421-7616 (toll-free)
- Parents United: (408) 453-7616

What else should you know?

Keep in mind that what looks like child abuse to an outsider isn't necessarily abuse. Unless you have close, prolonged contact with the family, you probably can't know for sure that a child has been abused — no matter how strong your suspicions are.

Traits of abusive parents

An abusive parent's background and behavior may give hints. Many abusive parents share certain characteristics. For instance, they tend to:
- have frequent bouts of depression
- demand too much from their children
- have suffered abuse themselves as children
- feel insecure and unloved and look to their children to give them the support and comfort they want
- believe their children exist mainly to satisfy their needs
- consider their children's needs unimportant
- project their problems onto their children and then deal with their frustration with these problems by attacking the children.

ABUSE OF AN OLDER PERSON

Older people at greatest risk for abuse are frail, white Protestant women over age 75 who have multiple physical, mental, and emotional problems and depend on others for nutrition, safety, and toileting.

This form of abuse involves the neglect, physical abuse, or emotional abuse of an older person. Emotional abuse may include ridicule, insults, verbal humiliation, threats, and isolation from the rest of the family or from the community.

Abuse of older persons has reached alarming proportions. Estimates range from 700,000 to 1 million cases of mistreatment annually in the United States alone.

Who's at risk?

Many older people become dependent on others because of poor health or financial problems. This makes them especially vulnerable to abuse. Older people at greatest risk are frail, white Protestant women over age 75 who have multiple physical, mental, and emotional problems and depend on others for nutrition, safety, and toileting.

The greater the person's disability, the more vulnerable he or she is to abuse or neglect by caregivers. Usually, the abuser is a close relative, such as a spouse or an adult child. (See *What causes abuse of an older person?*)

The most dangerous day
The first day of the month is a particularly dangerous time for older people who live with adult children or other caregivers. They may be forced to sign over their Social Security checks or other retirement checks to the caregivers.

What are the symptoms?
The abused older person isn't always easy to identify. Many victims won't admit they're abused for fear that they'll lose their only means of support.

Also, symptoms that may hint at abuse can be misleading. For example, older people's skin is fragile, so injuries can occur with normal activity. Or a condition that suggests mistreatment may actually represent the progression of a disease.

But you *should* be suspicious if an older person has multiple bruises or cuts in various stages of healing — especially if the injuries are on the upper arms, back, buttocks, or thighs. Also note unusual hand or foot positions, rope burns, or bruising in the corners of the mouth. These symptoms can mean that the person has been restrained for a long time.

Other symptoms to watch for
The abused or neglected older person may also have the following symptoms:
- bed sores
- dehydration
- malnourishment
- puncture wounds
- welts
- broken bones
- oversedation, grogginess, or listlessness
- poor hygiene
- lack of needed medical attention
- fear of a family member or other caregiver.

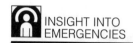

INSIGHT INTO EMERGENCIES

What causes abuse of an older person?

Not all experts agree on why an adult abuses an older person. Some believe that violence is a learned pattern in certain families and that people who were abused as children may later abuse their parents in revenge.

Outlet for stress?
According to another theory, the abusive person is under so much stress — for example, from a job or children — that he or she can't care for the older person properly and ends up abusing or neglecting the person.

What should you do?

If you suspect an older person is being abused — or if *you* are the victim of this abuse — call your local police, adult protective services agency, or elder abuse hot line. To find these numbers, look in your telephone book. In many localities, you can find these numbers in the "Guide to Human Services" section (often called the "Blue Pages").

Those who come in contact with older people in the course of their work may be *required by law* to report their abuse. For instance, if you work in a hospital, boarding house, or nursing home, you *must* report confirmed abuse cases to the authorities.

How is abuse of an older person treated?

An older person who's at risk for serious injury may be separated from the abuser by the adult protective services agency and placed with other relatives, friends, a shelter, or a nursing home.

What else should you know?

Often, abuse of an older person can be prevented by increasing his or her independence and relieving family tensions through respite care. Community resources can be a big help. Check your local telephone book for home health care agencies, visiting nurse or homemaker services, day-care programs, and respite care facilities. These services are geared to older people who function at various levels and can provide a social outlet to reduce their isolation.

Other sources of support

Welfare or family service agencies can provide additional support and may even offer financial aid. Other community resources, such as support groups for families of people with Alzheimer's disease, give family members a chance to share information and vent their frustrations.

If you suspect an older person is being abused, call your local police, adult protective services agency, or elder abuse hot line.

ABUSE OF A SPOUSE

Experts estimate that as many as one-third of Americans may be victims of abuse by their spouses or sexual partners. Spouse abuse can include not just physical battering but also verbal harassment, sexual abuse, social isolation, and home imprisonment.

The typical victim

Women are the classic victims of spouse abuse because they're usually physically weaker than men. Often, they're socially and economically dependent on them too. (See *Profile of the abusive man.*)

Sometimes the man is the abused partner. Like most abused women, most abused men are passive and have low self-esteem.

What are the symptoms?

The victim of spouse abuse may have frequent "accidents." Her clothes may be blood-stained, and she may seem anxious, panicky, and agitated. She may have difficulty sleeping and may have an eating disorder. And she may complain of physical ailments like:

- headache
- abdominal pain or upset stomach
- a choking sensation
- chest pain
- back pain
- joint pain
- muscle ache
- dizziness.

Physical injuries to watch for

Abuse may cause the following injuries:

- multiple bruises and cuts in various stages of healing on the face, neck, breasts, abdomen, back, and genitals
- broken bones
- dislocated joints
- cigarette burns
- rope burns
- other unusual or oddly shaped injuries.

Behavior clues

A person's behavior may suggest that she's being abused. Watch for:

- withdrawal, passivity, or indifference
- a belief that she brought the abuse on herself
- avoidance of eye contact
- frequent sighing
- crying or becoming tearful
- talking about someone she knows who's been abused.

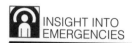 INSIGHT INTO EMERGENCIES

Profile of the abusive man

Men who abuse their partners commonly share several traits. Read on for the details.

Public image vs. private behavior

Many abusive men have successful careers. Some are sensitive, charming, affectionate, or seductive toward their partners in public.

However, in private they may abuse drugs or alcohol and, when alone with their partners, abusive men typically are:

- jealous
- possessive
- impulsive
- impatient
- angry
- intimidating.

A tendency to blame others

Many abusive men fail to recognize their behavior as inappropriate. Some feel threatened and demeaned by women. They may blame their partners for everything that goes wrong in their lives or may claim that their partners have betrayed them.

Childhood experiences

Many abusive men witnessed or experienced abuse while growing up. They may describe their fathers as weak and their mothers as domineering.

What should you do?

If *you* are the victim of spouse abuse, call the National Domestic Violence Hotline at 800-799-7233 for help. If you're in immediate physical danger, call the local police or an emergency number, such as 911. If you need to get to a shelter, look under "Women's shelters" in your telephone book. In many localities, you can find these numbers in the "Guide to Human Services" section (often called the "Blue Pages").

Taking legal steps

Be aware that spouse abuse may constitute assault and battery. Only the victim can bring charges. If you're being abused by your spouse, you may be able to obtain a restraining order from the local courthouse to keep the abuser away from you.

You can also contact the police after the abuse has occurred and file a report — even if you don't want to file criminal charges against your partner at the time. This documentation can be used as evidence for future legal actions, if necessary.

Helping someone else

If someone you know is the victim of spouse abuse, you can get advice by calling the National Domestic Violence Hotline at 800-799-7233. Or for the number of a local hot line, look in your telephone book.

How is spouse abuse treated?

Someone who's in immediate danger will need a suitable place to stay. If she can't stay with a relative or friend, a social service agency can help her find temporary housing. If all else fails, she'll be referred to a shelter for battered women.

A social service agency can also make the victim aware of community resources and the legal actions she can take. Although many victims return to the abusive partners after the immediate crisis, some are able to get out of the abusive relationship and stay with relatives or friends until they get back on their feet.

Getting counseling

Many victims of spouse abuse are referred for counseling, especially those who seem suicidal or have been subjected to prolonged abuse. If the abusive partner agrees to counseling, couple therapy might be

> *If you're in immediate danger of physical abuse, call the police or 911. To find a shelter, look under "Women's shelters" in the telephone book.*

recommended — but usually not until both partners have received individual therapy for several months.

What else should you know?

If an abused spouse decides to return to her abuser, you can't stop her. But you can help her develop a plan of action to use when abuse seems imminent or after it has occurred. Planning ahead will increase her chance of escaping to a safe place, with her children if she has any. Here are some steps you can advise her to take.

Decide where to go and how to get there

■ Choose a method of transportation. If she has a car, help her select a safe place to hide an extra set of keys. (Make sure she chooses a place her abuser won't find.) If she doesn't have a car, she can hide fare money and a bus schedule or the telephone number of a taxi company.

■ Choose possible destinations. Have her list the names and telephone numbers of people she can go to in an emergency. If she's unsure whether she can stay with someone, she can call from the hospital to double check. Also, help her list the addresses and telephone numbers of shelters in her area. She can hide the list with her taxi fare, bus schedule, or car keys.

Other important advice

■ Pack a few belongings. If possible, she should keep a few belongings at one of the "safe" homes on her list. Or, if she has a car, she can keep a change of clothes and a few personal items in the trunk, in case she needs to make a quick escape.

■ Save some money. Encourage her to start saving small amounts of money, if possible. She can keep the money in her hiding place.

■ Gather important papers. Help her make a list of important papers she'll need if she leaves home. She can hide these papers along with the items mentioned above.

■ Find someone who will call the police. Suggest that she confide in a neighbor, if possible, who can call the police if sounds of violence occur.

Encourage the abused spouse to start saving small amounts of money, if possible, and keep it in a special hiding place.

ALCOHOL INTOXICATION

Alcohol intoxication comes from drinking too much alcohol. Immediate risks of intoxication include impaired coordination and judgment, which can lead to accidents and injuries. Severe alcohol intoxication can be fatal.

Over the long term, alcohol abuse can cause permanent damage to organs and, eventually, death. (See *How alcohol damages the body.*)

A fetus whose mother drinks during pregnancy may be born with fetal alcohol syndrome. This condition can cause facial abnormalities, slow growth, and mental retardation.

How much is too much?
The amount of alcohol considered "too much" depends on a person's tolerance. Various factors affect tolerance, including:
■ gender — as a rule, men can tolerate more alcohol than can women
■ amount of body fat
■ amount of alcohol a person is accustomed to drinking.

Who's at greatest risk?
Young people drinking for the first time are at special risk for severe alcohol intoxication. That's because many are inexperienced drinkers and enjoy taking risks.

A fetus has much to lose, too, if the mother drinks during pregnancy. The infant may be born with fetal alcohol syndrome, which can cause facial abnormalities, slow growth, and mental retardation. The greatest risk to a fetus may come from alcohol use during the first 3 months — before the woman may even know she's pregnant.

What are the symptoms?
At first, the intoxicated person feels exhilarated. Later, he or she shows impaired speech, poor coordination, and poor judgment.

Sometimes nausea and vomiting are the first symptoms of intoxication. You may also notice a strong alcohol odor on the person's breath, along with slurred speech, swaying, and an unsteady gait. The person may be aggressive or violent.

Other symptoms to watch for
Severe alcohol intoxication can also lead to:
■ reduced body temperature
■ slowing or stoppage of breathing
■ seizures
■ coma.

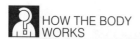

How alcohol damages the body

Habitually consuming too much alcohol is bad for the body in many ways.
- It damages the heart, lungs, liver, and digestive and nervous systems.
- It can make existing diseases worse.
- It can lead to or aggravate emotional and mental disorders.
- It can cause accidents. In fact, accidents that occur during intoxication account for many of the injuries seen in hospital emergency departments.

Heart and lung problems

Alcohol abuse can cause heart disease and predispose a person to lung disease. Alcoholics are at special risk for:
- irregular heartbeats
- chronic lung disease
- high blood pressure
- tuberculosis
- pneumonia.

Liver problems

Alcohol abuse may cause:
- alcoholic hepatitis, a type of liver inflammation
- cirrhosis, or widespread destruction of liver cells
- fatty liver, in which fats build up in liver cells.

Digestive problems

Alcohol abuse is responsible for many digestive disorders, including:
- long-term diarrhea
- cancer of the esophagus
- inflammation of the esophagus
- inflammation of the pancreas
- esophageal varices, or enlarged veins in the esophagus, which may bleed and cause death
- stomach ulcers and irritation
- bleeding in the digestive tract
- poor absorption of nutrients.

Nervous system problems

Long-term alcohol abuse can lead to:
- alcoholic hallucinations
- alcohol withdrawal delirium (also called delirium tremens, or "DTs"), which causes hallucinations, tremors, sweating, fever, and a fast pulse
- Korsakoff's syndrome, an irreversible memory impairment related to thiamine (vitamin B_1) shortage — a shortage caused by alcohol abuse
- seizures (convulsions)
- bleeding within the membranes covering the brain
- Wernicke's encephalopathy, a type of brain degeneration from alcohol-related thiamine shortage
- beriberi, a thiamine-shortage disease that can lead to paralysis, fatigue, diarrhea, swelling, and heart failure.

Mental and emotional problems

Long-term alcohol use is linked to:
- depression
- lack of motivation
- poor functioning at work and in social settings
- abuse of other substances, such as drugs
- suicide.

Other complications

Alcohol abuse can also cause:
- low blood sugar
- leg and foot sores
- inflammation of a man's prostate gland
- fetal alcohol syndrome (in newborns of alcoholics), which causes slow growth, mental retardation, and facial abnormalities
- potentially fatal interactions with drugs, even over-the-counter ones like Tylenol.

Sometimes the person seems alert but later doesn't remember events that occurred while he or she was intoxicated. These episodes, called *blackouts,* are serious warning signs of alcohol abuse that shouldn't be ignored.

What should you do?

 WHEN SECONDS COUNT

If the person is unconscious, check for a pulse and breathing. If you can't feel a pulse, can't see the chest rise or fall, and can't hear or feel the flow of air from the mouth or nose, it means the heart has stopped beating and the person isn't breathing. To avert death, have someone call for medical help immediately. Then start CPR, if you know how to perform it. *(See Performing CPR on an adult,* page 579.)

Also seek medical help promptly if a person passes out after heavy drinking and is difficult or impossible to arouse.

 Be sure not to let an intoxicated person fall asleep on his or her back.

Don't leave the person alone unless your safety would be at risk if you stayed.

What to do if the person is violent or hostile

If an intoxicated person seems violent or hostile, your priority is to protect yourself and others. Here are some ways to get the situation under control.

- Stay calm.
- Don't make threats.
- Limit eye contact.
- Listen attentively and respond with empathy.
- Ignore verbal abuse.
- Try to take the person's car keys.

Never try to intervene with a person who's hostile or violent. Instead, get to a safe place and call the police.

How is alcohol intoxication treated?

If the person lacks a pulse or isn't breathing, the emergency medical team will take steps to get the person's heart beating again and re-store breathing. To do this, they might try advanced life support methods, such as:

- inserting a breathing tube

Don't try to intervene if the intoxicated person seems violent or hostile. Get to a safe place and call the police.

■ giving emergency drugs

■ using such equipment as a defibrillator to get the heart beating again.

What else should you know?

In the hospital, a person with long-term alcoholism may be monitored for withdrawal symptoms or alcohol withdrawal delirium, sometimes called the "DTs." He or she may be referred to Alcoholics Anonymous (AA).

As the person tries to recover from alcoholism, health care workers may recommend that family members get involved in the person's rehabilitation. This can help reduce family tensions.

Help for the family

Family members can also turn to self-help groups — Al-Anon for spouses and Alateen for children of alcoholics. (See *If a loved one has a drinking problem*.)

ALLERGIC REACTION TO A BITE OR STING

An insect bite or sting can cause a severe allergic reaction called *anaphylaxis*. This life-threatening emergency leads to hives and breathing distress. Blood vessels may collapse, causing shock. Death can follow within minutes or hours of the sting.

The sooner the allergic reaction occurs, the more severe it will be. A delayed or persistent reaction may occur for up to 24 hours after the bite or sting.

What are the symptoms?

Typically, the person has feelings of impending doom or fright, along with:

■ hives

■ weakness

■ sweating

If a loved one has a drinking problem

If you need help coping with a loved one's drinking problem, here are some groups you can contact for assistance.

Help for family members

Al-Anon Family Group Headquarters
    P.O. Box 862
    Midtown Station
    New York, NY 10018
    (800) 356-9996
Alateen Family Group Headquarters
    P.O. Box 862
    Midtown Station
    New York, NY 10018
    (800) 356-9996
Mothers Against Drunk Driving (MADD)
    (800) 438-6233
Students Against Drunk Driving (SADD)
    (508) 481-3568

Help for alcoholics

If you're an alcoholic seeking help in recovering, contact:
Alcoholics Anonymous (AA) World Services
    P.O. Box 459
    Grand Central Station
    New York, NY 10163
    (212) 870-3400

- sneezing
- itchy, runny, or stuffy nose
- shortness of breath
- wheezing
- swelling of the face, neck, lips, throat, hands, and feet
- dizziness or light-headedness (from low blood pressure).

Other symptoms to watch for

Some people also have severe stomach cramps, nausea, diarrhea, urgent urination, and loss of bladder control. Some suffer irregular heartbeats or even go into shock.

Sometimes the respiratory system begins to fail. The person's throat begins to swell, and hoarseness, shortness of breath, and harsh, high-pitched breathing may occur.

Get medical help immediately if a person experiences a severe allergic reaction moments after being bitten or stung by an insect.

What should you do?

When seconds count

Get medical help immediately if a person has symptoms of anaphylaxis moments after being bitten or stung by an insect. Then check for a pulse and look, listen, and feel for breathing. If pulse and breathing are absent, start CPR, if you know how. *(See Performing CPR on an adult, page 579, Performing CPR on a child, page 585, or Performing CPR on an infant, page 590.)* Be aware that the person's swollen airway may make CPR difficult.

If the person has had a previous allergic reaction to an insect bite or sting, check for an anaphylaxis kit, and help administer the Adrenalin. (See *Using an anaphylaxis kit.*)

Keep the person quiet. If possible, help him or her to an upright position to make breathing easier. If dizziness, faintness, or nausea occurs, have the person lie down with the feet slightly elevated.

> Don't hesitate to call for medical help immediately if you suspect anaphylaxis.
>
> Be sure not to wait until an emergency occurs to familiarize yourself with an anaphylaxis kit.
>
> Never leave home without your anaphylaxis kit if you're allergic to insect bites or stings.

How is the allergic reaction treated?

The person must receive a shot of Adrenalin immediately to reduce

Using an anaphylaxis kit

If you have ever had a severe reaction to an insect bite or sting or another substance, you have probably obtained an anaphylaxis kit to use in an emergency. The kit contains everything you need to treat an allergic reaction:

- a prefilled syringe containing two doses of Adrenalin
- alcohol swabs
- a tourniquet
- antihistamine tablets.

If an insect bites or stings you, use the kit as follows. Also, notify the doctor immediately, or ask someone else to call.

Get ready

Take the prefilled syringe from the kit and remove the needle cap. Hold the syringe with the needle pointing up. Then push in the plunger until it stops. This will expel any air from the syringe.

Next, clean about 4 inches (10 centimeters) of the skin on your arm or thigh with an alcohol swab. (If you're right-handed, clean your left arm or thigh. If you're left-handed, clean your right arm or thigh.)

Inject the Adrenalin

Rotate the plunger one-quarter turn to the right so that it's aligned with the slot. Insert the entire needle — like a dart — into the skin, and push down on the plunger until it stops. It will inject 0.3 milliliters of the drug for an adult or a child over age 12. Then withdraw the needle.
Note: The dose and administration for babies and for children under age 12 must be directed by the doctor.

Remove the stinger

Quickly remove the insect's stinger if you can see it. Use a dull object, such as a fingernail or tweezers, to pull it straight out. Don't pinch, scrape, or squeeze the stinger. This may push it farther into the skin and release more poison. If you can't remove the stinger quickly, stop trying. Go on to the next step.

Apply the tourniquet

If you were stung on your *neck, face,* or *body,* skip this step and go on to the next one.

If you were stung on an *arm* or a *leg,* apply the tourniquet between the sting site and your heart. Tighten the tourniquet by pulling the string, as shown in the picture below.

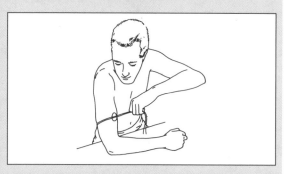

After 10 minutes, release the tourniquet by pulling on the metal ring.

Take the antihistamine tablets

Chew and swallow the antihistamine tablets. (For children age 12 or under, follow the dosage and administration directions supplied by your doctor or provided in the kit.)

What to do next

Apply ice packs, if available, to the affected area. Avoid exertion, keep warm, and see a doctor or go to a hospital immediately.
Important: If you don't notice an improvement within 10 minutes, give a second injection by following the directions with your anaphylaxis kit. If

(continued)

Using an anaphylaxis kit *(continued)*

your syringe has a preset second dose, don't depress the plunger until you're ready to give the second injection. Proceed as before, following the instructions to inject the Adrenalin.

Other instructions

■ Keep your kit handy to ensure emergency treatment at all times.

■ Ask your pharmacist for storage guidelines. Find out whether the kit can be stored in a car's glove compartment or whether you need to keep it in a cooler place.

■ Periodically check the Adrenalin in the preloaded syringe. If the solution is pinkish brown, it needs to be replaced.

■ Make a note of the kit's expiration date. Then renew the kit just before that date.

■ Dispose of the used needle and syringe safely and properly.

airway swelling. The shot is repeated every 5 to 20 minutes, as needed. If the person is conscious and has normal blood pressure, Adrenalin is injected into a muscle or under the skin. If the person is unconscious, the drug is given intravenously.

If the person's heart stops beating, treatment includes lifesaving measures like CPR. If the person goes into shock, treatment may include intravenous fluids and intravenous drugs.

Ensuring breathing

The person is also observed for symptoms of throat swelling, such as:

■ high-pitched breathing

■ hoarseness

■ shortness of breath.

If these symptoms occur, a breathing tube is inserted or the doctor may make an incision in the windpipe (called a *tracheotomy*) to permit breathing. Oxygen is given too.

Other therapy

Other therapy depends on how the person responds to treatment. After the severe emergency is over, the person typically receives other drugs, such as:

■ longer-acting Adrenalin to relieve breathing distress

■ steroids and Benadryl to ease breathing

■ Aminophyllin to treat airway spasms.

What else should you know?

Even if you don't know someone who's allergic to bites and stings, it's worthwhile to take the time and effort to learn CPR. People don't realize they're allergic until the first time they're bitten or stung.

ALLERGIC REACTION TO A DRUG

All drugs can cause side effects. But some people are extremely sensitive to one or more drugs and experience what's called an *antigen-antibody immune reaction*.

This drug reaction may take one of three forms:
- mild, possibly consisting solely of hives or a rash
- more severe, such as a fever and swollen glands
- life-threatening — a sudden, severe reaction called *anaphylaxis*. (See *How anaphylaxis occurs*.)

When distress may arise

A severe allergic reaction can produce physical distress within seconds or minutes after the person takes the drug. The sooner the reaction starts, the more severe it will be. Death may occur within minutes. A delayed or persistent reaction may occur for up to 24 hours.

What are the symptoms?

Typically, the first symptoms of anaphylaxis are:
- a feeling of fright or impending doom
- hives
- weakness
- dizziness
- light-headedness
- irregular heartbeats
- sweating
- sneezing
- shortness of breath
- wheezing
- itchy nose

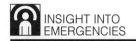 INSIGHT INTO EMERGENCIES

How anaphylaxis occurs

An anaphylactic reaction can occur only in someone who has been previously exposed, or sensitized, to the drug or other substance, called the *antigen*.

After this first exposure, the body produces antibodies that bind to receptors on special cells called *mast cells*.

Deadly chemicals

The next time the person is exposed to the antigen, an *antigen-antibody immune reaction* may occur.

Blood pressure crisis

This reaction triggers the release of powerful chemicals, which impair the person's circulatory system and drastically lower the blood pressure. Death may follow quickly.

- swelling inside the nose
- swelling of the face, lips, throat, hands, and feet
- swelling of the throat and airway, causing hoarseness, shortness of breath, and harsh, high-pitched breathing
- severe stomach cramps
- nausea
- diarrhea
- urgent urination
- loss of bladder control.

The person receives an immediate shot of Adrenalin to ease airway swelling. He or she may also need CPR, oxygen, and a breathing tube.

What should you do?

WHEN SECONDS COUNT

Get medical help immediately. Check the person for a pulse and look, listen, and feel for breathing. If pulse and breathing are absent, start CPR, if you know how. *(See Performing CPR on an adult,* page 579, *Performing CPR on a child,* page 585, or *Performing CPR on an infant,* page 590.)* Be aware that the person's swollen airway may make CPR difficult.

Keep the person quiet. Help him or her to sit upright to ease breathing. If dizziness, faintness, or nausea occurs, have the person lie down with the feet slightly elevated. If the person has an anaphylaxis kit, help give the injection.

Don't hesitate to ask someone to call for immediate medical assistance if *you* are experiencing a severe drug reaction.

Never leave home without your medical identification — and your Adrenalin — if you have a history of severe allergic reactions.

How is the allergic reaction treated?

The person needs an *immediate* shot of Adrenalin, which may be repeated every 5 to 20 minutes. This drug reduces swelling in the throat and airway. If the person hasn't lost consciousness and has normal blood pressure, the drug is injected into a muscle or under the skin. If the person is unconscious, it's given intravenously.

If the person's heartbeat and breathing have stopped, treatment includes lifesaving measures like CPR. If symptoms of shock occur, the doctor may order intravenous fluids and intravenous drugs.

The medical team also observes for symptoms of throat swelling — high-pitched breathing, hoarseness, and shortness of breath.

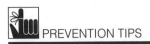 PREVENTION TIPS

How to avoid another episode of anaphylaxis

If you've had one anaphylactic reaction, no doubt you'll want to avoid a repeat. An obvious way to do this is to stay away from the drugs, foods, or other substances you're allergic to (called *antigens*).

Stay out of dangerous places
Avoid settings in which you're likely to encounter these substances. For instance, if you're allergic to insect bites or stings, avoid open fields and wooded areas during the insect season.

Of course, you can't completely avoid the possibility of being stung, so always keep an anaphylaxis kit on hand. The kit contains Adrenalin, an antihistamine, and a tourniquet.

Know your drug enemies
Some drugs are more likely than others to cause severe reactions. Knowing which drugs these are may save your life or that of a loved one.

Watch out for antibiotics
Penicillin and other drugs used to treat infection are common culprits. A person who's had a severe reaction to penicillin (or any antigen, for that matter) will react to this antigen in all forms. For example, if you've had an anaphylactic reaction to a penicillin tablet, you'll also have a reaction after a penicillin injection.

You must also avoid drugs derived from penicillin, like Amoxil, Geocillin, and Ticar, as well as cephalosporins. The latter group includes Ceftin, Keflex, Keflin, Mephoxen, and Rocephin.

Beware of other drugs
Other drugs that sometimes cause allergic reactions include:
- pain relievers, such as aspirin and ibuprofen (Motrin and Advil)
- water pills (diuretics)
- insulin
- serum proteins, such as gamma globulin
- vaccines — especially diphtheria, pertussis, and tetanus (DPT), given mainly to infants.

Get desensitized
What happens if you *must* receive a drug you're allergic to? Careful *desensitization* may help you avoid a severe reaction. In this treatment, the doctor either administers gradually increasing doses of the antigen or gives you steroids before administering the allergy-causing drug.

Take special precautions
If you know you're allergic to a certain drug or other substance, always wear medical identification jewelry or carry a card identifying your allergy. You can get more information by writing or calling:
Medic Alert
Turlock, CA 95381-1009
(800) ID-ALERT

Keep your doctor informed
Tell the doctor or nurse about any drug sensitivities or allergies you have. This is especially important if you're scheduled for diagnostic tests. The contrast dye used in some tests can trigger an acute allergic reaction in susceptible people.

If they develop, the person may need a breathing tube or an incision in the windpipe (called a *tracheotomy*) to permit breathing. Oxygen is given too.

Drug therapy
After the severe emergency is over, the person typically receives such drugs as:
- longer-acting Adrenalin to relieve breathing distress
- steroids and Benadryl to ease breathing
- Aminophyllin to treat airway spasms.

What else should you know?
Penicillin is a common cause of anaphylaxis. In fact, 1 to 4 of every 10,000 persons who take this drug get anaphylaxis. (See *How to avoid another episode of anaphylaxis,* page 29.)

ALLERGIC REACTION TO FOOD

Specific foods can cause allergic reactions in susceptible people. These reactions range from mild discomfort to life-threatening symptoms. Certain foods are more likely than others to cause allergic reactions. (See *Avoiding common food culprits.*)

The deadliest reaction
In *anaphylaxis*, the most sudden, severe allergic reaction, a person develops hives and breathing distress within a few minutes of eating the offending food. Then the blood vessels may collapse, and the person may go into shock. In fact, anaphylaxis can be fatal within minutes. However, a delayed or persistent reaction may occur for up to 24 hours. The sooner the reaction occurs after the food is eaten, the more severe it is.

What are the symptoms?
Typically, the person has feelings of impending doom or fright. Other common symptoms include:
- hives

In the most severe allergic reaction, a person develops hives and difficulty breathing minutes after eating the offending food. The person may go into shock and die within minutes.

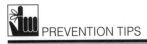

PREVENTION TIPS

Avoiding common food culprits

If you have food allergies, you'll need to be scrupulously careful about avoiding the foods that set off a reaction. Read on for advice.

Prime suspects
The following foods most commonly cause life-threatening allergic reactions:
- beans, including soybean products like tofu
- chocolate
- eggs
- fruit, especially strawberries and citrus fruits (including tomatoes)
- milk
- nuts and seeds
- seafood, especially shellfish.

Watch for food allergies in infants
Food allergies often start during infancy so, if possible, avoid giving these foods to your infant. Fortunately, many people outgrow food allergies.

Is mere avoidance enough?
If you have a food allergy, avoiding your food culprits may not be enough. You may have to prevent contact between these foods and other foods you eat.

Why? Some people can get severe reactions just from eating a food that *touched* a food they're allergic to. For instance, one teenager with a severe allergy to peanut butter nearly died from eating a chocolate candy simply because it had touched a peanut butter candy.

Keep safe and unsafe foods apart
Keep that cautionary tale in mind when storing, handling, and preparing food for yourself and others. For example, if your child has a severe allergy to peanuts, never dip the peanut butter knife into the jelly jar when making peanut butter and jelly sandwiches.

- weakness
- sweating
- sneezing
- itchy, runny, or stuffy nose
- shortness of breath
- wheezing
- swelling of the face, neck, lips, throat, hands, and feet
- dizziness or light-headedness (from low blood pressure).

Other symptoms to watch for
Some people also have severe stomach cramps, nausea, diarrhea, urgent urination, and loss of bladder control. Some suffer irregular heartbeats or even go into shock.

Sometimes the respiratory system starts to fail — a life-threatening condition that causes:
- swelling of the throat

- hoarseness
- shortness of breath
- harsh, high-pitched breathing.

What should you do?

 WHEN SECONDS COUNT

Call for medical help immediately. Then check the person for a pulse, and look, listen, and feel for breathing. If pulse and breathing are absent, start CPR at once, if you know how. (See *Performing CPR on an adult,* page 579, *Performing CPR on a child,* page 585, or *Performing CPR on an infant,* page 590.) If an anaphylaxis kit is available, help administer the Adrenalin. (See *Using an anaphylaxis kit,* pages 25 and 26.)

If the person is conscious, keep him or her quiet. If possible, help the person to an upright position to make breathing easier. If dizziness, light-headedness, or nausea occurs, have the person lie down with the feet slightly elevated.

How is the allergic reaction treated?

The person must receive a shot of Adrenalin immediately to reduce airway swelling. The injection may need to be repeated every 5 to 20 minutes. If the person is conscious and has normal blood pressure, Adrenalin is injected into a muscle or under the skin. If the person is unconscious, Adrenalin is given intravenously.

If the person's heart stops beating, treatment may include CPR. Someone who has gone into shock may receive intravenous fluids and intravenous drugs.

Ensuring breathing

The medical team also observes the person for symptoms of throat swelling — high-pitched breathing, hoarseness, and shortness of breath. If they occur, a breathing tube is inserted or the doctor may make an incision in the windpipe (called a *tracheotomy*) to permit breathing. The person also receives oxygen.

After the severe emergency passes, the person may receive these other drugs:
- longer-acting Adrenalin to reduce breathing distress
- steroids and Benadryl to ease breathing
- Aminophyllin to treat airway spasms.

If the person's throat starts to swell, a breathing tube is inserted or the doctor may make an incision in the windpipe to permit breathing.

What else should you know?

For a person who experiences a milder allergic reaction to food, the doctor may recommend an elimination diet to find out which foods are causing symptoms. First, the person eliminates the most likely food suspects. Then, if symptoms improve, each of these foods is put back into the diet, one at a time, in a form the person won't recognize. If symptoms then recur, the doctor presumes that the person is allergic to the food that has just been introduced.

Safe foods

Instead of an elimination diet, the doctor may put the person on a diet of relatively nonallergenic foods. Such foods include:
- rice
- spinach
- lettuce
- carrots
- beets
- lamb
- lemons
- pears
- grapefruit
- gelatin
- tapioca pudding.

An elimination diet can help identify which foods are causing symptoms. The most likely food suspects are eliminated from the diet first.

ALTITUDE SICKNESS

Altitude sickness can occur during mountain climbing or when traveling in an unpressurized aircraft. It's caused by the relatively low concentration of oxygen in the atmosphere at higher elevations. Typically, a person is susceptible to altitude sickness when traveling from near sea level to heights above 8,000 feet in less than 1 day.

Types of altitude sickness

Altitude sickness can take several forms:
- mountain sickness
- pulmonary edema — buildup of fluid in the spaces outside the lung's blood vessels
- swelling within the brain.

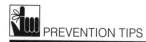
PREVENTION TIPS

How to avoid altitude sickness

If you're planning a trip to a higher elevation, sensible preparation and self-care can make the difference between a pleasant vacation and a disaster. Here are some guidelines to follow.

Get in shape

Get more exercise in the months or weeks before your trip to improve your physical condition.

Adjust your lifestyle

Don't drink alcohol during the trip — at least until you get used to the higher elevation.

Don't smoke at high altitudes, either. Smoking will put more stress on your already overburdened respiratory system.

Other instructions

■ If your trip will include mountain climbing, divide the climb into 2 days rather than 1. This will give your body time to adjust to the atmosphere.
■ Drink plenty of fluids. Being dehydrated increases your chance of getting sick.

What are the symptoms?

Any form of altitude sickness may cause a feeling of panic, chest pain, and tightness in the throat. Other symptoms vary with the form of the illness.

For instance, *mountain sickness* causes:

■ headache
■ confusion
■ shortness of breath on exertion
■ nausea
■ vomiting
■ diarrhea
■ extreme fatigue
■ decreased appetite
■ difficulty sleeping.

Pulmonary edema caused by high altitude produces some combination of these symptoms:

■ increasingly severe shortness of breath on exertion
■ inability to breathe deeply or comfortably except when sitting or standing
■ noisy, gurgling sounds when breathing
■ weakness
■ rapid pulse
■ persistent cough, which may be dry or produce frothy, bloody sputum.

A person with *brain swelling* caused by high altitude typically has these symptoms:

- increasingly severe headache
- rapid mood swings
- hallucinations
- muscle weakness
- uncoordinated movements
- confusion, possibly progressing to stupor or coma.

What should you do?

WHEN SECONDS COUNT

Check the person for a pulse and look, listen, and feel for breathing. If pulse and breathing are absent, call for medical help. Then begin CPR at once, if you know how. *(See Performing CPR on an adult, page 579 or Performing CPR on a child, page 585 or Performing CPR on an infant, page 590.)*

Get the person to a lower altitude and to a doctor or hospital as soon as possible. Provide oxygen, if available. Stay calm, and try to keep the person calm. Anxiety is catching, and panic can worsen shortness of breath.

How is altitude sickness treated?

Treatment depends on the severity of the illness. The person may receive a pain reliever for headache and anti-nausea drugs for nausea.

Someone with mountain sickness usually gets better with bed rest after being moved to a lower altitude. If the person chooses to stay at the higher elevation, it will take 1 to 3 days to get used to the reduced oxygen in the atmosphere.

With pulmonary edema, moving the person to a lower altitude should cause dramatic improvement. Typically, the person receives oxygen by mask.

As with other forms of altitude sickness, brain swelling usually subsides once the person reaches a lower altitude. The doctor may prescribe complete bed rest and oxygen administration. If these treatments don't bring improvement, intravenous steroids may be prescribed to reduce swelling.

What else should you know?

If you're planning to travel to a higher elevation, prepare yourself for the different atmosphere you'll encounter. (See *How to avoid altitude sickness*.)

AMPUTATION

Amputation occurs when a finger, a toe, an arm, or a leg is severed in an accident. Accidental amputation may be complete or partial. In *complete amputation,* the body part is totally severed from the body. In *partial amputation,* the body part remains connected to the body by soft tissue.

Accidental amputation usually results from an accident while operating factory or farm equipment, power tools, or a motor vehicle. At home, a person may partially sever a finger while using a knife or kitchen appliance. (Of course, a limb or part of one may be removed deliberately during surgery; this is called *surgical amputation.*)

The usual cause of accidental amputation is an accident involving factory or farm equipment, power tools, or a motor vehicle. At home, a person may sever a finger while using a knife or kitchen appliance.

What are the symptoms?
Amputation of a leg or an arm can quickly lead to heavy bleeding by damaging large blood vessels. Any type of amputation may cause:
- dizziness or light-headedness
- increased anxiety
- fast pulse
- rapid breathing
- pale skin
- loss of consciousness.

What should you do?

WHEN SECONDS COUNT
Get medical help immediately. Check the person for a pulse and look, listen, and feel for breathing. If the person isn't breathing and has no pulse, start CPR, if you know how. (See *Performing CPR on an adult,* page 579, *Performing CPR on a child,* page 585, or *Performing CPR on an infant,* page 590.)

While waiting for help to arrive, or if emergency medical services aren't immediately available, take the following steps.

Protect yourself
- Put on disposable latex gloves to guard against diseases that may be carried in the blood. If gloves aren't available, use a waterproof material, such as a plastic bag, plastic wrap, or several layers of gauze pads.

Try to stop the bleeding

■ Apply direct pressure with a clean or sterile dressing. (See *How to stop the bleeding*, page 38.) If the dressing becomes soaked with blood, don't remove it. Instead, place another dressing over it and press more firmly. Use your whole hand or both hands, if necessary. Continue to apply pressure until the bleeding slows or stops.

■ Elevate the injured part above heart level to help stop the bleeding. If possible, immobilize the part with a splint. You may need to improvise a splint using materials at hand, such as a wooden board, cardboard, a broom, rolled newspapers or magazines, a rolled blanket, a stick, an oar, an umbrella, or a pillow.

■ If the bleeding continues, apply pressure to a pressure point above the injury. A pressure point is a site over a bone where an artery lies close to the skin. For instance, if part of the arm has been severed, apply pressure to the brachial pressure point on the inside upper arm. To find this point, grasp the middle of the person's upper arm; then press your fingers toward your thumb, creating an inward force from opposite sides of the arm. (For more information on pressure points, see *Using pressure points to stop bleeding*, pages 76 and 77.)

Be sure to keep applying direct pressure as you apply pressure to the pressure point.

■ If the wound is still bleeding heavily despite pressure application, you'll need to use a tourniquet at a location slightly above the injury site.

✖ Don't loosen the tourniquet.

■ If the arm has been amputated at the shoulder, you won't be able to apply a tourniquet. Instead, apply firm pressure to the stump with dry gauze or your hand. When the bleeding stops, push the sterile gauze into the wound. Then place a folded towel over the wound. Wrap the towel around the person's body and tie over a pad under the opposite arm. Next, center a bandage over the padded wound. Wrap the bandage across the chest and behind the back and tie it under the opposite armpit, over a pad.

✖ Be sure not to cover the injured limb (for example, with clothing). It must be kept in plain view.

Preserve the severed part

■ Wrap the severed part in dry sterile gauze, a clean washcloth, or a towel.

■ Place the wrapped severed part in a plastic bag. Then put the bag

To help stop the bleeding, elevate the injured part above heart level. If possible, immobilize the part with a splint.

How to stop the bleeding

After an accidental amputation, the priority is to control bleeding from the person's stump. To do this, you must apply a snug dressing. Follow these instructions.

Apply a dressing

■ First, cover the end of the stump with gauze. Then position the stump in the center of a triangular bandage. The inside of the person's arm or leg should rest against the base of the bandage.
■ Bring the point of the triangle over the stump and then over the top of the injured arm or leg.
■ Then cross the ends over the fold of the bandage. Then bring the ends around the limb and cross them underneath.

Tie the ends together

■ Next, bring the ends of the bandage to the top of the limb and tie them together, as shown in the illustration below. Fold the point of the triangle over the knot and tuck it under.

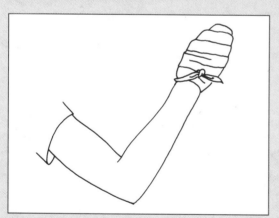

Elevate the limb

■ If the pressure dressing doesn't stop the bleeding, elevate the arm or leg. If the bleeding persists, apply pressure to a pressure point. (See *Using pressure points to stop bleeding,* pages 76 and 77.)

When and how to apply a tourniquet

As a last resort, you may need to apply a tourniquet to stop the bleeding. Follow these steps.
■ Get a bandage at least 2 inches (5 centimeters) wide to use as the tourniquet.

Position the bandage

■ Place the bandage just above the stump. Don't let it touch the stump edges. If the stump is in or just below a joint, such as the knee, elbow, or wrist, place the bandage just above the joint.
■ Wrap the bandage tightly around the limb twice. Then tie a half-knot.

Attach a stick

■ Place a short, strong stick or similar object on top of the knot. Then tie two more overhand knots on top of the stick.
■ Twist the stick to tighten the tourniquet until the bleeding stops.

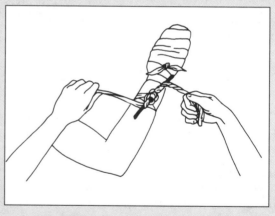

■ Secure the stick in place with the loose ends of the tourniquet, a strip of cloth, or similar material. *Don't loosen the tourniquet.*

Get medical help

■ Get the person to the hospital at once.

How to care for the severed part

The care the severed part receives in the first few minutes after an injury can mean the difference between successful reattachment and permanent loss of a body part. To improve the odds for successful reattachment, take the following steps.

Rinse the part
Rinse — don't scrub — the severed part with clean water. Don't use an antiseptic solution.

Wrap and pack the part
Wrap the severed part in dry sterile gauze or any other clean cloth that's available. Place the wrapped part in a plastic bag or a waterproof container, such as a glass or cup. Then put the bag or container on a bed of ice. *Don't bury it in the ice.*

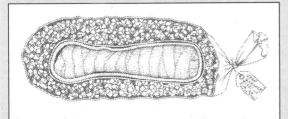

Get medical help
Get the person and the severed part to the hospital immediately.

Important precautions
■ Don't wrap the severed part in a wet cloth or dressing. This could cause the part to swell and soften, making reattachment more difficult.
■ Don't try to connect the severed part to the person's body — say, by cutting a small skin "bridge." Instead, place the part in a natural position and wrap it as described above.
■ Keep in mind that a severed part must be cooled right away. Otherwise, it probably won't survive longer than 6 hours. Even with proper cooling, it must be reattached within 18 hours.

in a plastic or foam-insulated container such as a cooler. Place a separate plastic bag filled with ice or ice water in the container, and rest the wrapped part on it to keep it cool. (See *How to care for the severed part*.)

⊗ Don't place the severed part under ice, in water, or on dry ice or formaldehyde.

⊗ Avoid covering the severed part directly with ice because this could cause frostbite. Usually, a frostbitten part can't be reattached.

⊗ Never decide that a severed part isn't worth saving. Let the doctor determine whether it can be reattached.

How is amputation treated?

The medical team takes steps to control bleeding and to replace lost blood and fluids. Then they consider reattaching the severed part. Thanks to advances in microsurgery, reattachment of severed body parts has become more successful. If reattachment or reconstruction is possible, the medical team tries to preserve usable joints.

If the injury has caused extensive damage to bone, tissue, or nerves in the remaining part of the limb, all or part of it may need to be amputated surgically. The surgeon creates a stump that will be fitted with a prosthesis, or artificial part.

What else should you know?

The prognosis for victims of accidental amputation has improved with modern medical management, advanced surgical techniques, early rehabilitation, better artificial limb fitting, and improved prosthesis design. But amputees still face problems, such as the inability to completely regenerate severed nerves and thus allow movement of body parts. That's why surgeons are seeking new methods for reattaching severed parts.

ARM PAIN

Arm pain may be sharp or dull, constant or intermittent. Sometimes the person can't move the arm or feel sensations as well as before.

Arm pain can come from many causes and take many forms. It can affect the entire arm or just the forearm or upper arm. It may come on suddenly or gradually.

What are the symptoms?

Symptoms of arm pain vary a great deal. For example, the pain may be:

- sharp or dull
- burning or numbing
- shooting or penetrating
- constant or intermittent.

Sometimes the arm looks deformed and the person can't move it or feel sensations as well as before.

What should you do?

If the person injured the arm in a recent accident, check for other injuries. If you suspect severe injuries, get medical help at once.

If you think that the arm may be broken, apply basic first aid, such as compresses and splinting. (See "Fractures [broken bones]," page 251.) Then elevate the arm and apply ice. Have the person see the doctor promptly.

> Don't give the person with a suspected arm fracture any drugs (including mild pain relievers like aspirin), and don't give anything to eat or drink.

If the person complains of pain in an arm that's already splinted, it may mean the splint is too tight. A tight cast or dressing can also cause pain by impeding circulation or movement in the arm. Have the person consult the doctor to correct the problem.

How is arm pain treated?

Treatment depends on the cause of the arm pain. For instance, a broken bone may be splinted, casted, or pinned. A strain or contusion requires anti-inflammatory drugs, such as aspirin. At first, cold compresses are used, then warm compresses.

What else should you know?

Besides broken bones, many disorders can cause arm pain. For example, such pain may mean angina — chest pain caused by heart disease. Usually, someone with angina also is short of breath and feels sweaty and apprehensive.

Sometimes arm pain is an extension of the chest pain caused by a heart attack. (See *When does arm pain mean a heart attack?*)

Other reasons for arm pain

Lifting weights too vigorously can cause arm pain by rupturing the biceps, a muscle in the arm. With this injury, the arm is usually weak, swollen, and deformed.

A muscle contusion, such as from a blow or bumping the arm, may cause widespread arm pain along with bruising and swelling. A muscle strain can cause mild to severe pain with movement. A tumor of the arm can cause constant, penetrating arm pain that gets worse at night.

In children, the most common causes of arm pain are broken bones, muscle sprain, muscular dystrophy, and arthritis.

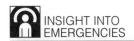 INSIGHT INTO EMERGENCIES

When does arm pain mean a heart attack?

Although arm pain is seldom an emergency, pain in the left arm or extending down both arms occasionally signals a heart attack.

What to do

Get medical help at once for a person who has left arm pain plus any of these other heart attack symptoms:

- deep, crushing chest pain
- weakness
- pale skin
- sweating
- nausea or vomiting
- fast pulse
- shortness of breath
- feeling of apprehension or impending doom.

ASTHMA ATTACK

Asthma is a lung disease that causes recurrent attacks, or episodes of troubled breathing. During an attack, small airways in the lungs called *bronchioles* overreact to certain types of stimulation (asthma triggers). The breathing passages then become inflamed and clogged, and the muscles around the bronchioles go into spasm. This restricts air flow in the respiratory system and makes breathing difficult.

Although asthma can occur at any age, about half of the cases are first diagnosed in children under age 10. (See *Coping with your child's asthma.*)

What are the symptoms?
Asthma typically occurs intermittently in the form of attacks. Between the attacks, the person may have few or no symptoms.

An attack may start dramatically, with many severe symptoms all at once. But sometimes the attack comes on slowly, with breathing gradually becoming more troubled. The person grows increasingly short of breath, with a worsening cough, wheezing, and chest tightness or some combination of these symptoms. The person may be unable to speak more than a few words without pausing for breath.

As the person exhales, you may hear wheezing or whistling. But don't expect to hear these sounds during a severe attack.

As the person exhales, you may hear wheezing or whistling. But don't expect to hear these sounds during a severe attack.

Typical position during an attack
Typically, the person sits up and leans forward during the attack, struggling to breathe. However, a child under age 2 may not assume this position and may not seem especially anxious. An infant may even lie on his or her back, smiling and playing with toys, despite the asthma attack.

Other symptoms to watch for
During an asthma attack, the person may also have:
- a fast pulse
- rapid breathing
- a choking sensation
- profuse sweating

An asthma attack may start dramatically, with many severe symptoms all at once. But sometimes the attack comes on slowly, with breathing gradually becoming more troubled.

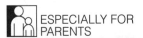

Coping with your child's asthma

Having a child with asthma can be a nerve-wracking experience. But the more you know about the condition, the more you can help your child gain some control over it. This will ease anxiety in all members of your family.

Learn about the condition
Try to find out what causes your child's asthma attacks, and then take steps to avoid these triggers. Also learn how to recognize the signs of an impending attack and what to do when an attack occurs. Ask the doctor or nurse to provide written material you can read at home.

Follow the treatment plan
To help prevent acute asthma attacks, teach your child to avoid asthma triggers, eat a well-balanced diet, and drink plenty of clear fluids — especially water. Make sure your child takes medicine exactly as prescribed. If the child is too young for self-administration, help him or her to take it.

Have your child exercise wisely
Make sure your child follows the doctor's advice about exercise. Although moderate exercise usually promotes good health, a child with asthma may need to avoid certain types of exercise. Also ask the doctor whether your child should take medicine before exercise to prevent an asthma attack.

Report drug side effects
Call the doctor if side effects of the medicine occur. If your child is taking Aminophyllin or Slo-Phyllin, report:
- nausea
- diarrhea

- vomiting
- fast pulse
- pounding heartbeat
- dizziness
- headache
- difficulty sleeping
- tremors
- rapid breathing
- flushed skin.

If your child is taking Orasone, report:
- acne
- purplish streaks on the skin
- pain in the back or ribs
- bloody or black, tarry stools
- vomiting
- easy bruising
- wounds that won't heal
- personality changes
- fever
- sore throat
- weight gain.

Stay calm during an attack
If your child has an acute asthma attack, *don't panic*. The calmer you are, the more active a role you can take in caring for your child. What's more, keeping cool and collected — and fighting off your child's anxiety — can mean a faster recovery for your child.

Many children can halt an acute attack by taking asthma medicine by inhaler. If the doctor has prescribed this treatment, have your child use the inhaler as soon as warning signs appear. If the attack doesn't start to subside, call the doctor and follow the instructions closely.

(continued)

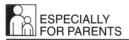

ESPECIALLY
FOR PARENTS

Coping with your child's asthma *(continued)*

Keep an upbeat outlook
Don't be gloomy about your child's health. Asthma doesn't cause permanent lung damage and is seldom fatal. And it won't prevent your child from living a full life — if you and your child accept the condition and work closely with the doctor, pharmacist, and other health care providers. Remember, Jackie Joyner Kersee has asthma, and she won an Olympic medal.

- exhaustion
- faintness
- restlessness
- agitation
- a cough (which usually sounds tight and dry).

What should you do?

Have the person rest, take prescribed asthma medicine (usually an inhaler), and sit up. (See *How to use an inhaler.*) If sitting upright proves uncomfortable for the person, try another position that eases breathing. Urge the person to relax as the medicine goes to work and to drink fluids to help clear the congested lungs. Often these measures alone will halt the attack.

If exercise seems to have caused the asthma attack, have the person sit down, rest, and sip warm water. This slows the breathing and opens the airways.

Don't force the person to lie down because this position could further hamper breathing.

When to call the doctor

If these measures don't ease the attack, call for emergency medical assistance at once and report all details of the attack. Try to calm the person, especially a child.

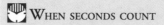 WHEN SECONDS COUNT

Get medical help at once if the person with asthma symptoms seems confused and sluggish, if the skin turns blue, or if the person pulls

How to use an inhaler

If you have asthma, the doctor will probably instruct you to take your prescribed asthma medicine with an inhaler. This device delivers a consistent amount of the drug into your lungs so that you receive the entire dose.

To reap the full benefits of your asthma medicine, you must use the inhaler correctly. Following these guidelines can make your drug therapy more effective.

Step 1: Remove the mouthpiece

Remove the mouthpiece and cap from the bottle. Then remove the cap from the mouthpiece.

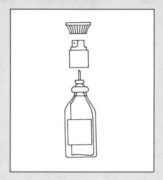

Step 2: Assemble the inhaler

Turn the mouthpiece sideways. Look for a small hole on one side of the flattened tip. To assemble the inhaler, fit the metal stem of the bottle into the hole.

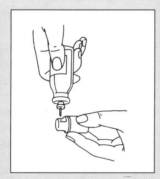

Step 3: Exhale through pursed lips

Exhale fully as you purse your lips. Then hold the inhaler upside down, as you see here. Close your lips and teeth loosely around the mouthpiece.

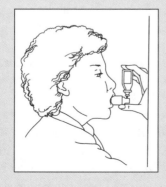

Step 4: Inhale and release a dose

Tilt your head back slightly. Take a slow, deep breath. As you do, firmly push the bottle against the mouthpiece *once* to release one dose of the medicine. Keep inhaling until your lungs feel full.

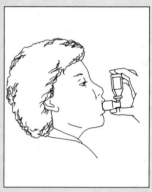

Step 5: Remove the mouthpiece

Remove the mouthpiece from your mouth, and hold your breath for a few seconds.

Step 6: Exhale through pursed lips again

Purse your lips and exhale slowly. If the doctor has instructed you to take more than one dose, wait at least 1 minute, and then repeat steps 3 through 6.

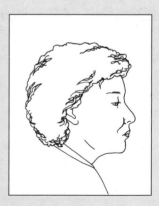

Step 7: Rinse your mouth

Rinse your mouth and gargle. Then drink a few sips of water.

(continued)

How to use an inhaler *(continued)*

Step 8: Clean your inhaler
Clean the inhaler every day. Take it apart and rinse the mouthpiece and cap under warm running water for 1 minute or immerse them in alcohol.

Shake off the excess fluid, let the parts dry, and then reassemble them. This helps to prevent the mouthpiece from clogging.

Using a holding chamber
Talk to your doctor about using the inhaler with a valved holding chamber, such as the Aero-Chamber. This device can help you use the inhaler more easily and effectively — especially during an acute asthma attack, when your lung power is reduced and your coordination may be impaired. Here's how to use it.

Step 1: Insert the mouthpiece into the chamber
Remove the protective cap from the inhaler and the mouthpiece of the chamber. Inspect the inside of the holding chamber for foreign objects. Then insert the mouthpiece of the inhaler into the holding chamber, as you see here.

Step 2: Place the chamber in your mouth
Shake the holding chamber and inhaler vigorously three or four times. Then place the chamber in your mouth and close your lips. Spray one puff from the inhaler into the chamber and start to inhale slowly.

Step 3: Inhale slowly and deeply
Keep breathing in slowly and deeply through your mouth until you've taken a full breath. (If you breathe in too quickly, the device will signal you by whistling.) Hold your breath for 5 to 10 seconds.

Step 4: Remove the inhaler from your mouth
Remove the inhaler from your mouth, exhale, and replace the protective cap on the holding chamber.

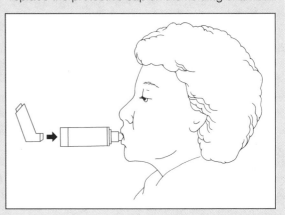

up the chin and shoulders to expand the chest and draw in air. These are signs of impending respiratory failure — a dire condition.

Be sure not to wait too long to get medical help. If the attack is severe and prolonged or if the person has a fever or chest pain, seek medical help immediately.

How is an asthma attack treated?
If the asthma attack doesn't stop, the person may need to be hospitalized. (See *"Not my kid!"*) Treatment may include drugs (for example, inhaled or injected beta-adrenergic agonists), oxygen, and

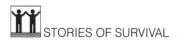

STORIES OF SURVIVAL

"Not my kid!"

My husband Darryl and I thought we were prepared to handle any emergency. I work in a doctor's office and have watched the nurses handle countless emergencies. And Darryl is one of those calm, cool, and collected types who never gets frazzled.

Asthma strikes

Then our toddler, Jamie, developed asthma. The doctor prescribed a nebulizer to keep Jamie's wheezing under control. The nebulizer sent medicine into Jamie's lungs through a mouthpiece shaped like an alligator's snout. He actually looked forward to his treatments.

The nebulizer seemed to be working so well that we thought Jamie might have outgrown his asthma. But one night, as we sat watching TV, Jamie began to cough and couldn't stop. "Mommy," he sputtered between gasps, "I...can't...breathe."

I can handle this

"OK," I thought, "I can handle this." I gave him another nebulizer treatment, 2 hours earlier than he was supposed to have it. Not only did the treatment not help, but Jamie seemed to get even worse.

Darryl wanted me to call the doctor, but I held off. I didn't want to bother someone I worked with; he might think I couldn't handle the crisis. Of course, he would have been right. How foolish I was.

Or can I?

I felt myself becoming more and more anxious and as a result, less able to make rational decisions. I didn't know *what* to do.

I pounded on Jamie's back the way I had seen visiting respiratory therapists do it to lung patients. I gave him cough medicine to try to stop the coughing. I even sat with him in the bathroom with the hot water running full blast to humidify his air. Nothing worked, and I was a wreck. Jamie still struggled to breathe.

Thank goodness for Darryl. He put his hand on my arm and said simply and quietly, "Marta, calm down. Jamie will be fine. Now, what would you tell a parent to do in this situation?"

Now I treat him like he's not my kid

I stopped in my tracks. "What would I tell a parent?" Why, of course — call the doctor. I should have done it long ago, I realized. But when your child is sick — not someone else's kid, but *yours* — you just don't make good decisions all the time.

The doctor told us to bring Jamie to the hospital right away. Two hours in the emergency room calmed Jamie's breathing — and my nerves.

Jamie's fine now, his wheezing better controlled than ever. And me? Well, I don't take asthma for granted any more. When Jamie has an asthma attack now, I take a deep breath myself and treat him like he's not my kid. What else can a good mother do?

AfterWords

Marta was right: She should have called the doctor sooner. Each year, thousands of asthmatics in the U.S. die because they don't seek help soon enough. When someone you know suffers an asthma attack that doesn't respond readily to home treatments, call the doctor — sooner, not later.

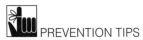

Avoiding asthma attacks

Asthma can't be cured, but it can be controlled. If you have asthma, following these guidelines may reduce the frequency of acute attacks.

Identify your asthma triggers

Try to identify — and avoid — the substances and conditions that cause your asthma attacks. The doctor can help you identify your asthma triggers. Common triggers include:

- pollen
- dust
- mold
- animal dander
- feathers
- insect parts
- certain foods, beverages, and drugs
- fumes and vapors
- cosmetic sprays, such as from perfumes and deodorants
- tobacco smoke
- car exhaust
- smog
- sudden temperature changes
- overexertion, such as from too much exercise or physical activity
- emotional factors like anxiety, stress, fear, anger, and laughing too hard.

Use drugs properly

Take prescribed asthma medicines regularly, exactly as the doctor has directed. A person with asthma may take:

- Nasalcrom, which prevents the allergic reaction that makes the throat close up
- Atrovent, which blocks the buildup of mucus in the airways
- bronchodilators, such as beta-adrenergics and Theo-Dur.

Many people also take steroids to reduce airway inflammation. Many asthma medicines are available as inhalers or nebulizers as well as in pill or liquid form.

Other instructions

If your asthma causes you to have trouble sleeping, don't take sleeping pills or sedatives because they may make your breathing slow or troubled. If coughing keeps you awake at night, prop yourself up on extra pillows.

Make sure the doctor knows about other drugs you're taking, including nonprescription ones.

Learn self-care

Become familiar with the warning symptoms of an impending asthma attack — coughing, chest tightness, breathing changes, and wheezing. If these symptoms occur, use your inhaler (if prescribed) to stop the attack from getting worse.

Then try to relax. Sit up in a chair, close your eyes, and breathe slowly and evenly. Start to tighten and relax the muscles in your body, beginning with your face. (Remember not to hold your breath while doing this.) First relax the muscles in your face, and then relax the muscles in your arms, hands, legs, and feet. Finally, let your whole body go limp.

Breathe through pursed lips

To regain control of your breathing, do the pursed-lip breathing exercises you've been taught. Be sure to keep your lips pursed as if whistling while breathing out slowly. Keep doing these exercises until you're no longer breathless. Don't gasp for air.

Lean forward to stop a coughing spell

To halt a coughing spell, lean forward slightly with your feet on the floor. Breathe in deeply and hold your breath for 1 or 2 seconds. Then, cough twice

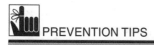
PREVENTION TIPS

Avoiding asthma attacks *(continued)*

into a tissue, first to loose mucus and then to bring it up.

If your asthma attack gets worse even after you've taken these steps, call the doctor.

Consider getting a peakflow meter
Talk to the doctor about using a peakflow meter to help control your asthma. This device measures the force with which you exhale — which declines during an asthma attack. By charting your peak flow, you can learn your baseline exhalation force. Then, if you notice it decreasing, you can take steps to prevent an asthma attack.

Other points to remember
■ Drink at least 6 eight-ounce glasses of water every day. This will loosen the secretions in your airways, helping you to cough them up.
■ Install air conditioning in your home and car.
■ On days when you're especially busy, rest often. Don't schedule more activities than you can tolerate.
■ Get moderate daily exercise, such as walking, swimming, or cycling. When used as part of an asthma management program, moderate exercise can help prevent asthma attacks.

intravenous therapy. If an infection is the suspected cause of the attack, the doctor may prescribe antibiotics.

Treating status asthmaticus
A person who doesn't respond to hospital treatments and still has blocked airways may be experiencing a life-threatening condition called *status asthmaticus.* This sudden, severe, prolonged asthma attack calls for aggressive drug therapy. Some people also need fluids, oxygen, and a special machine to aid their breathing.

Desensitizing treatments
If the person's asthma attacks seem to be triggered by a known substance (called an *allergen*), the doctor later may recommend that a small amount of the offending substance be given in a series of injections. This treatment helps to desensitize the person's immune response to the substance.

What else should you know?
Asthma can be extrinsic (caused by a source outside the body), intrinsic (caused by a source inside the body), or a combination of both. *Extrinsic (allergic) asthma* is caused by sensitivity to external substances that can cause asthma. Such substances include pollen,

animal dander, household dust or mold, feather pillows, and food additives containing sulfites. (See *Avoiding asthma attacks,* pages 48 and 49.) Extrinsic asthma usually starts during childhood and is accompanied by related disorders, such as eczema and allergies.

In *intrinsic asthma,* the allergen isn't obvious. Typically, a severe respiratory infection precedes an intrinsic asthma attack. Irritants, emotional stress, fatigue, harmful fumes, and changes in environmental temperature and humidity may worsen this type of asthma.

Other asthma triggers
Sometimes an asthma attack is brought on by ingesting aspirin, nonsteroidal anti-inflammatory drugs (such as Indocin), or the yellow food dye tartrazine. Exercise, too, can cause asthma attacks in some people; that's because heat and moisture loss in the upper airways can cause the throat to close up.

B

BACK PAIN

Nearly 80% of us experience back pain at one time or another. Back pain is second only to the common cold as a cause of time lost from work.

For some people, back pain strikes once, goes away, and never comes back. But others live with chronic back pain for years — or even decades.

The back is especially vulnerable to injury because of its structure, flexibility, and natural curve. Back pain usually strikes in the lower back, called the *lumbosacral area.*

Understanding the causes
Often, back pain comes from minor injuries like muscle sprain or strain. But just about any activity — especially bending, stooping, and lifting — can cause back pain or make it worse. (See *How to protect your back when lifting,* page 54.)

Other common causes of back pain include:
- herniated disk (often called "slipped" disk) — rupture of the disk, or cushioning structure, between two adjacent bones, or vertebrae, of the spine
- injury to the spine or spinal cord
- menstrual cramps
- osteoarthritis — a joint disease that causes stiffness and pain
- loss of calcium from the bones (osteoporosis).

Less common causes
Back pain sometimes results from:
- appendicitis
- kidney infection
- kidney stones
- inflammation of the pancreas
- tumor of the spine
- perforated ulcer
- growth outside the uterus of tissue usually found in the uterine lining (endometriosis)

Often, back pain is caused by minor injuries like muscle sprain or strain. But just about any activity can cause back pain or make it worse.

■ dissecting abdominal aortic aneurysm — ballooning of a section of the artery called the aorta, which may then rupture.

What are the symptoms?

Depending on the cause, back pain may be acute or chronic, constant or intermittent. It may affect only the back or may spread along the spine or down both legs. In some people, rest relieves back pain; in others, rest has no effect. Other symptoms may be present too.

Symptoms of a herniated disk

This disorder can cause either gradual or sudden low back pain. The pain may start in the back and spread to the buttocks and legs. Activity, coughing, and sneezing make the pain worse. Rest makes it better.

Symptoms of lower back strain

This injury causes aching back pain and tenderness, along with muscle spasm when the person moves to the side. Bending the spine makes the pain worse; rest relieves it.

Symptoms of appendicitis

Sometimes this life-threatening disorder causes pain in the back. Other symptoms may include nausea, fever, appetite loss, and vomiting.

Symptoms of endometriosis

This illness causes pain in the lower back, severe cramping pain in the lower abdomen and, in some people, constipation. The back pain gets worse just before or during menstruation.

Symptoms of a tumor of the spine

Cancer from another part of the body that spreads to the spine may produce low back pain. Typically, the pain starts suddenly, is accompanied by cramping muscle pain, and doesn't get better with rest.

Myeloma — a tumor that originates in bone — can cause back pain too. Usually, the pain starts abruptly and worsens with exercise. The person may also have fever, joint pain and swelling, and weight loss.

Symptoms of acute inflammation of the pancreas

Although this life-threatening condition usually causes pain in the upper abdomen, some people also have pain in the back and flank.

A "slipped" disk can cause gradual or sudden low back pain. The pain may start in the person's back and spread to the buttocks and legs.

Other symptoms include nausea, vomiting, fever, pale skin, and fast pulse.

Symptoms of a perforated ulcer

A perforated ulcer causes abrupt pain in the center of the abdomen, which may spread to the back. Other symptoms may include shallow breathing with grunting, fever, fast pulse, and dizziness.

Symptoms of a kidney infection

This disorder causes worsening pain in the flank and lower abdomen, along with back pain or tenderness, high fever, chills, nausea, vomiting, and frequent, urgent urination.

Symptoms of kidney stones

The person with this disorder typically has pain in the flank and pubic area. The pain may be excruciating if the stones travel down one of the tubes that carry urine from the kidneys to the bladder. If the stones are higher up in the kidneys, the pain is constant and dull.

Symptoms of a dissecting abdominal aortic aneurysm

This emergency may initially cause low back pain or dull abdominal pain. More often, though, it causes constant upper abdominal pain.

What should you do?

Anyone who has severe, persistent, or recurrent back pain should see a doctor.

WHEN SECONDS COUNT

Call for medical help immediately if the person has:
- acute, severe back pain that's not relieved by rest
- severe abdominal pain that spreads to the back.

Acute, severe back pain could mean a potentially fatal dissecting abdominal aortic aneurysm. Severe back pain that spreads to the abdomen may signal a perforated ulcer or acute inflammation of the pancreas.

Don't give the person with severe back pain anything to eat or drink, and don't give him or her any drugs.

To increase comfort, elevate the person's head and place a pillow under the knees. While waiting for the ambulance to arrive, urge

Call for medical help immediately if the person has severe back pain that's not relieved by rest or severe abdominal pain that spreads to the back.

How to protect your back when lifting

Bending or stooping to lift an object — or a child —is a common cause of back pain. If you already have back pain, these motions can make it worse. To avoid back pain and flare-ups, learn the right way to lift.

Step 1: Bend your knees
Keep your back straight, and bend your knees until you can comfortably hold the object you're going to lift.

Step 2: Straighten your knees while lifting
Lift by slowly straightening your knees, keeping your back straight and letting your legs bear the strain.

Take precautions
Be sure to test the weight of the object before lifting it, and get help if you need it.

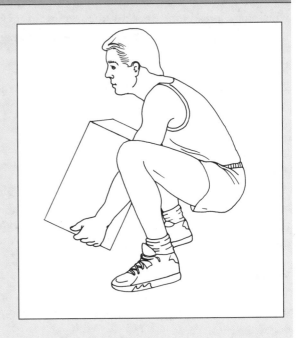

the person to take deep breaths or use another method to relax.

For less acute back pain, call the doctor. He or she may order blood tests and X-rays to try to find the cause of the pain.

How is back pain treated?
The treatment for severe back pain depends on the cause. A person with a dissecting abdominal aortic aneurysm, appendicitis, or a perforated ulcer must have emergency surgery.

Less acute or chronic back pain has no standard treatment. However, the doctor will probably recommend exercises, application of warm or moist heat, and cautious use of anti-inflammatory drugs like aspirin, Tylenol or other forms of acetaminophen, and Advil or other forms of ibuprofen.

What else should you know?
Here are some self-care measures that may ease chronic back pain:
■ Apply heat or cold to the painful area.

Exercises for chronic low back pain

If you have chronic low back pain, the exercises shown here may help you feel better. When doing these exercises, keep these tips in mind:

- Breathe in slowly through your nose, and breathe out slowly and completely through your mouth.
- Start gradually, doing each exercise just once a day at first. Then, every day do the exercise one time more than the day before, until you're doing it 10 times.
- Exercise moderately. Expect mild discomfort, but stop if you feel pain.

Doing a back press

Lie on your back with your arms on your chest and your knees bent. Press the lower part of your back to the floor while tightening your abdominal muscles and buttocks. Count to 10, then slowly relax.

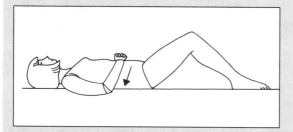

Doing a knee bend

Stand with your hands on the back of a chair for support. Keeping your back straight, slowly bend your knees until you're in a squatting position. Return to your starting position.

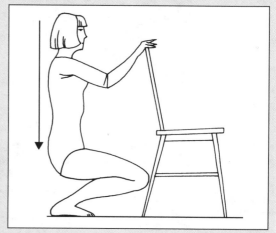

Doing a knee grasp

Lie on your back with your knees bent. Bring one knee to your chest, grasping it firmly with both hands. Then lower your knee. Repeat with the other knee, then with both knees, as shown here.

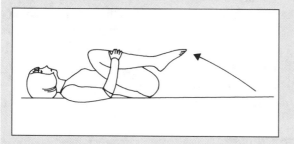

PREVENTION TIPS

How to avoid bee stings

Even if you're not allergic to bee stings, it makes sense to avoid attracting a bee's attention. Anyone can experience a swollen throat and difficulty breathing if stung in the throat. Here are some guidelines that can help you avoid getting stung.

Avoid becoming a target

- Don't wear fragrant cosmetics during insect season.
- Avoid wearing bright colors and going barefoot outdoors.
- Stay away from fruits and flowers that attract bees.
- Use insect repellent if you're planning to spend time outdoors.

Look before you sip

- Don't drink sweet beverages from a can outdoors, especially at the end of the summer, when bees are most aggressive.
- If you see bees landing on bottles or cans that contain fruit juice or some other sweet drink, warn others not to drink from them.

- Wear a corset or other lower back support.
- Sleep on a special mattress or backboard. To keep your spine straight, use a single flat pillow under your head (but not your shoulders) or no pillow.
- Take muscle relaxants, as prescribed.
- Place a pillow under your knees when resting in bed to increase comfort and relieve pressure on your back.
- Sit only in a firm, high-backed chair. Sit up straight, and keep your feet flat on the floor. If you must sit for long periods, use a cushion to support the small of your back.
- Learn the proper way to lift.
- Do back-strengthening exercises. (See *Exercises for chronic low back pain,* page 55.)

Alternative treatments

Some people also get relief from alternative methods, such as biofeedback and transcutaneous electrical nerve stimulation. Ask the doctor or nurse for more information on these techniques.

BEE STINGS

Although bee stings are usually harmless, they can be lethal to someone who is severely allergic to them. Unfortunately, most people with severe allergies aren't aware of them and so aren't prepared to treat themselves when they're stung. They can die within minutes of a single sting. (See *How to avoid bee stings.*) Even someone who isn't allergic can die if stung by hundreds of bees at once. Luckily, such massive multiple stings are uncommon.

Stinging insects include bees, wasps, yellow jackets, and hornets. (See *How to tell a bee from a wasp.*)

What are the symptoms?
Bee stings can be quite painful at first, causing tenderness, immediate swelling, and redness. The stinger may stick out of the person's skin.

People who are allergic to bee stings may experience a dangerous reaction called *anaphylaxis.* This reaction usually occurs within a few seconds to 20 minutes of the sting. (See *Recognizing warning signs of anaphylaxis,* page 58.)

Symptoms of anaphylaxis include:

- rash or hives
- dizziness
- weakness
- rapid breathing and pulse
- nausea and vomiting
- swelling of the face, neck, and tongue
- bluish or gray skin
- chest tightness
- closing up of the throat
- difficulty breathing or weak breathing with high-pitched sounds
- forceful coughing.

During anaphylaxis, some people are unable to cry, cough, or breathe. Breathing difficulty can lead to unconsciousness and seizures.

What should you do?

 WHEN SECONDS COUNT

If the person has hives or other symptoms of anaphylaxis, get medical help immediately. If a bee sting kit is available, read the directions and help the person inject the Adrenalin. Keep the stung body part below the level of the person's heart. (See "Allergic reaction to a bite or sting," page 23.)

Never ignore early symptoms of anaphylaxis.

Scrape the stinger off the skin with a credit card, your fingernail, or the blade of a knife.

Don't squeeze or pull on the stinger because you might inject more venom.

Important: If a friend or family member has had an anaphylactic reaction after a bee sting in the past, urge him or her to wear a medical identification bracelet and obtain a bee sting kit to use in an emergency. Encourage the person to learn how to use the kit *before* his or her life depends on it.

How to tell a bee from a wasp

How can you tell stinging insects apart? Here are some clues.

Bees: Heavier and hairier

Bees are heavier and hairier than wasps and yellow jackets.

The honeybee and bumblebee have rounded bellies, but the bumblebee (measuring about 1 inch [2.5 centimeters]) is longer.

Death after stinging

The honeybee and bumblebee have a lot to lose by stinging: they leave their stingers in their victims, then fly off and die.

Wasps and yellow jackets: Slender survivors

Wasps and yellow jackets have slender bodies and long abdomens. Unlike honeybees and bumblebees, they keep their stingers after they use them, so they can sting repeatedly.

PREVENTION TIPS

Recognizing warning signs of anaphylaxis

Normally, a bee sting is nothing to worry about. But if you or someone you're with is stung and then experiences any of the symptoms below, seek medical help immediately by calling 911 or your local emergency phone number.

Danger signs
- rash
- hives
- dizziness
- weakness
- flushed skin
- fast pulse
- rapid breathing
- swelling of the face, neck, lips, or tongue
- closing up of the throat
- bluish or gray skin
- forceful coughing
- wheezing
- abdominal cramps
- diarrhea.

What to do if the reaction is mild

Wash the sting site with soap and water, then apply ice for 15 to 20 minutes to prevent swelling. To ease itching and swelling, use an over-the-counter topical steroid cream, such as hydrocortisone. Relieve minor itching by applying a washcloth moistened with cold water. Give the person aspirin or Tylenol to relieve pain.

How are bee stings treated?

Someone with symptoms of anaphylaxis needs emergency treatment to restore breathing and circulation. In less severe reactions, the stinger is scraped off and the site is cleaned with soap and water. Then ice is applied for 15 to 20 minutes to prevent swelling.

Other treatments depend on the person's symptoms. The doctor usually prescribes antihistamines and corticosteroids to treat hives, aspirin or Tylenol to relieve pain, and a tetanus shot if the person hasn't had one recently.

What else should you know?

Bee stings to the mouth or eye are more dangerous than stings in other areas because facial swelling may make breathing difficult. Also, multiple stings usually cause more severe reactions than single stings. Now that the more aggressive Africanized ("killer") bees have reached the southern border states of the United States, the incidence of multiple stings is more likely to increase.

Bites from an animal

Although seldom fatal, animal bites do pose some danger. In the United States, about 60% to 90% of animal bites come from dogs; about 10% come from cats.

Dog bites commonly occur on the arms, legs, head, and neck. Cat bites usually aren't as serious as dog bites. However, cats' sharp teeth are capable of causing deep puncture wounds that damage muscles, tendons, and bones. Because these tissues have a limited blood supply, the risk of infection is greater than with dog bites — about 30% to 50%. A person who is *scratched* by a cat may develop an illness called cat-scratch fever. (See *What can you catch from a scratch?*)

When rabies is a threat

Many animals carry the rabies virus in their saliva and can transmit it by biting or by licking an open wound. Rabies is rare in the United States, but it's always fatal unless treated.

The risk of getting rabies from a dog is only 5% to 10%. Bats, skunks, and raccoons are responsible for nearly all rabies cases in the United States. (See *Protecting yourself from rabies,* page 60.)

What are the symptoms?

Dog bites may cause injuries ranging from bruises and superficial scratches to severe crush injuries, deep puncture wounds, and tissue loss. The person may have bleeding, pain, tenderness, swelling, and decreased sensation at the bite site. A large dog usually causes a more severe wound than does a smaller dog.

Cat bites cause small, deep puncture wounds.

What should you do?

A person who has been bitten on the face should get immediate medical attention.

Protect yourself

■ Before providing first aid for other bites, put on disposable latex gloves to guard against disease organisms that can be carried in the blood. If gloves aren't available, use a waterproof material, such as a plastic bag, plastic wrap, or several layers of gauze pads. Or, ask the person to help you by holding the bandages against the wound.
■ Immediately before and after you provide wound care, wash your hands with soap and water, if possible.

Wash, rinse, and dress the wound

■ If the bite isn't bleeding heavily (as with a puncture wound), wash the wound with soap and water for 5 to 10 minutes. Let it bleed a little to help flush out the bacteria.

 Don't scrub the wound — you could bruise the tissue.

■ Next, rinse the wound with running water under pressure. If Betadine antiseptic cleanser is available, dilute it with water and use it to rinse the wound.

What can you catch from a scratch?

About 3 to 10 days after being scratched by a cat, a person may start to show symptoms of a gland infection called *cat-scratch fever.*

How to recognize symptoms

Symptoms of cat-scratch fever include:
■ mild fever
■ tender, raised bumps on the skin
■ painful, swollen lymph glands
■ headache
■ extreme fatigue
■ reddened skin.

Disappearing act

No treatment exists for cat-scratch fever. It resolves on its own within several months.

PREVENTION TIPS

Protecting yourself from rabies

Suspect an animal has rabies — and stay away from it — if it shows these symptoms:
- excessive salivation
- uncoordinated movement
- unusually aggressive or docile behavior
- other abnormal behavior; for example, a nocturnal animal like a raccoon appearing in your backyard in the daytime.

Help capture the animal
If you suspect the animal is rabid, try to locate its owner. If it's a wild animal, try to determine its location.

Then call the police or animal control department, who will try to capture the animal. After it has been captured, it will be observed for rabies.

Important precautions
- Don't approach any animal that shows symptoms of rabies.
- Don't try to catch a potentially rabid animal by yourself.
- Don't kill the animal. Let the appropriate authorities examine it.
- Don't touch a dead animal. You could be infected by its tissues or saliva.
- Never try to touch a wild animal — especially a raccoon — and warn children not to go near one. Be aware that rabid animals may seem tame because the illness can make them docile.

Help prevent the spread of rabies
To keep your household pets safe from rabies, have them vaccinated. Also, be sure to keep their immunization schedule up to date.

■ To control bleeding, apply pressure with dry, sterile gauze. Cover the gauze with a sterile gauze dressing. Then seek medical attention.

How are animal bites treated?
Animal bites on the face call for immediate medical attention; the person may need stitches.

All bite wounds and scratches are washed thoroughly with soap and water. The person may also need a tetanus-diphtheria shot. Depending on the wound location, the person may need surgery to repair damage.

Checking for rabies
If you witnessed the animal bite, tell authorities where the incident occurred and the name of the animal's owner. If it was a wild animal, tell them the animal's location at the time of the bite.

Authorities will try to capture the animal and then confine it for

10 days of observation. If it appears rabid, it will be killed and its brain tissue tested for rabies.

Who needs rabies shots?
If the animal can't be found or identified, or if it's found to be rabid, the person will need to get a series of rabies shots. These shots aren't as painful as they used to be since a new vaccine was introduced in the early 1980s.

What else should you know?
In North America, dog vaccinations have significantly reduced the risk of rabies. Bites from wild animals — such as skunks, foxes, raccoons, and bats — account for 70% of all rabies cases.

The risk of developing rabies is highest if the bite is on the face (60%). A bite on the leg carries a 10% risk.

BITES FROM A HUMAN

More people are bitten by human beings than by any other animal except dogs and cats. Human bites can cause severe injury to the skin, the soft tissues under the skin, and even the blood vessels.

In fact, human bites are more dangerous than any other mammal bites. Why? The human mouth contains a multitude of bacteria and viruses that can infect humans, including herpes simplex virus, cytomegalovirus, syphilis, and tuberculosis. (See *Can you get AIDS from a bite?* page 62.)

The human mouth contains a multitude of bacteria and viruses that can infect humans. That's why human bites are more dangerous than any other mammal bites.

What are the symptoms?
Bleeding from a human bite may be scant or profuse. If the bite also causes a puncture wound or tear, bleeding occurs right away and bruising and swelling arise later.

Other symptoms to watch for
If the bite isn't treated promptly, infection can occur. Symptoms of infection include:

■ pus

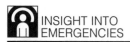

Can you get AIDS from a bite?

Authorities don't know of anyone who has gotten AIDS from a bite.

However, if you've been bitten by someone who tests positive for the human immunodeficiency virus — the virus that causes AIDS — get tested for the virus immediately and again 3 and 6 months later.

- swelling
- redness.

What should you do?

Seek immediate medical attention for a human bite that breaks the skin. Such a bite may transmit bacteria or a virus, causing infection.

Protect yourself

■ Before providing first aid, put on disposable latex gloves to guard against diseases that may be carried in the blood. If gloves aren't available, use a waterproof material, such as a plastic bag, plastic wrap, or several layers of gauze pads. Or, ask the person to help you by holding the bandages against the wound.

■ Just before and after you provide wound care, wash your hands with soap and water, if possible.

Wash, rinse, and dress the wound

■ If the wound isn't bleeding heavily, wash it with soap and water for 5 to 10 minutes to help prevent infection. Then rinse it with running water.

Never scrub the wound because you could bruise the tissue.

Be sure not to put an antiseptic or a home remedy on the wound unless the abrasion is on the surface and doesn't break the skin. For such an abrasion, apply an over-the-counter antibiotic ointment, such as Baciguent or Polysporin.

■ Next, apply pressure to stop the bleeding. Cover the wound with sterile gauze and a bandage.

■ Make sure the person gets prompt medical attention for more wound cleaning, antibiotics and, possibly, a tetanus shot and stitches.

Don't tape the wound or seal it in any way. Doing so increases the chance of infection.

How are bites from a human treated?

If the bite has broken the skin, the medical team evaluates the extent of the injury. Then they clean and rinse the wound again. They may also collect some drainage from it for a wound culture to determine which bacteria may be present.

The doctor may cut away dead tissue, especially for a hand wound.

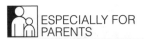

Coping with your child's biting

At different ages, children bite for different reasons. Your child may be either the biter or the victim.

When a baby bites
Babies bite when teething or when exploring objects. Once a baby's teeth start to come in, don't allow the baby to bite you.

Discourage biting during breast-feeding
Biting and breast-feeding can be a painful combination. Discourage your baby from biting your breast. Don't laugh or make loud noises if your baby bites you — he or she might think biting is entertaining and repeat it for amusement.

Instead, immediately stop breast-feeding. Place your finger between the baby's mouth and your breast to break the seal, if necessary. Withholding your breast will help teach your baby not to bite.

If a bite from your baby breaks the skin on your breast or nipple, seek medical attention.

When a toddler bites
Toddlers bite when teething and to vent feelings of aggression. A child age 16 months doesn't understand that biting hurts the other person.

Break the biting habit
If your toddler bites another child, firmly say "No" and temporarily separate him or her from other children. With your guidance, by the time the child is a preschooler, he or she will understand that biting other people isn't acceptable.

When a school-age child bites
A school-age child shouldn't be expressing aggression through biting. But if your child *is* doing this, find out why and seek help in handling the cause.

Inform authorities
If your child is bitten, seek treatment for the bite. If the incident took place at school, be sure to notify the school authorities.

When an adolescent bites
If your teenager bites someone in a fight, seek professional help for your child in managing anger or in nonviolent conflict resolution. Also, find out if the school, your church, a local hospital, or a community group offers courses in handling aggression.

Seek treatment
If your teenager is the victim of a bite, don't hesitate to have the bite treated.

A wound on the face may require stitches. Other treatment may include antibiotics and a tetanus shot to help prevent infection.

What else should you know?
Because most bites occur during a fight, hand bites are most common. (See *Coping with your child's biting*.) These bites are especially dangerous because they can cause infection and permanent paralysis of the hand or fingers.

The worst type of hand bite is the clenched-fist injury, which happens when the fist strikes the teeth. This bite often causes:

- a cut over a finger joint
- a broken bone
- a dislocation
- tendon damage.

BITES FROM AN INSECT

Besides transmitting diseases, insect and spider bites can cause respiratory failure and death.

At the very least, insect and spider bites can be annoying. At worst, they can cause respiratory failure and death. What's more, many insects and spiders can transmit diseases. For example:
- the mosquito can transmit malaria
- the wood tick and dog tick can transmit Rocky Mountain spotted fever
- the deer tick can transmit Lyme disease. (See *How to recognize ticks and spiders.*)

Bites from the black widow spider and the brown recluse spider can cause a whole-body reaction that leads to shock, stoppage of breathing, and death. This reaction may come from either a toxin released during the bite or an allergy to the bite.

What are the symptoms?

Any insect or spider bite may cause pain and swelling, with a stinger left in the skin or a visible bite or puncture mark. Other symptoms vary because specific poisons act on specific areas of the body.

Symptoms of tick bites

Painless at first, a tick bite may cause itching at the site. If the tick isn't removed or the head is left in the body, the site will become irritated and, possibly, infected.

Some people get *tick paralysis*, a whole-body reaction, after the tick bite. They may suffer weakness, pain in the feet or legs, or respiratory failure.

Symptoms of deer tick bites

Because the deer tick is only as big as the period at the end of this sentence, its bite produces no sensation. Within a few days, a bull's-

How to recognize ticks and spiders

Knowing how to spot certain ticks and spiders can protect you from potentially dangerous bites. This guide helps you to recognize dangerous insects.

Deer tick

This tick is one of several ticks that can transmit disease to humans. The deer tick, common throughout the United States, is responsible for transmitting Lyme disease.

The deer tick matures in stages. Between the larval and adult stage, it's as small as a pencil point. Growing to $\frac{1}{8}$ inch, the deer tick seeks a host. Once it attaches to a host, it swells to five to seven times its original size.

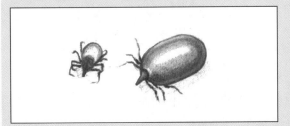

Wood tick

This flat, brown-speckled tick is found in woods and fields throughout North America. It attaches to humans and feeds on their blood. Like spiders, the wood tick has eight legs. It may inject a poison that can cause acute paralysis or transmit Rocky Mountain spotted fever, a potentially lethal disease.

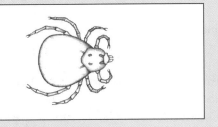

Brown recluse spider

This small, light brown spider, found in the south central part of the United States, injects a poison that causes its victim's blood to clot.

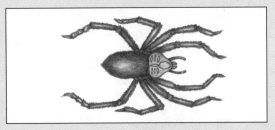

Black widow spider

The female is coal black with a red or orange hourglass mark on its underside. (The male doesn't bite). Its venom affects the nerves and muscles of a human victim.

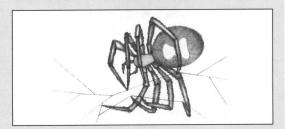

Identifying the symptoms of Lyme disease

Lyme disease comes from a bite by a deer tick. If you live in an area with a large deer population, make sure you're familiar with the symptoms of Lyme disease. Untreated, the disease progresses in three stages. Here are the symptoms to look for in each stage.

Stage one

The person may have a bull's-eye rash, often at the site of the tick bite. The rash may feel hot and itchy and may grow to more than 19 inches (48 centimeters) in diameter. Several days before the rash appears, a persistent sore throat and dry cough may develop.

From rashes to blotches

Within a few days, more skin lesions may come out. A rash may appear on the cheeks, the eyes may become inflamed, or widespread hives may occur.

In 3 to 4 weeks, the rash is replaced by small red blotches, which last several weeks. The person constantly feels fatigue and may have an intermittent headache, fever, chills, achiness, and swollen glands.

More serious symptoms

Less often, the person experiences more serious problems, such as:
- irritation of the membranes covering the brain and spinal cord
- muscle and bone pain
- hepatitis.

Stage two

Several weeks to months later, nervous system problems occur. They may last from a few days to a few months. Paralysis of the facial muscles is especially noticeable. Heart abnormalities may develop during this stage too.

Stage three

This stage begins weeks to years after the tick bite, with muscle or bone pain leading to arthritis. Joint swelling is pronounced, especially in the large joints — hips, knees, elbows, and shoulders.

Chronic arthritis

Recurrent bouts of arthritis may subside into chronic arthritis. Bone and cartilage may suffer severe erosion.

---

eye rash may appear. Then, over the next few weeks, months, or even years, severe symptoms may occur. (See *Identifying the symptoms of Lyme disease.*)

Symptoms of black widow spider bites

These bites cause an immediate sharp, stinging pain, followed by a dull, numbing pain. The bitten area begins to swell and tiny red bite marks appear. About 10 to 40 minutes after the bite, the person's stomach muscles become rigid and severe abdominal pain occurs. Both problems subside within 48 hours. Muscle spasms of the arms and legs also occur.

Some people may suffer a whole-body reaction to a black widow spider bite. Symptoms include:

- extreme restlessness
- dizziness
- sweating or chills
- pallor
- seizures (especially in children)
- nausea
- vomiting
- headache
- swelling of the eyelids
- hives
- itching
- fever.

Symptoms of brown recluse spider bites
Unlike bites from black widow spiders, those from brown recluse spiders cause little or no pain at first. But pain gets worse over time. About 2 to 8 hours after the bite, a small, red puncture wound forms a small blister. The center becomes dark and hard 3 to 4 days later. In 2 to 3 weeks, a sore develops.

Some people have whole-body reactions, which can cause:
- fever
- chills
- nausea
- vomiting
- fatigue
- muscle pain
- pinpoint red spots on the skin.

Symptoms of spider, scorpion, and tarantula bites
These bites may cause severe symptoms, especially pain. Expect to see puncture marks and some redness and swelling at the site. The person may have muscle pain and cramps in the arms, legs, shoulders, and back. Although symptoms usually subside after 6 to 12 hours, some people experience life-threatening symptoms.

Other symptoms to watch for
After *any* insect or spider bite, watch for the following symptoms, which signal a whole-body reaction from a toxin or an allergic reaction:
- weakness
- extreme restlessness
- nausea

After an insect or spider bite, watch for symptoms of a life-threatening reaction, such as fever, chills, nausea, and pinpoint spots on the skin.

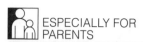 ESPECIALLY FOR
PARENTS

What to do if your child is bitten

An insect bite or sting that doesn't bother an adult may cause considerable alarm in a child. By staying calm, you can help to calm your child.

Keep the child calm

Keeping your child calm will slow absorption of the poison into the bloodstream. Speak quietly and reassuringly, and try not to share your fears.

Get immediate care for a scorpion bite

Because they're smaller, children may react more strongly to toxins that affect the nervous system. That's why a child who has been bitten by a scorpion (which looks like a miniature lobster) must get immediate medical attention. Death, although rare, is possible.

■ vomiting

■ dizziness

■ difficulty breathing, which may signal respiratory failure.

What should you do?

 WHEN SECONDS COUNT

If the person has symptoms of a whole-body reaction, call for medical help immediately. Check for a pulse and look, listen, and feel for breathing. If pulse and breathing are absent, start CPR, if you know how. *(See Performing CPR on an adult, page 579, Performing CPR on a child, page 585, or Performing CPR on an infant, page 590.)*

Treatment for less severe bites depends on the specific insect or spider that has inflicted the bite. A mild reaction is no cause for alarm and can be treated at home with cold compresses and Tylenol or other forms of acetaminophen. (See *What to do if your child is bitten*.)

Removing a tick

First, cover the tick and surrounding skin with heavy mineral oil and wait for 30 minutes. Typically, the mineral oil will suffocate the tick, which responds by backing out of the skin. If that doesn't work, firmly grasp the tick at its head with tweezers, and then slowly and gently pull the tick out. Clean the wound with an antiseptic or rubbing alcohol.

If the tick's head remains embedded in the skin, get the person to a doctor to have it removed.

> ⊗ Be sure not to pull a tick out with your hand; this action could leave the tick's head embedded in the skin.
>
> ⊗ Don't try to remove the tick with a lighted match or cigarette.

What to do for a minor bite

To relieve minor discomfort from an insect bite, apply ice or ice water to the bite. This stops the swelling, decreases pain, and slows absorption of any toxin. Or, you can apply a paste from baking soda and water or a cloth dampened with aloe vera juice.

What to do for a spider bite

If you suspect someone is having an allergic reaction to the bite of a spider, scorpion, or tarantula, call for medical help immediately. Tie

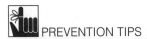

PREVENTION TIPS

How to avoid Lyme disease

If you live in an area that has many deer, you probably coexist with many deer ticks. Taking precautions when going outdoors can help you avoid getting Lyme disease from a deer tick bite. Here are some guidelines to follow.

Keep your distance
- Avoid areas with large deer populations.
- Stay out of long grass. It's more likely to harbor hungry ticks.
- Stick to trails when hiking.

Dress properly
- Wear light-colored, long-sleeved shirts.
- Tuck long pants into socks. This makes it harder for the ticks to reach you and makes it easier for you to see the ticks.
- Always wear shoes and socks outdoors; don't go barefoot.
- Check your clothes and skin for deer ticks often when outdoors.

Take precautions when you get home
- After hiking, brush or comb your hair. Brush hiking companions with a broom or towel, and have them brush you.
- After a trip to a wooded or grassy area, check for ticks before you bathe.
- When checking yourself and others for deer ticks, remember — they're tiny and easy to overlook. But if you see what looks like a speck of dirt on your skin, try to brush it off gently. If it's truly dirt, this action will remove it, but if it's a tick that's already bitten, it won't brush off.

Keep your children safe
- Routinely check your children for ticks if they play outdoors. Before they bathe or shower, check the backs of their necks and other out-of-the-way places, like behind their knees and ears.
- Remember that even in a lovely, tree-lined play area at your child's preschool, your child can be exposed to ticks. And don't overlook everyday exposure. For instance, if your backyard has signs of deer visitors, be especially diligent about checking your child daily for ticks.

a tight band around the bitten limb between the bite location and the person's heart. Then apply a cold pack or ice to the bite. Splint a bitten arm or leg, and keep it lower than the person's heart. Stay with the person until help arrives.

Never delay getting medical help; call the doctor immediately if you're concerned about an allergic reaction.

How are insect bites treated?
Someone who is having a severe allergic reaction needs lifesaving emergency measures, such as CPR. The victim of a toxic spider or scorpion bite needs medical care to receive antivenin.

A person with symptoms of Lyme disease may receive an antibiotic. Typically, adults get tetracycline and children get penicillin. When given in the early stages of Lyme disease, these drugs can minimize later complications. In the late stages, high-dose penicillin given intravenously may be effective. (See *How to avoid Lyme disease,* page 69.)

What else should you know?
If you're allergic to insect bites, take special precautions to avoid exposure to insects. Be sure to carry an antidote kit and, if possible, receive desensitization or immunization from the doctor.

BLACK STOOLS

Sometimes black stools are harmless and result from ingesting licorice, iron supplements, or a bismuth preparation.

A person who passes black or dark stools may be bleeding from somewhere in the upper digestive tract. The usual source of such bleeding is the esophagus, stomach, or small intestine. (See *What stool color says about the bleeding source.*) Swallowed blood (for example, from a nosebleed) can also cause dark stools.

If the person's stools are tarry as well as black, this indicates *significant* bleeding in the digestive tract, not just trace amounts of blood. Doctors call black, tarry stools *melena.* When severe, melena may indicate a life-threatening emergency.

When black stools are harmless
Sometimes, black, tarry stools are harmless. Called false melena, these stools may appear in a person who has ingested:
- black licorice
- a bismuth preparation (such as Pepto-Bismol)
- iron, as in a mineral supplement.

What are the symptoms?
Besides passing black stools, the person may have other symptoms, such as:
- vomiting of blood
- bright red bleeding from the rectum
- dizziness and weakness (from shock caused by blood loss).

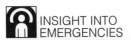
INSIGHT INTO
EMERGENCIES

What stool color says about the bleeding source

Usually, *black, tarry stools* indicate that the person is bleeding from the upper part of the digestive tract. *Bright red stools,* in contrast, mean the person is bleeding from the lower digestive tract. (However, in some disorders, black, tarry stools may alternate with bright red stools.) This chart links stool appearance with specific bleeding sources in the digestive tract.

STOOL APPEARANCE	POSSIBLE SOURCE OF BLEEDING
Black and tarry	▪ Esophagus (food tube) ▪ Stomach ▪ Small intestine
Bright red or dark mahogany	▪ Colon ▪ Esophagus, stomach, or small intestine if blood loss is rapid and massive

What should you do?

A person with unexplained black stools should consult a doctor promptly so that the stools can be tested for hidden blood. Someone who passes a large amount of black, tarry stools needs immediate medical attention; he or she is at risk for going into shock from massive blood loss.

Don't ignore black, tarry stools. They often warn of a serious medical condition.

How are black stools treated?

The doctor usually recommends bed rest to keep the person comfortable. To find out what's causing the abnormal stools, the doctor may order the following diagnostic tests:
▪ blood studies
▪ gastroscopy — passage of a thin, flexible tube into the digestive tract to look for the bleeding source

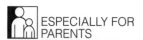

ESPECIALLY FOR PARENTS

What it means if your child passes unusual stools

At different stages of development, a child may pass black or dark red stools for different reasons.

Black stools in a newborn
A newborn may pass black, tarry stools from swallowing blood during birth.

Black or dark red stools in an older child
The most common reasons for black, tarry stools or dark red stools in an older child are:

- stomach ulcer

- inflammation of the stomach lining (typically, from a viral or bacterial infection)
- a pouch in the lining of the small intestine (called *Meckel's diverticulum*).
- ingesting Pepto-Bismol or another drug that contains bismuth.

What to do
Unless you know there's a harmless explanation for your child's unusual stools (such as Pepto-Bismol use), consult a doctor promptly.

- X-rays of the upper digestive tract.

If the person is bleeding seriously enough to experience shock, the doctor may order intravenous fluids and blood products. Most people also need supplemental oxygen.

What else should you know?

Black, tarry stools often come from a stomach ulcer that has penetrated into a blood vessel, causing massive, life-threatening blood loss. (See *What it means if your child passes unusual stools.*) Black, tarry stools may be the first sign of such bleeding.

The person with a peptic ulcer may also have other symptoms, including:

- bloody stools
- nausea
- vomiting, possibly of blood
- gnawing, burning, or sharp stomach pain.

If the person starts to go into shock, he or she may develop:

- a fast pulse
- rapid breathing
- cool, clammy skin
- dizziness and weakness from low blood pressure.

BLEEDING

In a healthy adult, the circulatory system — the network of blood vessels that carries nutrient fluids throughout the body — contains about 10 pints of blood. Losing a small amount of blood usually doesn't cause problems. But losing 2 pints or more is life-threatening.

Is it external or internal?
Blood loss can be external or internal. An example of *external bleeding* is when you cut yourself and the cut bleeds. *Internal bleeding* occurs when a blood vessel ruptures and bleeds into the surrounding tissue. Causes of internal bleeding include:
■ a blow to the abdomen, chest, or head
■ a broken bone
■ a puncture wound, such as a gunshot or stab wound.

What are the symptoms?
In *external bleeding*, symptoms depend partly on whether the person is bleeding from an artery, a vein, or a capillary. (See *Where is the blood coming from?* page 74.)

Symptoms of *internal bleeding* may not surface for hours or even days after the injury. Sometimes internal bleeding causes obvious symptoms, such as a bruise, or produces symptoms that correspond to the injury site. Here are some examples.
■ A head injury may lead to bleeding from the ears, nose, or mouth.
■ A chest or abdominal injury may cause the person to vomit or cough up blood.
■ A stomach ulcer could cause vomiting of blood that looks like coffee grounds.
■ A punctured lung may cause the person to vomit pale, frothy blood.
■ Bleeding in the urinary or digestive tract could lead to blood in the urine or stools.
■ Abdominal bleeding may cause a swollen, rigid, painful abdomen.

Symptoms of shock may also indicate internal bleeding. Suspect shock if the person has these symptoms:
■ excessive thirst
■ restlessness or anxiety
■ weakness
■ pale, wet, cool skin

Losing a small amount of blood usually doesn't cause problems. But losing 2 pints or more is life-threatening.

Where is the blood coming from?

The body has three types of blood vessels: arteries, veins, and capillaries. Arteries carry blood away from the heart. Veins carry blood toward the heart. Capillaries are tiny vessels that carry blood from small arteries called arterioles to small veins called venules. Bleeding can come from an artery, a vein, or a capillary.

When an artery bleeds

Blood from an artery is bright red. Because arterial blood comes straight from the heart, it may pulse or spurt from the body. Hard to control, arterial bleeding is usually a medical emergency.

When a vein bleeds

Blood from a vein is dark red and flows steadily. Blood loss from a cut vein can range from minor to severe. Because veins are closer to the skin surface than arteries, bleeding is more likely to come from a vein than an artery.

When a capillary bleeds

Most capillaries lie close to the skin. If you suffer a shallow cut from a knife, for example, what escapes is capillary blood. Capillary blood is scant, bright red, and tends to ooze from the wound.

- weak, rapid pulse
- fast, irregular, and shallow breathing.

Other symptoms to watch for
Bleeding may also cause dizziness, light-headedness, and passage of dark or red-streaked stools.

What should you do?

With external bleeding, your first priority is to stop the bleeding so a clot will form. Once formed, the clot acts as a barrier against continued bleeding and promotes healing. Next, get appropriate medical care for the victim.

If the person is bleeding heavily, call for medical help right away. Then try to stop the bleeding by applying direct pressure.

WHEN SECONDS COUNT

If the person is bleeding profusely, call for medical help right away. Then try to stop the bleeding. To do this, put on disposable latex gloves to guard against diseases that may be carried in the blood. If gloves aren't available, use a waterproof material, such as a plastic bag, plastic wrap, or several layers of gauze pads. Apply direct pressure to the wound using a clean cloth, a gauze pad, or your bare hand if no dressing is available. Press firmly for 10 to 15 minutes. (See *Applying pressure to a wound.*)

Applying pressure to a wound

Usually, you can stop bleeding by applying direct pressure to the wound, as you see here.

If the wound keeps bleeding, add another dressing while maintaining pressure on the wound.

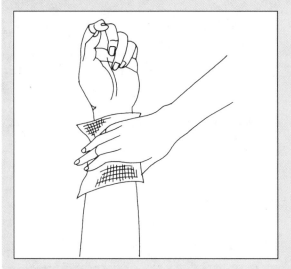 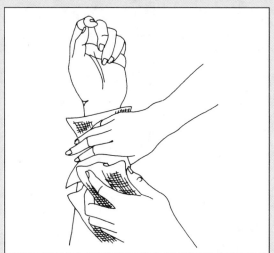

If the bleeding starts again when you release the pressure, don't remove the original dressing. Simply apply a clean dressing on top of it and keep applying pressure.

Don't move the person until you have taken steps to stop the bleeding. The exception is when the person is in immediate danger, such as from fire or a explosion.

If the injury has severed a body part, you'll need to care for the severed part properly as well as stop the bleeding. (See "Amputation," page 36.)

Elevate a bleeding limb
If the bleeding is coming from the person's arm or leg and you don't think the bone is broken, raise the injured limb slowly and gently until it's just a bit above heart level. This will help slow the bleeding.

When to use indirect pressure
If direct pressure and elevation don't stop the bleeding, try indirect

Using pressure points to stop bleeding

Pressure points are locations over a bone where an artery lies close to the skin. The body has 26 pressure points — 13 on each side — located along main arteries.

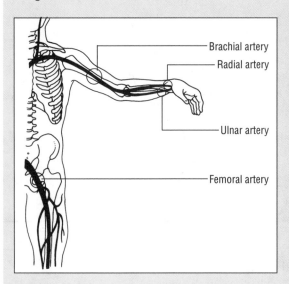

- Brachial artery
- Radial artery
- Ulnar artery
- Femoral artery

How it works
Applying pressure to the right pressure point can stop severe bleeding from a wound if direct pressure alone doesn't work. Why? Pressing the artery against the bone slows the flow of blood to the wound.

When to use a pressure point
Use a pressure point only if a wound keeps bleeding even though you have applied direct pressure. As you keep applying direct pressure to the wound with one hand, press against the nearest pressure point with your other hand. You'll be able to feel the artery because it pulsates.

Important precautions
Only someone skilled in first aid should use pressure points to stop bleeding. That's because if you don't find the exact location of the pulse point, applying pressure is useless. Also, this method can be dangerous because it cuts off circulation to the

pressure — pressing on a pressure point. (See *Using pressure points to stop bleeding.*)

Tourniquet: A last resort
If the combination of direct and indirect pressure doesn't stop the bleeding, you may need to apply a tourniquet. But remember that a tourniquet is a last resort because it cuts off blood supply to tissues that need it. Apply one only in extreme circumstances, when you're certain the limb must be sacrificed to save the person's life.

Once the tourniquet is in place, bandage the wound securely and get the person to a hospital immediately.

Other steps to take
■ If the person starts to show symptoms of internal bleeding (de-

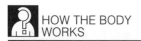

HOW THE BODY
WORKS

Using pressure points to stop bleeding *(continued)*

affected area. Use it only if direct pressure and limb elevation don't stop the bleeding.

Keep using direct pressure

And remember — using pressure points is *not* a substitute for direct pressure. If you use a pres-sure point, make sure to apply direct pressure to the bleeding site at the same time.

The illustrations on this page show the locations of important pressure points to use for wounds of certain parts of the body.

ELBOW OR LOWER ARM WOUND

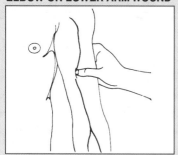

HAND WOUND

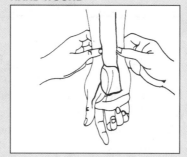

LOWER LEG WOUND

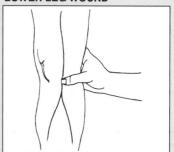

scribed on page 73), call for medical help immediately. Then have the person lie down and elevate the lower legs.

- If the person has a chest injury, keep him or her in a sitting position.
- If the person has suffered a head injury, elevate the head.
- Keep the person warm. Stay with him or her until the ambulance arrives.

 Don't give the person anything to drink.

How is bleeding treated?

If the person has external bleeding, medical personnel may give intravenous fluids and blood transfusions to replace lost blood and fluids. They also treat the victim for shock, clean and dress the wound, and set any broken bones. They may need to give antibiotics and a tetanus shot to help prevent infection.

For internal bleeding, the person may need surgery to repair the injury as well as intravenous fluids and blood transfusions. If a peptic ulcer is causing the bleeding, the doctor may prescribe ulcer medicine, such as antacids.

What else should you know?

Someone with internal bleeding — especially from a head injury — may have only a headache for a few days. The headache comes from increasing pressure within the skull as blood leaks into the layers of the brain. This is a dangerous condition, so urge the person to get medical attention at once.

BLOODY STOOLS

A person who passes bloody stools or has rectal bleeding is probably bleeding from the lower part of the digestive tract. Bloody stools may be the first symptom of such bleeding.

Sometimes, bloody stools result from a massive, rapid blood loss from the *upper,* rather than lower, part of the digestive tract. When this happens, though, the person usually vomits blood before passing bloody stools.

Understanding the causes

Many disorders can cause bloody stools. Inflammation of the large intestine (colitis) and hemorrhoids are among the most common.

What are the symptoms?

Bloody stools may range from formed, blood-streaked stools to liquid, bloody stools that appear bright red, dark mahogany, or maroon. Frequently, bloody stools develop suddenly after abdominal pain.

Symptoms of colitis

The person with colitis may have bloody diarrhea along with:
- severe, cramping pain in the lower abdomen
- dizziness and weakness
- a tender, swollen abdomen.

Symptoms of ulcerative colitis

In this disorder — a chronic inflammation of the colon — the bloody

Many disorders can cause bloody stools. Among the most common are inflammation of the large intestine and hemorrhoids.

diarrhea may contain mucus, and the person may have:

- mild-to-severe abdominal cramps
- fever
- loss of appetite
- nausea
- vomiting
- a rapid pulse.

Symptoms of hemorrhoids

Bloody stools may occur with either external or internal hemorrhoids. A person with an external hemorrhoid typically has pain when defecating, resulting in constipation.

Internal hemorrhoids, less painful than the external type, usually produce a more chronic bleeding with bowel movements. Eventually, the person may show symptoms of anemia — such as weakness and fatigue — caused by blood loss.

Other symptoms to watch for

If the person loses a great deal of blood through the stools, he or she may have symptoms of shock, such as:

- a rapid, slow, or weak pulse
- dizziness and weakness (from low blood pressure)
- anxiety followed by apathy, confusion, and sluggishness.

Occasionally, an intestine is injured when a person undergoes endoscopy, a diagnostic test of the digestive tract.

What should you do?

Get medical attention at once for someone with bloody stools. Internal bleeding can be life-threatening if enough blood is lost.

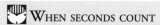 **WHEN SECONDS COUNT**

If you detect symptoms of shock, such as a rapid pulse, dizziness, or a change in the person's mental state, immediately call for emergency medical help. Have the person lie down, and elevate his or her feet on a rolled-up blanket, towel, or coat.

⊗ Don't delay seeking medical attention just because the person may be embarrassed by the symptoms.

How are bloody stools treated?

A person who requires hospitalization is put on bed rest. The medical team watches for symptoms of shock and measures the person's fluid intake and urine output. To prevent shock, the doctor may order intravenous fluids and blood transfusions.

To find out what's causing the bloody stools, the doctor may order the following diagnostic tests:
- blood tests
- stool specimens
- X-rays of the digestive tract
- endoscopy — passage of a flexible tube into the lower digestive tract.

What else should you know?
Bloody stools may also come from:
- colon cancer
- a bleeding disorder
- presence of a toxic substance
- certain diagnostic tests. Occasionally, an intestine is inadvertently injured when a person undergoes a procedure like endoscopy, in which a flexible tube is passed into the digestive tract to help diagnose a disorder. This can lead to potentially severe complications.

BLOODY URINE

Bloody urine can come from many different kidney and urinary tract problems. These include infection, injury, and tumors.

Blood in the urine is seldom visible to the naked eye. More often, it's discovered only when a person's urine is examined under a microscope — say, as part of a routine physical exam.

When the blood is found this way, the underlying condition probably isn't an emergency. In fact, it may not even warrant treatment. (See *When is bloody urine harmless?*)

When blood means trouble
But sometimes bloody urine *does* signal serious trouble — especially when it's visible to the naked eye. Bloody urine can be a symptom of many different kidney and urinary tract problems. These include:
- infection
- injury
- blockage in a blood vessel

- a cyst, or multiple cysts
- a tumor
- a kidney stone
- prostate infection. (See *Conditions that can cause bloody urine,* page 82.)

Some body-wide illnesses can also cause bloody urine. Whatever the underlying cause, though, anyone who sees bright red blood in the toilet is apt to become alarmed.

What are the symptoms?

Because bloody urine can result from so many different disorders, the accompanying symptoms can vary widely. But suspect an emergency if the person has bloody urine along with:

- difficulty urinating
- pain
- vomiting
- fever.

What should you do?

Seek medical care right away for anyone who has visible blood in the urine. If the person also has pain, fever, or vomiting, assume the situation is an emergency.

How is bloody urine treated?

First, the medical team makes sure the person can breathe, has a steady heartbeat, and has no other immediate threats to life. Then they run tests to find out what's causing the problem. Depending on what the tests uncover, treatment may range from medications to surgery.

What else should you know?

A little blood in the urine may come from exercising vigorously, such as running a marathon. That's because over time, hard exercise can injure the urinary tract enough to rupture tiny capillaries, causing blood-tinged urine. Eating fruits or vegetables like blackberries, rhubarb, and beets can also turn your urine red.

"Red diaper" syndrome

If your baby's diapers are stained red, stay calm. The cause may be one of these harmless conditions:

- Urate crystals. Urine normally contains urates, which are salts of

When is bloody urine harmless?

Blood in the urine isn't always an emergency or even a problem. Some people live with it for years or for their entire lives.

Benign condition
These people have what's called *benign hematuria.* They don't develop kidney damage and don't seem to have any long-term kidney problems.

Two types of benign hematuria
Doctors talk about two types of benign hematuria. One kind is inherited, the other isn't. Both typically are discovered in childhood. Other than having blood in the urine, everything else about the person's urine, blood, and kidneys is normal.

Why it's not treated
Because benign hematuria doesn't seem to cause any problems and no one knows why it happens, doctors don't recommend any treatment. Sometimes it disappears on its own.

At risk for kidney stones?
Some people with benign hematuria have a high level of calcium in their urine. They may be at increased risk of developing kidney stones later in life.

INSIGHT INTO EMERGENCIES

Conditions that can cause bloody urine

Many conditions can result in blood turning up in a person's urine, even though it may not be visible to the naked eye. Here's a partial list of causes.

Bladder disorders
- Bladder infection (cystitis)
- Bladder injury
- Bladder stones
- Bladder tumor
- Formation of pouches in the bladder

Kidney disorders
- Acute kidney inflammation
- Blocked vein in the kidney
- Kidney blockage
- Kidney infection
- Kidney injury
- Kidney stones
- Kidney tuberculosis
- Kidney tumor
- Polycystic kidney disease

Prostate problems
- Prostate enlargement
- Prostate infection

Other disorders
- Appendicitis
- Blood clotting problems
- Endocarditis (a heart infection) that causes a tiny clot to get stuck in the kidney
- Inflammation of the blood vessels (vasculitis)
- Injury to the urethra
- Lupus
- Schistosomiasis, a parasitic infection
- Sickle cell anemia
- Vaginal infection that spreads to the urinary tract

Medical tests and treatments
- Diagnostic tests, such as kidney biopsy
- Treatments in which instruments are used in the urinary tract
- Drugs, such as blood thinners, Cytoxan (a cancer-fighting drug), and Mintezol (used to treat pinworms, roundworms, and trichinosis)

uric acid. When urates cool to room temperature, as they might on a diaper, reddish crystals form.

■ Normal bacteria. The main bacteria in a newborn's digestive tract, *Serratia marcescens,* produces a red pigment that may stain a diaper.

Of course, if you're not certain whether the red in your infant's diaper is from one of these conditions or from something potentially serious, call the doctor.

BLUNT HEAD INJURIES

In blunt head injuries, the head suffers either a direct or an indirect blow that causes the brain to strike the inside of the skull. Usually, the blow is sudden and forceful, such as from a fall, a motor vehicle accident, or a punch. Blunt head injuries fall into two main categories: skull fractures and brain injuries.

Skull fractures
In these injuries, part of the skull — the head's bony structure — cracks or breaks. A skull fracture is a serious — even life-threatening — injury. The main peril isn't the broken skull bone itself but possible damage to the brain.

A skull fracture may be simple (closed) or compound (open) and may or may not displace brain structures. The most serious type of skull fracture is one in the base of the skull, called a *basilar fracture.*

Brain injuries
These injuries occur when a blow to the head jars the brain. Like other body tissues, the brain swells when injured. But unlike other tissues, the brain is confined by the rigid skull, which can't expand to accommodate much swelling. In response to swelling, pressure within the skull rises. Called *increased intracranial pressure,* this life-threatening condition limits the flow of blood to the brain.

A brain injury may be a concussion, contusion, or hematoma. These injuries vary in severity.
Concussion. By far the most common head injury, a concussion is a temporary loss of brain function. For more information, see "Concussion," page 150.
Contusion. This injury is a bruising of the brain. More serious than a concussion, it usually results from a more severe blow to the head. (See *How the brain gets bruised,* page 84.) A contusion may disrupt normal nerve functions in the bruised area, causing loss of consciousness as well as bleeding and swelling within the brain.
Hematoma. This is a localized mass of blood caused by a broken blood vessel. It's one of the most serious types of brain injury.

What are the symptoms?
A blunt head injury may cause any or all of the following symptoms:
- pain at the injury site

> *A skull fracture can be life-threatening. The main peril isn't the broken skull bone but possible damage to the brain.*

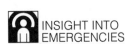

INSIGHT INTO EMERGENCIES

How the brain gets bruised

A hard blow to the head that sets the brain in motion can cause a contusion — bruising of the brain. What happens inside the brain depends on the type of force produced by the injury.

Coup injury
When a stationary object strikes the head of a person who is moving, the head's momentum stops suddenly.

Bruising at the point of impact
The sudden stop causes a coup injury. The brain is flung against the inside of the skull and gets bruised at the point of impact.

Contrecoup injury
During some head injuries, the brain rebounds against the opposite wall of the skull after the blow. For instance, in a motor vehicle accident, a person's forehead may rebound after striking a car windshield.

Bruising opposite the point of impact
Such rebounding causes a contrecoup injury. In this injury, the brain gets bruised in the area *opposite* the point of impact.

- headache
- confusion, drowsiness, or loss of consciousness
- skull deformity
- a bruise, lump, cut, or depression in the skull
- bleeding from the ears, nose, or mouth or from all three
- a scalp wound, which typically causes scalp bleeding
- leakage of clear or pinkish watery fluid from the person's nose or ear
- "raccoon" eyes (bleeding behind the eyes that shows as bruising around the eye sockets) and discoloration behind the ear; these symptoms show up several hours after the injury.

Symptoms of brain swelling
If the injured brain tissue starts to swell, the person may show the following symptoms 6 to 18 hours after the injury:

- nausea
- vomiting
- headache
- seizures
- loss of consciousness
- memory loss
- combative behavior
- vision disturbance
- loss of balance
- pupils of unequal sizes
- weakness or paralysis.

What should you do?

WHEN SECONDS COUNT

- Ask someone to call for medical help immediately.
- Check the person's airway, breathing, and pulse. If the person isn't breathing and has no pulse, start CPR immediately, if you know how. (See *Performing CPR on an adult,* page 579, *Performing CPR on a child,* page 585, or *Performing CPR on an infant,* page 590.) But *don't* open the airway by moving the person's head. Remember — a blow that causes a head injury can also injure the neck or spine. Moving the person's head could worsen a neck or spinal injury.

Stabilize the spine
- Place rolled blankets or similar materials on either side of the neck and torso.
- Tell the person not to move.

❌ Don't let the person's body bend or twist because this could worsen a neck or spinal injury.

Control bleeding

■ Next, check for severe bleeding. If the scalp is bleeding, apply direct pressure to the wound.

■ If you suspect a more serious head injury, *don't* use direct pressure because doing this could cause further damage to a fractured skull. Instead, apply pressure around the wound edges by making a dough-nut pad. To make this pad, obtain a narrow bandage, such as a roller bandage. Wrap one end of the bandage several times around four of your fingers to form a loop. Next, pass the other end of the bandage through the loop again and again until you've used the entire ban-dage.

Important: Protect yourself whenever you're exposed to another person's blood or other body fluids. This guards against diseases that may be carried in the blood, such as hepatitis and human immuno-deficiency virus. Latex gloves offer the best protection. If they aren't available, use any waterproof material — plastic bags or plastic wrap, for instance — or several layers of gauze pads or clothing.

Place the person in the proper position

■ If the person has vomited, roll him or her onto the side while stabilizing the neck against movement. A side-lying position helps prevent vomiting, drains the vomit, and keeps the airway open.

■ To help reduce bleeding, raise the head and shoulders as a single unit if you must move the person.

■ Stay with the person until professional help arrives.

❌ Don't raise the person's legs because this could cause pressure within the skull to rise.

❌ Be sure not to give the person anything to eat or drink.

How are blunt head injuries treated?

Depending on the type of injury, treatment may range from surgery to mere observation.

Treating a severe skull fracture

The person usually must have surgery to reduce the risks of infec-tion and further brain damage. After opening the skull, the surgeon raises or removes bone fragments that have been driven into the

If the fracture is at the base of the skull, the person may receive antibiotics to prevent brain infection, and steroids to reduce brain swelling.

brain. The person usually needs antibiotics and, if bleeding is severe, may need a blood transfusion.

If the fracture is at the base of the skull, the person may receive antibiotics to prevent brain inflammation and infection. The medical team closely observes the person for hematomas and bleeding within the brain. Surgery may be necessary to relieve either condition. The doctor also may give steroids to reduce brain swelling and minimize brain damage.

Treating a less serious skull fracture

Usually, a person who hasn't lost consciousness is observed in the hospital for at least 4 hours. The wound is cleaned, and a mild pain reliever, such as Tylenol, may be given. (Narcotics are avoided because they make it difficult to evaluate the person's nervous system. Aspirin is avoided because it may increase the risk of bleeding.)

If vital signs — pulse, breathing, and body temperature — are stable, the person may be discharged, along with written instructions for the family about what to look for over the next 24 to 48 hours.

Treating a contusion

The person with this injury may need immediate emergency treatment, such as:

■ opening the airway to establish breathing
■ inserting a tube in the airway to maintain breathing
■ intravenous fluids
■ restricted fluid intake to reduce brain swelling
■ drugs to reduce pressure within the brain
■ brain surgery to decrease pressure within the skull and help control bleeding.

What else should you know?

Even if the person didn't lose consciousness at the time of the injury, he or she must be watched for the next few days to detect delayed symptoms of brain damage.

Watch for delayed symptoms

Observe the person closely for:

■ loss of consciousness
■ a pulse rate that's slower or faster than normal
■ difficulty breathing

- seizures
- severe vomiting
- pupils of unequal sizes
- decreased arm or leg strength
- change in behavior
- overall ill appearance.

Call the doctor
If you notice any of these symptoms, make sure the person gets medical attention at once.

BLURRED VISION

For many people over age 40, blurred vision is a fact of life — inconvenient but no more worrisome than gray hair. This type of blurred vision can usually be corrected by wearing glasses or contact lenses. (See *Understanding normal causes of blurred vision,* page 88.) For some people, the problem can be relieved through an operation called refractive surgery, a procedure that changes the curve of the cornea to improve vision.

Sudden warning
But blurred vision that comes on suddenly may warn of a dangerous medical problem — especially if the person has additional symptoms. Here are some examples:
- Flashing lights and floating spots with sudden blurring or clouding of vision could signal a condition called *retinal detachment.* In this emergency, the eye's image-receiving structure, called the retina, separates from the back of the eye.
- Blurred vision that comes on after a blow to the head could mean a *concussion.*
- Sudden blurred vision with a headache could indicate *very high blood pressure.*
- Pain, nausea, and vomiting along with blurred vision may indicate a potentially blinding eye disease called *closed-angle glaucoma.*

Blurred vision accompanied by numbness, tingling, or seeing flashing lights, floating spots, or halos often indicates a medical emergency.

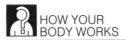

Understanding normal causes of blurred vision

Blurred vision that comes on gradually is usually a harmless effect of the shape of your eyeball.

The normal eye

In a normally shaped eyeball, as you see in the picture below, the cornea and lens work together to focus incoming light rays on the retina. When this happens properly, you have clear vision.

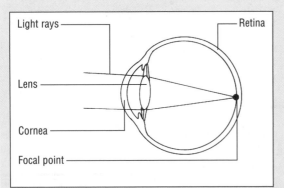

The farsighted eye

If you're farsighted, your eyeball is somewhat shortened, so your cornea and lens focus light rays behind your retina. This makes nearby objects blurry and distant objects clearer.

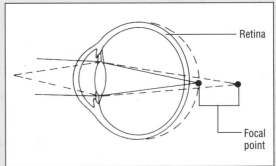

The nearsighted eye

If you're nearsighted, your eyeball is somewhat elongated, or football shaped. This means that your cornea and lens focus light rays on a point in front of your retina, as shown in the picture below.

Distant objects appear blurry and nearby objects seem clearer. Glasses or contact lenses can make your vision clear again by changing the location where light rays get focused.

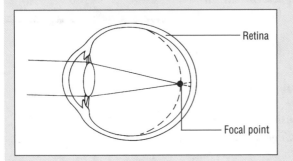

What happens when the lens becomes less elastic

Another harmless cause of blurred vision is a condition called *presbyopia*. In this condition, aging makes the lens of the eye less elastic, so it's less adept at getting shorter when focusing on nearby objects.

Eventually, presbyopia affects all of us as we age. That's why so many older people need bifocals or reading glasses.

What are the symptoms?

A *sudden* change in vision may indicate a serious condition, especially if it's accompanied by:

- numbness
- tingling
- seeing flashing lights, floating spots, or halos.

What should you do?

Anyone who experiences sudden blurring of vision — or *any* sudden vision change, for that matter — should call the doctor right away.

How is blurred vision treated?

Treatment depends on the underlying cause. Here are some examples:

- Someone with retinal detachment may need eye surgery to reattach the retina.
- A concussion may go away by itself, although the doctor will want to watch the person closely to be sure the brain doesn't swell.
- A person with high blood pressure needs immediate medicine to bring down the blood pressure.
- Someone with glaucoma needs medicine to reduce pressure inside the eye.

What else should you know?

Although sudden blurred vision is a possible symptom of glaucoma, this eye disease doesn't always cause blurred vision. Sometimes the person instead sees halos around lights or bright objects. Here's how the halo effect occurs:

The eye produces a fluid called *aqueous humor,* which normally moves from the back of the eye to the front of the eye through the pupil, then filters out through a tiny meshwork of fibers at the base of the iris (the colored part of your eye).

Glaucoma blocks that tiny meshwork, reducing the amount of aqueous humor that can escape from the eye. As a result, fluid builds up in the eyeball, increasing pressure within the eye and causing excess fluid to enter the cornea.

This excess fluid breaks light into a spectrum of color. To someone with glaucoma, this looks like a halo. If you begin seeing halos, report it to your eye doctor right away.

Someone with retinal detachment may need eye surgery. A person with high blood pressure needs immediate drug therapy to bring down the blood pressure.

BREAST DIMPLING

Breast dimpling is the puckering of breast skin over a mass or hardened tissue. Dimpling is most common in women over age 40, but it occasionally occurs in men.

Breast dimpling is usually a late symptom of a cancerous breast tumor just under the skin surface. But it can also come from an inflammatory breast mass, a breast abscess, an injury to the breast (which causes fatty tissue to become inflamed), or a bacterial breast inflammation called *mastitis.*

Other symptoms of cancer usually appear before breast dimpling.

What are the symptoms?

Other symptoms usually appear before the dimpling. But a breast self-exam may alert the person to a breast problem. A dimpled breast looks puckered in the affected area. To see the dimpling better, gently move or compress the breast against the chest wall.

Other symptoms to watch for

Symptoms that often go along with breast dimpling include:
- a recent change in breast shape
- swelling, redness, or warmth of the dimpled area
- an abnormal nipple — for instance, retracted, withdrawn, flattened, deviated, or facing inward
- nipple discharge.

If dimpling comes from a breast abscess, the person may also have a firm, irregular, and nontender lump and the glands under the arms may be swollen.

A breast injury can cause dimpled, red skin as well as bruising, tenderness, a hard lump in the breast, and a retracted nipple.

Mastitis can cause dimpling along with redness, warmth, swelling, pain, and tenderness of the breast. Seen in breast-feeding women, this infection usually comes from blocked milk ducts.

What should you do?

A person with breast dimpling should consult a doctor without delay.

How is breast dimpling treated?

The doctor performs a thorough breast exam and orders tests to find out what's causing the breast dimpling. The tests may include mammography, ultrasound, and biopsy (surgical sampling of breast tissue).

The type of treatment used varies with the cause of the dimpling. If the biopsy shows cancer, the treatment may be some combination of surgery, chemotherapy, and radiation therapy.

What else should you know?

In a child, *don't* assume breast cancer is the cause of breast dimpling. Breast cancer is rare in children, and breast dimpling usually comes from injury.

BREAST INFECTION

The most common type of breast infection is *mastitis,* an inflammation that mainly affects breast-feeding women. Typically, mastitis comes from bacteria — streptococcal (strep) or staphylococcal (staph) germs from the infant's skin, nose, or throat.

Mastitis usually begins 3 to 4 weeks after the woman starts breast-feeding. Factors that contribute to mastitis include:
- a crack in the nipple
- a blocked milk duct, caused by inadequate or infrequent breast emptying
- fatigue
- stress
- poor nutrition
- too little fluid intake.

Occasionally, a woman who isn't breast-feeding develops mastitis. The usual cause is an abscess under the nipple or, in a woman with fibrocystic breast condition, a ruptured breast cyst.

What are the symptoms?

Mastitis can cause:
- pain, warmth, redness, and tenderness of the breast
- an inverted, flattened, or deviated nipple
- cracked, sore nipples

Mastitis usually begins 3 to 4 weeks after a woman starts breast-feeding. Factors that contribute to this condition include a crack in the nipple, and too little fluid intake.

- an orange-peel or dimpled appearance of the breast skin
- swollen underarm glands
- flulike symptoms — chills, fatigue, muscle aches, and fever.

Symptoms of an abscess

If mastitis goes untreated, an abscess may form in the breast. This condition causes increased breast pain, swelling, redness and, occasionally, a pus-filled nipple discharge.

What should you do?

A woman with symptoms of mastitis should consult her doctor promptly. Timely treatment may help her avoid breast abscesses.

How is breast infection treated?

The doctor typically prescribes drug therapy, rest, good nutrition, and increased fluid intake. Wearing the right kind of bra and using the proper breast-feeding technique can help too. (See *Recovering from mastitis*.) A breast abscess usually must be drained.

Drug therapy

Drugs for mastitis include pain relievers to reduce pain and antibiotics to kill bacteria. Pain relievers help the woman to express milk from the breast more often and completely. Why? Pain inhibits the reflex that triggers the flow of milk from the breast. So reducing pain promotes milk flow. (See *Pain relievers you can take when breast-feeding,* page 94.)

The doctor may prescribe antibiotics for 10 days. Most women begin to feel better within 24 to 48 hours of starting antibiotic therapy. To help clear up the infection completely, though, the drug should be taken for the full 10 days. The woman shouldn't save some of the drug to use in case another infection occurs.

Getting rest

Fatigue and stress contribute to mastitis. Until the infection starts to resolve, the woman should stay in bed and rest as much as possible. If necessary, she should ask family members, friends, or others to share in family care and household chores.

Maintaining a good diet and sufficient fluid intake

A woman who wants to continue breast-feeding should eat a balanced diet and increase her caloric intake. Drinking plenty of water,

Recovering from mastitis

To help ensure your complete recovery from mastitis, follow these self-care guidelines.

Breast-feeding tips
■ Breast-feed your infant at least every 2 to 3 hours.
■ Start breast-feeding with the affected breast and continue with this breast until it feels completely soft.

Before you begin
■ Wash your hands and nipples gently before breast-feeding. This helps stop the infection from coming back.
■ Immediately before each feeding, apply a warm, wet washcloth or an ice pack to the affected area to decrease pain. Repeat this as often as desired.

During breast-feeding
■ Gently massage the affected area while you breast-feed. This helps the milk ducts to empty completely.
■ Rotate feeding positions to distribute stress evenly on your nipple.
■ Make sure your baby sucks correctly — with your areola (the nipple tip and the darkened circle of skin around it) well into the baby's mouth. This helps you avoid cracked nipples.
■ Don't wear a bra or other restrictive clothing when breast-feeding.

After breast-feeding
■ Express by hand or pump any milk your baby doesn't remove from your breast.
■ Air-dry your nipples carefully after each feeding. This toughens them and keeps them from staying damp for long periods.
■ If your nipples become cracked or dry, apply a vitamin-based skin ointment — for example, A and D Ointment.

Other instructions
■ Increase your daily water intake by several glasses.
■ When lying on the affected side, use pillows to support your breast.
■ When you're not breast-feeding, wear a bra that's supportive and well fitting but nonbinding. A bra that's too tight can contribute to a blocked milk duct, predisposing you to another bout of mastitis.
■ Call your doctor if you don't feel better after 48 hours of antibiotic therapy and breast-feeding. Also call if your infant develops diarrhea; this may mean your medicine needs to be changed.

juice, and milk are important too, especially if the woman is dehydrated from fever. But she should limit her intake of coffee, tea, and other caffeine-containing beverages. Caffeine can contribute to dehydration and disturb her sleep.

Draining an abscess
A single abscess close to the surface of the breast may be removed by withdrawing its contents with a needle. If the woman has several deep abscesses, the doctor may admit her to the hospital for breast incision and drainage. After removing pus from the abscess, the doctor leaves a drain in place for several days. Until the breast heals,

Pain relievers you can take when breast-feeding

Many drugs a breast-feeding woman takes can pass through her breast milk to her infant. If you have mastitis, though, you may need to take pain relievers to reduce your pain.

Be safe about pain relief
Fortunately, most breast-feeding women can take the pain relievers listed below, but check with your doctor first:
■ Advil, Motrin, or other forms of ibuprofen
■ aspirin after the first postpartum week
■ Tylenol or other forms of acetaminophen
■ Darvon.

Take special precautions
■ Call for emergency medical assistance if you have symptoms of an allergic reaction to a pain reliever, such as itching, hives, rash, or wheezing or other breathing problems.
■ Be aware that any of these drugs can upset your stomach. To help prevent this reaction, take them with food or milk.
■ Be sure to take all medicines, especially Darvon, only as directed. Darvon may cause drowsiness, constipation, nausea, vomiting, and general stomach upset. Also, watch for drowsiness and slowed breathing in your infant. If you notice any of these symptoms, stop taking this drug and call the doctor.

the woman can't breast-feed, but she can keep up her milk production by expressing her milk manually.

What else should you know?
Mastitis doesn't cause permanent breast damage or increase the risk for breast cancer or other breast disease. Also, the woman will be able to breast-feed other infants in the future if she wishes.

BREAST LUMP

A breast lump is any mass in the breast. Most breast lumps — nearly 85% — aren't cancerous. In fact, it's normal for the breasts to feel somewhat uneven because they contain hundreds of milk glands surrounded by fibrous tissue and fat. The breasts feel more uneven during or just before menstruation, when hormonal changes cause the milk glands to enlarge.

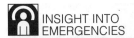
INSIGHT INTO
EMERGENCIES

What causes breast discharge?

Breast discharge may occur spontaneously or only when the nipple is pressed. It can come from either a normal or an abnormal cause.

Normal causes
During the breast-feeding period, a woman's breasts provide milk high in nutrients to nourish her baby. The milk produced during the first 3 days after birth, called *colostrum*, helps build the baby's immune system. Both milk and colostrum are normal for the breast-feeding woman.

Discharge after pregnancy
After pregnancy, some discharge from the breasts other than milk is also normal.

Abnormal causes
In breast-feeding women, an abscess of the breast is a common cause of discharge. It results from infection by bacteria that may enter through a crack in the skin.

Less common causes
Less commonly, breast discharge results from:
- a tumor of the breast duct or the pituitary gland
- reactions to drugs like female hormones or drugs used to control high blood pressure
- breast cancer
- cancer of the duct system — a slowly developing condition marked by a flaking, bleeding sore on the nipple, which progresses to a tumor.

A cancerous lump can't be distinguished from a noncancerous one without diagnostic tests. These tests typically include a biopsy, the removal of a tissue sample for viewing under a microscope. So anyone who finds a breast lump should call her or his doctor promptly. Yes, a man *can* get a lump in the breast.

What are the symptoms?
Depending on the cause of the breast lump, the person may have the symptoms described below.

Symptoms of fibrocystic breast condition
The most common cause of breast lumps, this condition produces one or more smooth, round, slightly elastic cysts. The cysts grow larger and become more tender just before menstruation. They may occur in fine, granular clusters in both breasts or as widespread, well-defined lumps of varying sizes.

Unlike cancerous lumps, the cysts are easy to move around with the fingers and are not fixed to underlying tissue. The nipples aren't retracted or dimpled, although they may have a sticky or clear watery discharge. (See *What causes breast discharge?*)

Classifying breast cancer

Doctors classify breast cancer according to cell appearance and tumor location. The doctor may refer to the following classification terms.

Types of cancer
- *Adenocarcinoma*, which occurs in the covering of an organ
- *Intraductal breast cancer*, which develops within the ducts — narrow tubes carrying secreted or excreted fluids
- *Infiltrating breast cancer*, which occurs in the tissue of the breast itself, not the connective or supporting tissue
- *Inflammatory breast cancer* (rare), which causes the skin over the lump to become swollen and inflamed, reflecting rapid tumor growth
- *Lobular carcinoma in situ*, which involves segments of glandular tissue
- *Medullary or circumscribed breast cancer*, which refers to a large tumor that grows rapidly.

Classifying the extent of cancer
A staging classification system is used to give a clearer understanding of the extent of the tumor. The most commonly used system is called the tumor-node-metastasis (TNM) system.

Symptoms of adenofibroma
This benign breast lump is extremely mobile and slippery to the touch. It feels firm, elastic, and round or lobed and has well-defined edges. It can vary from pinhead size to very large and often grows rapidly. The lump doesn't cause pain or tenderness.

Symptoms of breast abscess
An *acute* breast abscess causes a hot, tender mass with redness and an orange-peel appearance of the skin over the lump. The person may also have fever, chills, malaise, and generalized discomfort.

In *chronic* abscess, the lump is nontender, irregular, and firm. It's often accompanied by a retracted nipple and skin that's dimpled or looks like an orange peel.

Symptoms of breast cancer
A cancerous breast lump usually occurs singly and is fixed to the skin or underlying tissue. (See *Classifying breast cancer*.) Other symptoms may include:
- redness and tenderness of the breast
- breast dimpling
- nipple discharge (especially bloody discharge)
- a retracted nipple
- a deviated nipple that points to the area of the tumor
- a flattened breast contour

- swelling and an orange-peel appearance of the skin over the lump
- swollen underarm glands
- a breast sore or ulcer.

Symptoms of fat necrosis
This condition, caused by a breast injury, results in a rare, harmless mass. The mass may feel hard and fixed, like a cancerous lump. The breast may be tender, bruised, and red, with dimpled skin and a retracted nipple.

Symptoms of mastitis
In this disorder, the lump feels either firm and hard or tender and fluffy. (For other symptoms of mastitis, see "Breast infection," page 91.)

What should you do?
A person who discovers or suspects a breast lump should call the doctor. But don't panic — keep in mind that most breast lumps are harmless.

How is a breast lump treated?
To evaluate a breast lump, the doctor examines the breasts thoroughly and orders diagnostic tests — for instance, a mammogram, ultrasound, thermography (a heat-sensing method), or a biopsy of the lump.

What else should you know?
Women should examine their breasts monthly when they're least swollen — immediately after the menstrual period ends. Pregnant and postmenopausal women should choose one day of the month for the breast self-exam and perform the exam monthly. (See *How to examine your breasts,* pages 98 and 99.)

Regular self-exams are especially important for women at high risk for breast cancer, such as those who:
- have had cancer in one breast
- have a family history of breast cancer
- have never given birth
- had their first child after age 30
- began menstruating early
- experienced menopause late.

A person who discovers a breast lump should call the doctor. But don't panic. Most breast lumps are harmless.

(Text continues on page 100.)

How to examine your breasts

Women discover about 90% of cancerous breast lumps themselves, so it's important to learn and practice breast self-exam techniques.

When is the best time?

Examine your breasts once a month. If you haven't reached menopause, the best exam time is just after your menstrual period. If you're past menopause, choose any convenient, easy-to-remember day each month — the first of the month, for example. Here's how to proceed.

Observe your breasts

■ Undress to the waist, and stand or sit in front of a mirror with your arms at your sides. Observe your breasts for any change in their shape or size. Look for any puckering or dimpling of the skin.
■ Raise your arms and press your hands together behind your head. Observe your breasts as before.

■ Press your palms firmly on your hips and observe your breasts again.

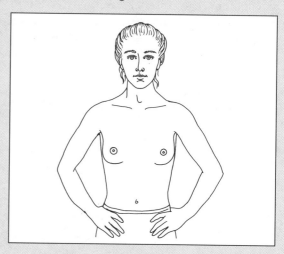

Examine your left breast

■ Next, lie flat on your back. This position flattens and spreads your breasts more evenly over your chest wall. Place a small pillow under your left shoulder, and put your left hand behind your head.
■ Examine your left breast with your right hand. Use a circular motion and progress clockwise until you've examined every portion. You'll notice a ridge of firm tissue in the lower curve of your breast. This is normal.

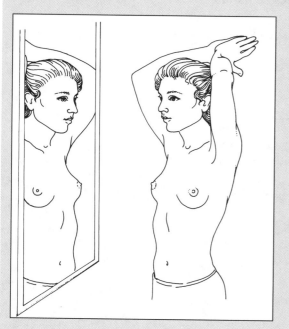

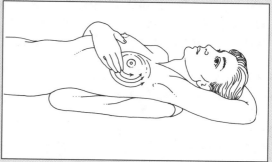

How to examine your breasts *(continued)*

Check under your arms
■ Check the area under your arm with your elbow slightly bent. If you feel a small lump that moves freely under your armpit, don't be alarmed. This area contains your lymph glands, which may get swollen when you're sick. Check the lump daily. Call the doctor if it doesn't go away in a few days or if it gets larger.

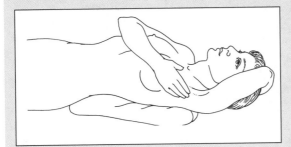

Check for discharge
■ Gently squeeze your nipple between your thumb and forefinger, and note any discharge.

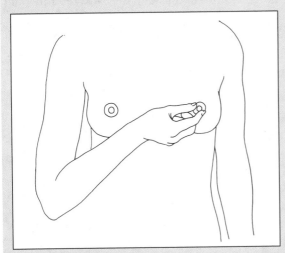

Check your right breast
■ Repeat these steps on your right breast, using your left hand.

Examine your breasts while bathing
■ Finally, examine your breasts while you're in the shower or bath, lubricating your breasts with soap and water. Using the same circular, clockwise motion, gently inspect both breasts with your fingertips.

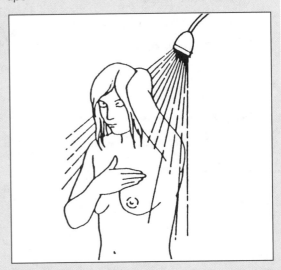

What to do if you feel a lump
If you feel a lump, don't panic — most lumps aren't cancerous. First, note whether you can easily lift the skin covering it and whether the lump moves when you do.

Then, call your doctor. Be prepared to describe how the lump feels (hard or soft) and whether it moves easily under the skin.

Chances are, the doctor will want to examine the lump. Then he or she can advise you about what treatment (if any) you need.

Get regular medical check-ups
Although breast self-exams are important, they're not a substitute for examination by your doctor. Be sure to see your doctor once a year, or twice a year if you're considered at high risk for breast cancer.

BREAST PAIN

Pain in the breast usually indicates benign (harmless) breast disease or premenstrual syndrome. It's *seldom* a symptom of cancer.

Some women experience breast pain only before their menstrual periods. Others get it intermittently or constantly. Before menstruation, hormonal changes increase blood flow to the breasts, causing breast pain or tenderness. (See *A look inside the breast.*)

During pregnancy, hormonal changes may lead to breast tenderness and throbbing, tingling, or prickling sensations.

Breast pain in males

A boy or man can get breast pain too. (See *Why some males get breast pain,* page 102.)

What are the symptoms?

Breast pain may be:
- sharp or dull
- stinging, shooting, stabbing, throbbing, or burning.

Breast pain may get worse when the breast is touched. It may affect one breast or both. Sometimes it occurs only with rest, sometimes only with movement. It can spread to the back, the arms, and even the neck.

After a breast injury, such as a surface cut or bruising, breast pain is likely to be superficial. Severe pain may come from a crack in the nipple, inflammation of the milk ducts or areola, or a growth that irritates sensory nerve endings.

Other symptoms to watch for

A *breast abscess* causes breast tenderness, redness, and warmth as well as pain. The woman may have a fever, chills, and other flulike symptoms.

A breast cyst that enlarges rapidly may cause acute pain in one breast. *Mastitis* (an inflammation of the breast) may cause severe pain in one breast, plus red, warm skin with an orange-peel appearance.

In women with a condition called *fibrocystic breasts,* breast pain may precede menstruation and disappear after it ends. Later in the course of this condition, breast pain and tenderness may be con-

> Some women have breast pain before menstruation and during pregnancy. Before menstruation, hormonal changes increase blood flow to the breasts, causing pain or tenderness.

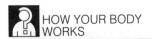

HOW YOUR BODY WORKS

A look inside the breast

Before puberty, a girl's breasts resemble a boy's. Then, at puberty, when the ovaries start producing estrogen and progesterone, the breast ducts, lobules, and fibrous tissue start to increase rapidly in number. Fat tissue accumulates too.

The mature breast

The mature breast contains glandular tissue, fibrous tissue, and fat. Except during pregnancy and lactation, breast size depends on the amount of fat and fibrous tissue present, not the amount of glandular tissue.

How hormones affect the breast

The breast is extremely responsive to hormonal stimulation. During the menstrual cycle, glandular breast tissue varies somewhat. These changes can make the breasts slightly fuller and more tender during the middle and later stages of the cycle. That's why many women complain of tender breasts just before their periods start.

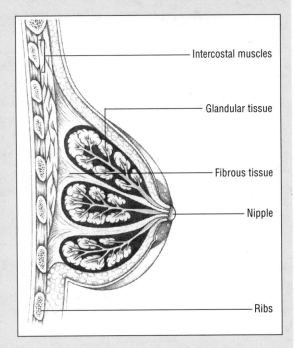

Intercostal muscles

Glandular tissue

Fibrous tissue

Nipple

Ribs

stant. Symptoms of premenstrual syndrome — headache, irritability, bloating, and abdominal cramps — may be present too.

What should you do?

First, perform a breast self-exam (see *How to examine your breasts,* pages 98 and 99). Although breast cancer doesn't usually cause breast pain, it's always a good idea to check for lumps.

Breast tenderness can be an early sign of pregnancy. If you think you could be pregnant, take a home pregnancy test or call the doctor or clinic to arrange an office test.

If you can't readily identify the cause of your breast pain, call your doctor — especially if you feel a lump.

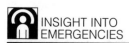

INSIGHT INTO
EMERGENCIES

Why some males get breast pain

In boys and men, the usual cause of breast pain is gynecomastia — a temporary enlargement of the breasts. The enlargement is most common during puberty and old age.

Other causes
Other causes of male breast pain are:
- malnutrition
- abnormalities of the reproductive system
- liver disease
- a disorder of the pituitary gland, adrenal gland, or thyroid gland.

How is breast pain treated?

The doctor will try to find out what's causing your pain — first by examining your breasts and then, possibly, by ordering a mammogram. If you have a breast lump, you may need to have a breast biopsy (surgical removal of some breast tissue) to find out if the lump is benign or cancerous.

Treating fibrocystic breasts

If the doctor thinks your breast pain comes from fibrocystic breasts, he or she may advise you to cut down on your intake of caffeine and dietary fats and to take vitamin supplements. Some doctors also recommend water pills (diuretics) to reduce fluid retention and mild pain relievers to reduce discomfort. Wearing a well-fitting bra helps too, especially for women with large breasts.

What else should you know?

Birth control pills and hormone replacement therapy (such as estrogen) can cause swollen, tender breasts and sore nipples. If you develop these symptoms while taking such drugs, talk to your doctor about adjusting your dosage.

If you're large breasted, have you started wearing a different type of bra lately? Bras with underwires or side ribstays can cause the breasts to ache.

BURNS CAUSED BY CHEMICALS

Chemical burns occur when a caustic or corrosive substance comes in contact with the skin. They can come from touching, eating, inhaling, or injecting the following substances:
- an acid, such as battery acid
- an alkali, such as lye
- a vesicant, or blistering agent.

Sometimes fatal and often permanently disfiguring, chemical burns can cause tremendous physical and emotional suffering. Major chemical burns require painful treatment and a long rehabilitation.

Inhalation burns

Inhaling smoke or certain chemicals — especially in an enclosed space like a bathroom — can cause an inhalation burn, blocking the person's airway. Also, chemical irritants can disrupt normal lung function and allow fluids and protein to build up in the lungs. Without prompt treatment, a life-threatening condition called *adult respiratory distress syndrome* may occur. (See *When to get immediate medical help,* page 104.)

What are the symptoms?

An external chemical burn may make the skin red or discolored, raw, white, soft, mushy, or irritated. Tissues under the burn swell. The person may feel tremendous pain and general weakness, or he or she may feel no pain if the burn has completely destroyed nerve endings. Some people have trouble breathing or lose consciousness.

Symptoms of inhalation burns

The victim may have:
- facial burns
- difficulty breathing
- light-headedness
- nausea
- chest pain
- burning sensation of the eyes or the inside of the mouth
- swelling of the throat
- loss of consciousness.

Chemical burns occur when a caustic or corrosive substance comes in contact with the skin. They can come from touching, eating, inhaling, or injecting such a substance.

What should you do?

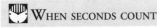 WHEN SECONDS COUNT

Call for medical help immediately. Feel for a pulse and look, listen, and feel for breathing by feeling for air over the nose and mouth and seeing if the chest rises and falls. If pulse and breathing are absent, start CPR, if you know how. (See *Performing CPR on an adult,* page 579, *Performing CPR on a child,* page 585, or *Performing CPR on an infant,* page 590.) But before starting CPR, make sure there are no caustic chemicals on the person's mouth or face.

Flush the skin

If the person has a pulse and is breathing, immediately start to flush the burned area with large amounts of water. Otherwise, the chemi-

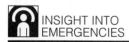 INSIGHT INTO
EMERGENCIES

When to get immediate medical help

Always seek immediate medical attention for a burn that:
- causes difficulty breathing
- affects more than one body part
- involves the person's head, neck, hands, feet, or genitals
- results from a chemical, an explosion, or an electric current.

Other precautions
Children and elderly people always need immediate treatment, unless the burn is very small.

cal will continue to burn as long as it touches the skin. Keep flushing for 15 to 30 minutes.

 Be sure not to flush the burn if it was caused by dry lime.

If a large area of the person's body came in contact with the chemical, gently hose the person with running water, if possible. Or place the person under a cool shower and rinse for at least 5 minutes. Be sure to brush any dry powder chemicals off the person's clothing before wetting. Otherwise, the water may activate the dry chemical, causing greater damage. (See *When not to flush a chemical burn*.) Also, make sure to protect yourself from exposure to the chemical.

 Don't place the person under a high-pressure flow of water. High pressure can worsen the burn by forcing the chemical deeper into the skin.

Remove the clothes
After the person has been rinsed with water for at least 5 minutes and the remaining chemicals have been washed away, start to remove the person's clothes. Also remove any jewelry that may cause constriction or keep the chemical in contact with the person's skin.

Before the final rinse, wash the person with a mild soap.

 Don't use soap if the burn came from an alkali or if you're not sure which chemical caused the burn. Soap increases pain and irritation from an alkali.

If the person was burned by an oven cleaner or a drain cleaner, rinse for several minutes and then call for emergency medical help.

 Be sure not to throw away the bottle label from the chemical that caused the burn. If available, send it to the hospital with the emergency rescue team.

Cover the person
After prolonged rinsing, you or the emergency rescue team should cover the burned area with a sterile dressing and then cover the person's entire body with a clean sheet. Then take the person to the nearest medical facility.

Treating an eye burn
Before you call for medical help, immediately begin flushing the

When not to flush a chemical burn

Usually, someone who has been burned by a chemical must rinse the area with copious amounts of water. But sometimes this does more harm than good because certain chemicals react when mixed with water. Read the chart below to learn when *not* to rinse and what to do instead.

CHEMICAL	HOW IT REACTS WITH WATER	HOW TO TREAT THE BURN
Dry lime	Becomes more corrosive	Wearing gloves, remove person's clothes and brush off lime; then flush burn with water for 30 minutes.
Sodium	May explode	Cover burn with oil.
Hydrofluoric acid	Causes continuing tissue destruction	Take person to hospital emergency department for calcium gluconate shot.

person's eye with large amounts of cool water. Flush for at least 15 minutes while holding the eye open. Direct the water toward the inside corner of the eye — the one nearer the nose. The water will then flow toward the outside corner. If both eyes have been burned, alternate the flow of water between them. If the eyes still burn after 15 minutes of flushing, resume the flushing. (See *How to flush the eye,* page 106.) Seek medical assistance as soon as possible.

How are chemical burns treated?
The medical team tries to maintain or restore the person's breathing and circulation. If pain and anxiety are making breathing difficult, they may administer an intravenous narcotic pain reliever.

Other treatments
Other treatments depend on how much of the person's body surface area was burned. The greater the burned area, the higher the risk of shock. When the burn covers 30% or more of the body surface, the person is at risk for heart and blood vessel collapse.

Fortunately, chemical burns typically affect a smaller area than other types of burns. If the burn covers 20% of the body surface area, the person will receive intravenous fluids to prevent shock. A person who has inhaled carbon monoxide needs intensive oxygen therapy. (See "Poison inhalation," page 409.) Other injuries are

How to flush the eye

If a chemical splashes into someone's eye, immediately flush the eye with water.

Use the right method
Have the person tilt the head toward the side of the splash, and then flush from the inner (nose) corner of the eye toward the outer corner. Hold the person's eye open while flushing. Continue to flush for at least 15 minutes.

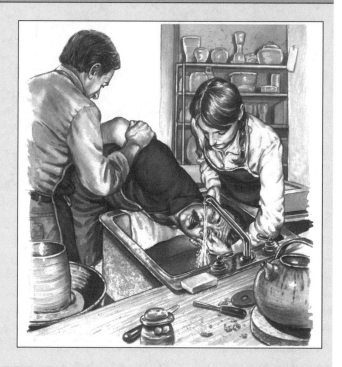

treated after the person's airway, breathing, and circulation have been ensured.

What else should you know?

Alkali burns — for example, from a drain cleaner — are more serious than acid burns. That's because alkalis penetrate deeper into the skin than acids and continue to burn longer.

Promote workplace safety

If you work around hazardous chemicals, learn first aid for a chemical spill. This information should also be posted in the workplace and made available to all workers.

BURNS CAUSED BY ELECTRICITY

Electrical burns come from contact with electric current, such as from touching faulty electrical wiring or a high-voltage power line. They can also come from being struck by lightning.

Even the relatively low current in most homes (110 volts) can be fatal. Children who chew on electrical cords are the typical victims of electrical burns at home. (See *Keeping your child safe,* page 108.)

How the current causes damage

The electric current burns the skin surface at the point where it enters the body (called the entrance burn). Then it causes massive internal damage as it travels through the body along blood vessels and nerves. Leaving the body, the current creates another surface burn at the exit site. Usually, this exit burn occurs where the body touches a surface or a metal object (called a ground). The longer the current takes to pass through the body and the higher its voltage, the greater the damage.

Burn severity also varies with the part of the body touched by the current. Moist, thin skin suffers more damage than thick, dry, calloused skin.

What are the symptoms?

During an electrical burn, the person suffers severe pain. Pulse and breathing may stop.

The skin may have extensive surface injuries. The entrance burn typically is charred, whitish yellow, and surrounded by blisters. The exit burn may be small and resemble the entry burn, or it may be much larger. Sometimes no pain occurs at either the entrance or the exit burn. (See *What happens in electrical burns,* page 109.)

If the person was struck by lightning, the skin around the entrance wound may be swollen, charred, or reddened. The burn pattern may resemble a tree branch.

Other symptoms to watch for

An electrical burn also may cause:
- irregular heartbeats
- stoppage of the heart
- rapid, shallow breathing or breathing cessation
- rapid pulse

Electrical burns result from contact with electric current, such as from touching faulty electrical wiring or a high-voltage power line. They can also come from being struck by lightning.

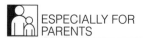

Keeping your child safe

Electrical outlets, cords, and appliances in your home pose a threat to your child's safety. Infants and toddlers are at highest risk for electrical burns. Remember — it takes just a few seconds for an active toddler to get into trouble.

Baby-proof your home

Start baby-proofing your home before your child turns 6 months old. This will help prevent calamity if your infant proves to be an early crawler.
Install inexpensive socket plugs in any electrical outlets you're not using.
Put hinged covers on electrical outlets that are in use. Store appliances like hair dryers safely out of children's reach when not in use.

Keep electrical cords out of reach

Use inexpensive tape to secure cords and keep them from dangling. This will help prevent electrical injuries and stop the child from yanking on the cord and getting injured if the appliance falls.

Unplug appliances that aren't in use. With appliances that have removable cords, always unplug from the outlet end rather than the appliance end.

Distract your child

If you see your infant heading for an electrical cord or outlet, try distraction, but don't make a fuss. If you do, your child could become curious about the forbidden hazard.
To discourage a toddler from playing with a cord, say "Ouch!" while pointing to the cord. This teaches the child that cords are dangerous and not for play.

Other precautions

If your preschooler persists in exploring an electrical outlet, teach him or her how to safely plug in appliances.
Teach an older child respectful use of electricity. Explain the risks of using radios, hair dryers, and other electrical appliances near water.

- damage to bones, joints, and tendons
- spinal injuries
- weakness
- paralysis
- seizures
- sluggishness, stupor, or loss of consciousness.

What should you do?

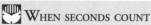

WHEN SECONDS COUNT

Immediately call 911 or the telephone number for your local emergency service (or send someone else to call). Then unplug the electrical appliance or turn off the electric current at its source. If the accident took place outdoors, call the power company first so they can shut off the power. (See *Protecting yourself during rescue,* page 110.)

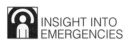

What happens in electrical burns

Electric current — whether machine-generated or natural (lightning) — can cause a wide range of injuries. When the current contacts the skin, three types of injury can occur:

- *heat burns* on the skin surface from the flames that accompany the current
- *arc* or *flash burns* from current that doesn't pass through the body
- so-called *true electrical injury* from current that does pass through the body.

Deeper damage

True electrical injury is more like a crush injury than a burn. Why? Heat burns usually destroy only the skin and underlying tissue, whereas electrical injury goes deeper, often destroying muscle tissue and affecting internal organs.

The most dangerous burns

Some electrical burns are more dangerous than others. Here are the factors that come into play.

Intensity of voltage and amperage

Lightning is measured in millions of volts and from 12,000 to 200,000 amperes. In contrast, common household electricity generates 110 or 220 volts. The higher the voltage, the greater the potential for damage.

Type of current

Alternating current (AC), such as household current, is much more dangerous than direct current (DC), such as from lightning or a car battery. Alternating current causes the muscles to contract violently. If a person has grasped a live wire, these contractions make it impossible for him or her to drop the wire.

Tissue resistance

Wet skin is much less resistant to electric current than dry skin. That's why a typical bathtub acci-

dent — when someone drops a low-voltage appliance into the water — often causes death.

Length of contact with the body

The longer the person touches the source of the electrical burn, the greater the damage. That's why it's so important to interrupt the current as soon as you can.

Current's route through the body

The most serious injuries occur from electric current passing through vital organs. For example, a current that moves from one hand to the other passes through the heart. This can cause a fatal irregular heartbeat or make the heart stop beating.

Complications of electrical burns

An electrical burn can damage the nervous system, heart and blood vessels, and kidneys. Organ damage may result from direct current or, as cells are destroyed, from interrupted blood flow. What's more, swelling tissue further disrupts the flow of blood. The following complications may occur.

Heart, brain, and spinal cord problems

- The heart's rhythm may be interrupted, possibly causing the heart to stop beating.
- Seizures, coma, and stoppage of breathing may occur if the central nervous system is affected.
- Weakness or even paralysis may result if the spinal cord is fractured.

Kidney failure and massive bleeding

- Massive lack of blood flow to the muscles causes release of large amounts of hemoglobin and myoglobin. These proteins then block the small tubes that make up the kidneys, destroying them and possibly leading to kidney failure.
- Later, the person may suffer massive bleeding, gallstones, and cataracts.

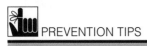 PREVENTION TIPS

Protecting yourself during rescue

If you're near someone who has been burned by an electric current, don't approach the person until the power has been turned off. Not only will this prevent you from getting injured, it will stop the flow of current into the person, helping to reduce burn severity.

What to do after an indoor accident

If the accident happened indoors, turn off the electricity in one of three ways:
- Shut off the fuse box or circuit breaker.
- Shut off the outside switch box.
- Unplug the appliance.

What to do if a power line is down
- Call the fire department or power company.
- Don't touch or try to move the downed wire.
- Keep others away from the wire.

 Never touch the person until the power has been shut off.

Next, check the person for a pulse and look, listen, and feel for breathing. If pulse and breathing are absent, start cardiopulmonary resuscitation, if you know how. (See *Performing CPR on an adult,* page 579, *Performing CPR on a child,* page 585, or *Performing CPR on an infant,* page 590.)

Be sure not to move the person if you think the neck or back has been injured. Doing this could make any spinal injury worse.

Cover the person and check for fractures
Cover the burned skin with a clean dressing or the cleanest cloth available. This protects the exposed nerve endings from a breeze blowing across them and increasing the pain.

The victim of a high-voltage injury may have suffered broken bones from violent muscle spasms. Check for symptoms of a fracture, as described in "Fractures (broken bones)," page 251. If you suspect a fracture, splint the broken bone before moving the victim. (For instructions, see *How to splint a broken bone or dislocated joint,* pages 596 to 606.)

Wrap the person in a coat or blanket to prevent heat loss. Then elevate the legs 8 to 12 inches (20 to 30 centimeters) as a precaution in case shock occurs. Cover the entry and exit burns with a clean dressing.

Don't put butter, margarine, or antibiotic ointment on a burn. These substances seal in the heat, causing further damage.

How are electrical burns treated?
In the hospital, the medical team tries to restore the person's breathing, pulse, and circulation, if necessary. To ensure breathing, they may need to insert an artificial airway or a breathing tube. If the burn impaired the person's heart function, they'll probably use a defibrillator to restore a normal heartbeat.

Other treatments
Other treatments may include:
- oxygen therapy
- a breathing machine
- intravenous fluids and water pills to help prevent kidney damage
- therapy for thermal burns if heat from the electric current made the person's clothing catch on fire

■ continuous heart monitoring (dangerous irregular heartbeats can arise *after* the heart appears stable)
■ surgery to repair damaged tissue

If the current passed through an arm or a leg, the limb is elevated to minimize swelling, which impedes the flow of blood and fluids through tissues. Swollen tissue can press on nerves and vessels; unless the swelling is reduced, tissue death and gangrene could set in.

What else should you know?

The total extent of tissue damage isn't apparent for 12 to 24 hours after an electrical burn.

The medical team tries to restore the person's breathing, pulse, and circulation, if necessary. They may need to use special measures, such as a breathing tube.

Burns caused by heat

Burns caused by heat (thermal burns) are the most common type of burn. They frequently come from:
■ house fires
■ motor vehicle accidents
■ children playing with matches,
■ improperly stored gasoline
■ space heater mishaps
■ electrical malfunctions
■ arson.

Other ways to get thermal burns include improper handling of firecrackers, scalding accidents, and kitchen accidents. In children, burns from heat, especially scalding, are sometimes traced to abuse.

Major burns require painful treatment and prolonged rehabilitation. Those that aren't fatal can cause permanent disability and disfigurement, leaving both emotional and physical scars.

How burns are classified

Burns are often classified as first-degree, second-degree, or third-degree.
■ A *first-degree* burn injures only the top layer of the skin, called the *epidermis*. Examples of first-degree burns are minor sunburn and burns from brief contact with a hot iron.
■ A *second-degree* burn damages both the top skin layer and the one

under it, called the *dermis*. Examples include deep sunburns and burns caused by hot liquids.

■ A *third-degree* burn destroys all skin layers and may damage muscles and bones beneath the skin. This type of burn commonly comes from a fire, electricity, and prolonged contact with a hot object. (See *How severe is the burn?*)

A first-degree burn injures only the top layer of the skin. In contrast, a third-degree burn destroys all skin layers.

What are the symptoms?

Symptoms vary with burn severity. *A first-degree burn* causes:
■ tenderness
■ redness
■ pain
■ slight swelling of the skin
■ no blisters.

    A *second-degree burn* causes:
■ pain, which may be excruciating
■ blisters
■ swelling
■ a moist or oozing surface
■ red, streaked, or splotchy skin.

    A *third-degree burn* can cause:
■ loss of consciousness
■ breathing distress (from lung injury due to smoke inhalation)
■ white, reddened, grayish, darkened, or charred skin
■ little or no pain (because the nerve endings have been destroyed)
■ peeling off of dead skin.

What should you do?

WHEN SECONDS COUNT

■ If you see a person who has suffered severe or extensive burns, first put out the flames to stop the burning or remove the person from the source of the burn.
■ Have someone immediately call 911.
■ Next, feel the person for a pulse and look, listen, and feel for breathing. If pulse and breathing are absent, start CPR, if you know how. (See *Performing CPR on an adult,* page 579, *Performing CPR on a child,* page 585, or *Performing CPR on an infant,* page 590.)
■ If the person is unconscious, gently roll him or her onto the side, unless you suspect a neck or back injury.
■ Wash your hands thoroughly. Put on latex gloves, if available, to help prevent infection.

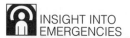

INSIGHT INTO
EMERGENCIES

How severe is the burn?

Burns are often classified by depth, although most burns are a combination of different degrees and thicknesses. Sometimes even an experienced doctor can't tell how severe a burn is until several days later.

First-degree burn

In this burn, damage is limited to the top skin layer, called the _epidermis_. The burn causes pain and redness.

Second-degree burn

The top skin layer and part of the layer under it, called the _dermis_, are damaged in a second-degree burn. The person has blisters, pain, and swelling.

Third-degree burn

This burn damages both the epidermis and the dermis. No blisters appear, but white, red, brown, gray, or black leathery tissue is visible.

Fourth-degree burn

Sometimes doctors refer to a fourth category, called a _fourth-degree burn._ Damage from this severe burn extends through deeply charred tissue under the skin to the muscle and bone.

This illustration shows the depth of first-, second-, and third-degree burns.

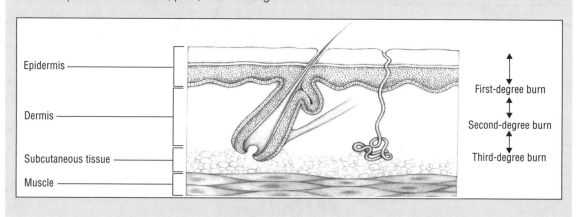

■ Keep the person lying down. Elevate a burned arm or leg. Keep the person's head and chest slightly lower than the rest of the body. If possible, raise the legs.

■ Cool the burned area quickly with cold running water. Apply towels soaked in cool water to any burns of the face, back, chest, or abdomen. Moisten the materials often to keep them cool. To prevent heat loss, cover the wet towels with sheets. (See _First-aid for burns,_ page 115.)

> ❌ Don't put ice or ice water on the burn.
>
> ❌ Be sure not to put ointments, salves, margarine, butter, creams, or sprays on the burn. These substances will increase pain.
>
> ❌ Never rupture any blisters over the burn.
>
> ❌ Don't let the person become chilled. Cover wet dressings with a dry sheet or blanket.
>
> ❌ Avoid letting burned surfaces touch. For example, use a clean towel or sheet to separate the underside of the person's arm from the side of the body.
>
> ❌ Don't give the person anything to eat or drink or any drugs.
>
> ❌ Be sure not to apply tight dressings. Burns often swell.

If you see a person who has suffered severe or extensive burns, first put out the flames to stop the burning, or remove the person from the source of the burn.

For a burn to the face or head

■ Because a person with facial burns may have suffered smoke inhalation injury, move him or her to fresh air. Have someone call for medical help immediately.

■ Check the person for a pulse and breathing. If pulse and breathing are absent, start CPR if you know how. If you detect a pulse and the person is breathing, position the person to make breathing more comfortable.

■ To treat a facial or head burn, apply soaked sheets, towels, or other wet materials to the area. Add more water to the materials often to keep them cool.

■ Then apply several layers of gauze to the burn. Make sure to put gauze behind the person's ears to separate the ears from the head.

> ❌ Don't cover the person's nostrils when applying gauze to the face or head because this makes breathing more difficult.

■ Next, make bandages from clean handkerchiefs or sheets. To make a *cravat, or triangular bandage,* fold a square piece of cloth diagonally so it resembles a necktie, or cravat. (You can improvise a triangular bandage from a clean cloth diaper, handkerchief, or torn sheet.) Loosely apply the bandage around the forehead to hold the gauze in place on the upper half of the face. Apply a second cravat bandage around the chin to hold the gauze in place on the lower part of the face. (For a *neck burn,* apply gauze in several layers.)

■ While dressing the burn, keep checking to see if the person has a clear airway and pulse and is breathing.

First-aid for burns

This chart provides a quick summary of what to do and what not to do for the main types of burns caused by heat.

TYPE OF BURN	DO	DON'T
First-degree	■ Apply cold water and dry sterile dressing.	■ Don't apply butter, margarine, salve, or ointment.
Second-degree	■ Immerse burned part in cold water if it's still burning. ■ Cover with sterile cloth.	■ Don't break blisters or remove shreds of tissue. ■ Don't use antiseptic preparations or sprays. ■ Don't use home remedies.
Third-degree	■ Get medical attention immediately. ■ Cover burned part with dry sterile cloth. ■ Watch person for trouble breathing.	■ Don't remove any charred clothing that's sticking to burn. ■ Don't apply ice to burn. ■ Don't use home remedies or drugs.

For a burn to the back
■ Apply gauze to the burned area in several layers. Be sure to cover all burned surfaces. Also cover the side of the person's body under the arm. If the arm and body are raw, put gauze between them so they won't touch.
■ Next, apply a triangular bandage over the gauze. Place the base of the bandage around the person's lower back and tie it in front.

For a burn to the chest
■ Apply gauze in several layers, making sure to cover all burned surfaces. Also put dressings on the side of the person's body under the arm, including the chest wall and armpit. If the arm and body are raw, put gauze between these areas so they don't touch.
■ Then make a triangular bandage that's large enough to tie at the back of the person's neck.
■ Split the point of the bandage. Place the base of the bandage around the person's waist and tie it in the back.

For a steam burn or scalding burn
■ If the burn is minor, apply cool, moist gauze or bandages.

- For a more serious burn, cover with a clean, dry dressing and get the person to the hospital at once.

For a minor burn
- If the burn hasn't broken the skin, immerse the burned part in cold running water or apply a cold compress. If you see broken blisters, apply cold running water only.
- Place a clean cloth or pad over the burn and bandage it loosely.
- If the burn is on the face, eyes, hands, feet, or genitals or if it covers an extensive area, get the person to a hospital as soon as possible. Other minor burns usually don't call for hospital treatment.

For a serious steam burn or scalding burn, cover with a clean, dry dressing and get the person to the hospital at once.

How are thermal burns treated?
Treatment depends on the severity of the burn.

Treating severe or extensive burns
The medical team takes steps to maintain the person's airway, breathing, and circulation. To ensure breathing, they may:
- insert an artificial airway or breathing tube
- administer oxygen
- attach the person to a breathing machine.

To help prevent shock, the medical team administers intravenous fluids. Massive fluid replacement usually continues for 24 hours after a severe burn. The person will be monitored not only for shock but also for respiratory complications, decreased body temperature, irregular heartbeats, and blood vessel problems.

Also, drugs are given to relieve pain — especially if the person is having trouble breathing because of pain and anxiety. Antibiotics and a tetanus shot may be given to prevent infection.

Treating moderate burns
These burns usually can be treated in the doctor's office or at home. After the emergency treatment described above, the burn is washed gently with lukewarm water and mild soap to prevent infection. Once the burn cools, a thin coat of antibiotic ointment, such as Baciguent, Polysporin, or Silvadene cream, may be applied. Then a sterile dressing is applied over the burn and secured by a strip of gauze. The doctor may give the person instructions for daily home care. (See *Caring for a moderate burn at home*.)

Caring for a moderate burn at home

If you have a moderate burn, the instructions below will help you avoid infection and other burn complications.

Keep the burn clean

- Once or twice a day, wash the burn with lukewarm water and mild soap.
- After washing the burn, apply a thin coat of antibiotic ointment, such as Baciguent, Polysporin, or Silvadene cream. Cover with a sterile dressing.

Treat the wound gently

- If you have trouble removing the old dressing, try soaking it in clean, lukewarm water.
- Don't pull or yank the old dressing off.

Other instructions

- If the burn is on an arm, a leg, a hand, or a foot, keep the part elevated to prevent swelling.
- Take an anti-inflammatory drug, such as aspirin or Motrin, to reduce pain and swelling.
- See your doctor within 1 to 2 days for a wound check.

Treating minor burns

The person may receive an anti-inflammatory drug, such as aspirin or ibuprofen (Advil or Motrin), to reduce pain and swelling. A dressing usually isn't needed.

What else should you know?

After discharge from the hospital, a person who has suffered a severe or extensive burn can aid healing by eating properly and caring for the burned parts of the skin. Here are some suggestions.

Dietary guidelines

- Eat well-balanced meals with adequate carbohydrates and proteins.
- Eat between-meal snacks.
- Include at least one protein source in each meal and snack.
- Avoid tobacco, alcohol and caffeine.

Skin care

- Wash new skin with mild soap and water.
- Apply a lubricating lotion — one that doesn't contain alcohol or perfume.
- Avoid bumping or scratching the new skin tissue.
- Don't wear tight-fitting or abrasive clothing.
- Never expose new skin to strong sunlight.

- Always use a sunblock with a sun protection factor of 20 or higher.
- Don't expose new skin to irritants, such as paint, solvents, strong detergents, or antiperspirants.
- If your new skin itches, take cool baths or apply an ice pack.
- Wear protective clothing during cold weather to prevent frostbite.

C

CALF PAIN

Pain in the calf or lower leg can come from various conditions relating to the skin, muscles, bones, blood vessels, or nerves. The type of pain experienced and the person's other symptoms may offer clues to the cause.

Thrombophlebitis: A common cause

Severe calf pain may mean *thrombophlebitis.* In this condition, a vein becomes inflamed and a blood clot (thrombus) forms. A clot may form in either a deep vein or a surface vein.

The clot may block the vein partially or totally, or it may break free and lodge somewhere else in the circulatory system. In *pulmonary embolism,* a deadly complication, the clot travels to the lungs.

Primarily affecting people over age 40 and hospital patients, clots in deep veins are more serious than those in surface veins because they tend to occur in larger vessels.

Other causes of calf pain

If the person recently injured or broke the leg, extreme pain, increased swelling, numbness, or tingling in the leg may mean a condition called *compartment syndrome.* This is a limb-threatening problem and requires immediate treatment. For more information, see *Understanding compartment syndrome,* page 169.

What are the symptoms?

In thrombophlebitis, symptoms usually depend on whether the clot is in a surface vein or a deep vein. A surface clot usually makes the vein hard and cordlike, warm, extremely sensitive to pressure and, possibly, red and swollen.

Although a deep-vein clot may produce no symptoms, it more commonly causes aching pain, fever, chills and, possibly, swelling and bluish discoloration of the leg. The pain may get worse when the person walks or flexes the foot upward.

Severe calf pain may mean that a leg vein has become inflamed and a blood clot has formed. The clot may then block the vein.

Treatment for a surface blood clot usually involves bed rest, elevating the leg, and applying warm, moist soaks.

What should you do?

Keep the person in bed and arrange for prompt medical attention. If the calf pain stems from a blood clot, moving around too much could cause the clot to break free and block other veins.

Be sure to give the doctor an accurate and complete description of the pain, including:

■ when and how it started
■ whether it's steady or intermittent
■ whether anything makes it better or worse.

Try to use descriptive words for the pain, such as "aching," "sharp," "cramping," "boring," "dull," "shooting," "throbbing," or "tingling."

WHEN SECONDS COUNT

Calf pain followed by shortness of breath may mean a blood clot in the lungs (pulmonary embolism). Get immediate medical help for this life-threatening emergency.

How is calf pain treated?

Treatment for a blood clot in a surface vein involves bed rest, elevating the leg, and applying warm, moist soaks. The doctor usually prescribes medicine to relieve pain and inflammation.

After the initial treatment, the person should make an effort to prevent future blood clots. (See *Taking steps toward healthier legs.*)

Wearing elastic stockings

The person will need to wear elastic support stockings called *antiembolism stockings*. In the hospital, a nurse will teach the person how to put on these stockings correctly. They must be applied *before* the person gets out of bed so the legs don't have a chance to swell.

Be sure not to let the person sit or stand for prolonged periods.

Don't allow the person who's taking blood thinners, such as Coumadin, to use sharp razors. These drugs increase the risk of bleeding, so a razor cut may cause profuse bleeding. Urge the person to use an electric shaver instead of a razor.

Never let the person take aspirin-containing drugs because they heighten the risk of bleeding.

What else should you know?

Although the cause of a deep-vein blood clot may be unknown, it

Taking steps toward healthier legs

If you have a blood clot in one of the veins in your leg, improving the circulation in your legs can promote healing and prevent complications, such as pain and swelling. Here's how you can have healthier legs.

Keep your legs elevated

When lying down, elevate your feet higher than the level of your heart. This helps gravity to move excess fluid out of your legs. When you sit — at your desk, for example — rest your feet on a footstool.

Watch your diet

Eating a healthy diet can improve the health of your circulatory system. Be sure to eat plenty of fresh fruits and vegetables and seafood.

Cut down on salt

Avoid salty foods, which can increase swelling. Examples of salty foods include:

- bacon
- ham
- corned beef
- smoked fish
- pickles
- potato chips
- crackers.

Read food package labels

When you shop, read the nutrition labels on food packages to find out how much fat and sodium the product contains. Then choose foods low in fat and sodium.

Eat healthy snacks

Choose fruit over packaged snacks. If you must eat processed snacks, look for low-sodium alternatives.

Prevent infection

Wash your legs daily with soap and warm water to remove germs that could cause infection. Avoid using bath powders that could dry your skin. Don't hesitate to call the doctor if you notice symptoms of a leg infection, such as redness and swelling.

Exercise regularly

Get involved in swimming or other pool exercises, such as walking or jogging in water. Or ask the doctor to recommend other exercises for your legs.

Choose proper clothing

Avoid tight garments that could cut off circulation in your legs, such as garters, girdles, and knee-high hosiery. Wear elastic support stockings all day, every day.

Watch for warning signs

Inspect your legs every morning. Call the doctor if you notice these warning signs of poor circulation:
- discolored skin — for example, brown or bluish red areas
- sores
- scales
- increased leg pain or swelling.

Follow your treatment plan

Take your blood thinner or other prescribed drugs exactly as the doctor directs. And be sure to keep all appointments for follow-up visits with the doctor.

usually results from damage to the lining of a vein, rapid blood clotting, and reduced blood flow. Factors that make the formation of a deep-vein clot more likely include:
- prolonged bed rest
- traumatic injury

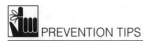
PREVENTION TIPS

How to avoid leg ulcers

When a blood clot blocks an artery or a vein in your leg, you have an increased risk of developing a leg ulcer. A leg ulcer is an area of dying skin.

Why a leg ulcer forms
A leg ulcer can form for a couple of reasons. First, when a blood vessel gets blocked, it can't deliver its usual supply of blood to the skin tissues in your leg. Those tissues then become malnourished and, possibly, damaged.

Pooling of blood
A leg ulcer can also result from blood that has pooled in your leg veins. You may notice the pooling as swollen ankles. The pooled blood puts extra pressure on the insides of your veins, further reducing the flow of blood that gets to your leg tissues. Over time, your skin may become fragile and more susceptible to infection. The result may be leg ulcers.

Ways to prevent leg ulcers
The best way to prevent leg ulcers is to improve the circulation in your legs. You can do that by wearing elastic support stockings called *antiembolism stockings.* By compressing your leg veins a bit, the stockings help stop blood from pooling in your lower legs.

Also, be sure to elevate your feet above the level of your heart when resting. The doctor may want you to elevate your feet for a certain amount of time each day.

Reduce the chance of injury
Try to avoid activities in which you could bruise or injure your legs. And take steps to reduce your risk of falling. For example:
- Install safety rails in the bathtub.
- Don't use throw rugs.
- Avoid prolonged sitting or standing.
- Wear low-heeled, nonskid shoes.

Check for symptoms
Check your legs every day for new symptoms of leg ulcers. If any part of your leg is swollen or painful or there are discolored skin areas, call the doctor.

Ways to promote healing
If you already have a leg ulcer, wearing antiembolism stockings will help it heal by improving blood circulation in your legs. Keeping your ulcer clean and germfree is important too. Wash your hands before and after changing your dressing or touching the wound. Change the dressing and apply medicine to the ulcer exactly as the doctor directs.

Be patient
Finally, be patient. It may take several months for your ulcer to heal. Call your doctor if it becomes larger, more painful, or foul-smelling.

- surgery
- childbirth
- use of oral contraceptives.
    Causes of a blood clot near the surface of the leg include:
- traumatic injury
- infection

- intravenous drug abuse
- irritation from intravenous drugs and diagnostic tests.

Watch for leg ulcers
Having a blood clot makes a person more likely to develop an additional problem: leg ulcers. See *How to avoid leg ulcers,* for an explanation of leg ulcers and ways to prevent and treat them.

CHEST INJURIES

Chest injuries — injuries to the heart, lungs, or ribs — may be blunt or penetrating. Blunt chest injuries typically result from motor vehicle accidents, such as when a person's chest strikes the steering wheel. They may also occur from explosions or sports accidents; for example, from being tackled in a football game or struck by a baseball bat. (See *How a blow injures the chest,* page 124.)

Chest injuries — blunt and otherwise — account for about one-fourth of all deaths from injuries in North America. (For information on penetrating chest injuries, see "Gunshot wounds," page 265, and "Stabbing," page 487.)

The victim of a blunt chest injury may experience:
- lung injuries
- a bruised heart
- broken ribs
- a broken breastbone.

What are the complications?
Blunt chest injuries can lead to such complications as:
- tears in the heart muscle
- compression of the heart by fluid or blood, called *cardiac tamponade*
- tears in the pulmonary artery
- rupture of one of the heart's chambers
- rupture or tear in the windpipe, air passages, or esophagus
- shock.

Chest injuries account for about one-fourth of all deaths from injuries in North America.

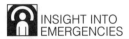

How a blow injures the chest

A blunt injury to the chest can occur when:
- a moving object strikes a person's chest
- a person's chest strikes a stationary object
- a massive object crushes the chest.

When a moving object strikes a person's chest

A moving object — for example, a baseball bat — hitting a person's chest may cause injuries like hemothorax (buildup of blood within the lining around the lungs) or a bruised lung.

Hemothorax

This chest injury may break ribs and tear major arteries. Blood then collects in the lung cavity.

HEMOTHORAX

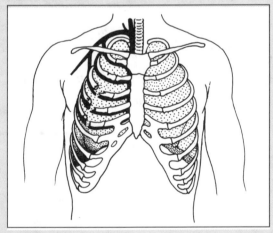

Bruised lung

In this injury, a forceful impact bruises lung tissue without tearing it. This causes swelling and bleeding in addition to bruising.

When a person's chest strikes a stationary object

When a person's chest hits a stationary object with great force — for example, someone hitting the steering wheel in a motor vehicle accident — severe damage to internal organs occurs.

CHEST STRIKING STATIONARY OBJECT

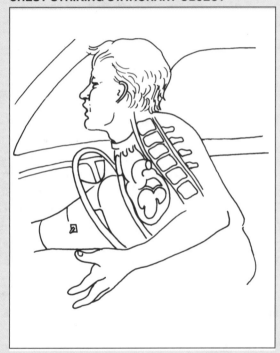

Bruised heart

In this injury, the heart is squeezed between the breastbone and the spine, bruising the heart muscle.

When a massive object crushes the chest

Crushing of the chest, such as when a car falls onto a mechanic who's working under it, forces blood from the heart to the veins of the head, neck, and upper chest. This injury can cause asphyxiation and death.

Lung injuries

Damage from a lung injury varies with the location and force of the blow. These injuries may lead to:

■ pneumothorax — buildup of air in the lining around the lungs. This can occur when a broken rib punctures a lung. In *open pneumothorax,* air in the chest cavity moves in and out but the lung doesn't expand. In *tension pneumothorax,* air is pulled into the chest cavity as the person inhales, but then it can't exit. This results in tension or pressure in the chest, which can impair heart and lung function and cause shock.

■ hemothorax — blood buildup in the lining around the lungs, which impedes breathing. Massive hemothorax is the most common cause of shock after a chest injury.

■ bruising of lung tissue. This condition decreases oxygen flow to the lungs, causing swelling and bleeding within the lungs.

Chest wall injuries

Blows to the chest that injure the chest wall may cause broken ribs and a condition called *flail chest.* In this injury, three or more adjacent ribs are broken in two more places, causing an unstable chest wall and abnormal breathing. (See *How flail chest disrupts breathing,* page 126.) Also, a broken rib may tear or rupture a very large blood vessel called the *aorta.* This condition nearly always causes immediate death. (See *Which ribs are most likely to break?* page 127.)

If the chest injury breaks a rib, the lung may suffer damage. If the breastbone breaks, the person may suffer persistent chest pain.

What are the symptoms?

Symptoms of blunt chest injury vary with the specific injury. For instance, if the injury breaks a rib, one or both lobes of the lungs may suffer damage. A broken breastbone may cause persistent chest pain, even at rest.

Symptoms of pneumothorax

The person with a pneumothorax may have:

■ severe shortness of breath

■ shallow, rapid breathing

■ extreme pain

■ bluish skin

■ agitation.

Symptoms of tension pneumothorax

A person with this injury may have:

■ severe shortness of breath

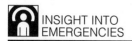

INSIGHT INTO
EMERGENCIES

How flail chest disrupts breathing

A blunt injury that hurts the chest wall may lead to *flail chest*. In this condition, chest movements as well as the breathing pattern are abnormal as the person breathes in and out. This abnormal opposite movement is called *paradoxical breathing*.

Inhalation
Injured chest wall collapses in.
Uninjured chest wall moves out.

Exhalation
Injured chest wall moves out.
Uninjured chest wall moves in.

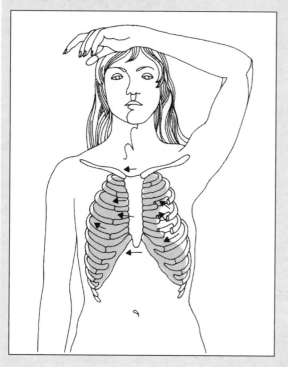

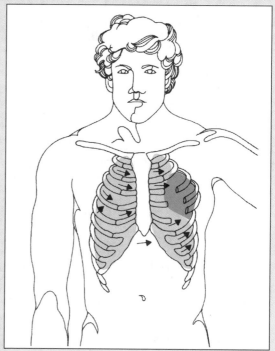

- enlarged neck veins
- rapid pulse
- restlessness
- acute chest pain
- bluish skin.

Symptoms of hemothorax

A hemothorax may cause:

- chest pain
- rapid breathing
- shortness of breath
- coughing up of blood
- bloody, frothy sputum
- a fast pulse
- dusky skin
- increased perspiration.

Symptoms of bruised lung tissue

Someone with a bruised lung may experience:

- coughing up of blood
- shortness of breath
- agitation
- anxiety
- rapid breathing.

Symptoms of flail chest

Flail chest may cause:

- extreme pain
- bruises
- abnormal chest movement, with part of the chest moving opposite the rest of the chest during breathing
- rapid, shallow breathing
- fast pulse
- bluish skin.

Symptoms of a broken rib

A broken rib may cause:

- tenderness and slight swelling over the fracture site
- shallow breathing
- pain that worsens with deep breathing and movement.

What should you do?

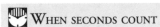 **W**HEN SECONDS COUNT

Call for medical help immediately — especially if the person has symptoms of shock (pale or bluish skin, a fast pulse, shortness of breath, dizziness, or weakness). Then check for a pulse and look, listen, and feel for breathing. If pulse and breathing are absent, start

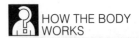 HOW THE BODY WORKS

Which ribs are most likely to break?

We have 12 pairs of ribs. The 5 pairs in the middle of the chest are most often broken. The upper 2 pairs, in contrast, seldom are broken because they're sheltered between the collarbone and the shoulder blades.

How the "floating ribs" bend

The "floating ribs" (the lower 2 pairs) also resist fracture. That's because they're not attached to the breastbone, so they're free to move in and out. Like the willow tree, they bend rather than break.

CPR if you know how. *(See Performing CPR on an adult,* page 579, *Performing CPR on a child,* page 585, or *Performing CPR on an infant,* page 590.)*

If the person has a pulse and is breathing, keep him or her sitting up with the head and shoulders elevated. Or place the person with the injured side down. Recheck the airway and breathing periodically until help arrives.

> *The person with suspected heart damage needs intensive care to detect irregular heartbeats and prevent shock.*

Other steps to take

Your next actions depend on the type and severity of the chest injury. For instance, if the person has symptoms of a broken rib, have him or her hold a pillow or other soft object against the rib.

 Never ignore symptoms of shock.

 Don't strap or tape the person's chest.

How are chest injuries treated?

The person needs immediate treatment to control bleeding and maintain breathing. For a *simple rib fracture,* the person usually rests in bed and receives mild pain relievers and heat application. For more *severe rib fractures,* the doctor may administer drugs to deaden nerves between the ribs and thus reduce pain. If the person is having serious trouble breathing, the medical team may need to insert a breathing tube.

Treating lung injuries

To treat *open pneumothorax,* the team inserts a tube into the person's chest to remove air from the lung cavity and reexpand the lungs.

For *tension pneumothorax,* the doctor inserts a needle into the chest to release pressure, and then inserts a chest tube to help restore normal pressure and reexpand the lungs.

For *hemothorax,* the person receives intravenous fluids for shock and blood transfusions to replace massive blood loss, if needed. A chest tube is inserted to remove blood from the chest.

The person with a *bruised lung* typically receives fluids, pain relievers, water pills and, if necessary, steroids to reduce inflammation.

For a *ruptured diaphragm,* a tube is inserted through the person's nose and stomach to reduce pressure within the stomach. Then surgery is done.

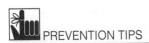

Avoiding blunt chest injuries

By taking a few simple precautions, you can prevent blunt chest injuries to yourself and your loved ones.

Make sure everyone buckles up
Everyone riding in a motor vehicle should use a seat belt every day on every trip. Infants up to age 6 months should be in a rear-facing, specially designed infant seat. Infants older than age 6 months should face forward in a safety seat designed for them. Safety seats have weight limits; review yours periodically.

Many children ages 6 to 8 are severely injured in motor vehicle accidents because they've outgrown booster seats but are too small for adult shoulder harnesses. Some experts recommend that these children sit in the rear of the vehicle, if possible.

Install your child safety seat correctly
Because many people don't use their child safety seats correctly, children are injured unnecessarily. Follow the directions that come with the safety seat. If you don't have the directions, call the company and ask for another set. Note the model number. (If the telephone number isn't on the safety seat, call 1-800-555-1212 and ask for the manufacturer's 800 number.)

Use your locking clip
If your vehicle has automatically adjusting shoulder harnesses, you must use a locking clip to buckle the child safety seat into the vehicle. The locking clip comes with the safety seat. If you have a secondhand safety seat that's missing the locking clip, you can purchase a clip at a hardware store.

How to buy a secondhand child safety seat
If you buy or borrow a secondhand child safety seat, be sure to ask if it's been used in a vehicle that was involved in an accident. Don't use one that has — it may no longer offer protection. If any cracks are visible, don't use the safety seat.

Use inflatable air bags
If you don't own a vehicle that has air bags, try to buy such a vehicle when you replace your current one. Air bags reduce the severity of blunt chest injuries by preventing the driver from hitting the steering wheel. However, infants and young children can be injured by passenger-side air bags. For this reason, always buckle young children in approved child safety seats in the back seat, if possible.

Wear the right sports equipment
Athletes can avoid blunt chest injuries by wearing the appropriate protection. For example, some Little League teams now use chest pads and lighter bats to prevent fatal chest injuries to very young players.

Treating flail chest
The lung is reexpanded and the person receives oxygen and intravenous drugs.

Treating heart injuries
The person with suspected *heart damage* needs intensive care to de-

tect irregular heartbeats and prevent shock caused by abnormal heart function. He or she receives oxygen and drugs to steady the heartbeat or to ease symptoms of heart failure.

A person with a *ruptured heart muscle* or another type of heart laceration requires immediate surgery. So does the person with an *aortic rupture* or *laceration* (if he or she survives long enough to get to the hospital).

What else should you know?

School-age children riding in motor vehicles can suffer blunt chest injuries if the vehicle's shoulder harnesses are too big for them. They're at particular risk for chest injuries if they're too big for a booster seat but too small for an adult shoulder harness. (See *Avoiding blunt chest injuries,* page 129.)

CHEST PAIN

Although chest pain doesn't always mean a heart attack, many lives are lost unnecessarily to heart attacks because people ignore chest pain and other symptoms and delay getting help.

Chest pain usually comes from a disorder of a structure in the chest or abdomen, such as the following:
- heart
- lungs
- chest cavity lining
- gallbladder
- pancreas
- stomach.

Does chest pain always signal a heart attack?

A major cause of chest pain is a heart attack. Chest pain occurs because the attack prevents the heart from getting enough oxygen.

Although chest pain doesn't always mean a heart attack, many lives are lost unnecessarily to heart attacks because people ignore chest pain and other symptoms and delay getting help. Most people who have fatal heart attacks die within 2 hours of the first symptoms.

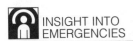

INSIGHT INTO
EMERGENCIES

Where does chest pain come from?

Not all conditions that cause chest pain require immediate treatment. However, someone with chest pain should seek medical attention at once. Only a doctor can tell if the pain signals a life-threatening condition. Here's a list of some serious and not so serious causes of chest pain.

Heart conditions
- Cardiomyopathy, or disease of the heart muscle
- Mitral valve prolapse, or floppy valve syndrome
- Heart attack

Respiratory problems
- Blastomycosis, a fungal condition affecting the lungs
- Bronchitis, or inflammation of the breathing passages
- Disease of the spaces between lung tissues
- Legionnaire's disease
- Lung abscess
- Lung cancer
- Pleurisy, or inflammation of one of the lung's membranes
- Pneumomediastinum, a condition in which a section of the chest cavity fills with air or gas
- Pulmonary hypertension, in which pressure in the pulmonary artery rises above normal
- Tuberculosis

Digestive tract problems
- Gallstones

- Hiatal hernia, in which a portion of the stomach juts upward through the diaphragm
- Spasm of the esophagus
- Stomach ulcer

Bone and muscle problems
- Broken rib
- Inflamed rib
- Muscle strain

Infections
- Coccidioidomycosis, a fungal disease caused by inhaling spores
- Nocardiosis, a bacterial infection that causes pneumonia
- Psittacosis, a bacterial infection transmitted to humans by birds
- Shingles, or herpes zoster

Other causes
- Sickle cell disease
- Anxiety
- Reaction to monosodium glutamate (MSG) in food

Other causes

Besides heart attack, chest pain can come from the following conditions:
- pneumonia and other lung disorders
- indigestion
- shingles
- muscle strain
- bone problems, such as a broken rib

Alone with chest pain: What should you do?

If you experience chest pain and no one is there to help, call 911 or the phone number for the local emergency services and explain that you think you may be having a heart attack. Then follow these instructions.

Get as comfortable as possible

■ Sit up or use a recliner, but don't lie down.
■ Prop yourself up on one or two pillows if that makes you more comfortable.
■ Loosen any tight clothing, especially around your neck.
■ Put on a coat or wrap yourself in a blanket to keep warm.

Other instructions

■ If you've been using prescribed nitroglycerin, take your medicine as directed.
■ Don't eat or drink anything.
■ If you can get to your door, unlock it so rescuers can get in. If you know you won't be able to get to the door, make sure to tell the emergency medical service when you call. This way, rescuers will know to bring the right equipment to open the door.

■ blood disorders, such as anemia
■ certain drugs, such as cocaine
■ anxiety. (See *Where does chest pain come from?* page 131.)

What's more, chest pain may be caused or worsened by exertion, deep breathing, or eating certain foods. The pain may be sharp and may recur, but it usually lasts only a few seconds. Nonetheless, chest pain *always* warrants a call to the doctor.

What are the symptoms?

Chest pain may arise suddenly or gradually. It may be steady or intermittent, mild or severe. It can range in character from a sharp, shooting sensation to a feeling of heaviness, fullness, or indigestion.

When to suspect a heart attack

Knowing the symptoms of a heart attack — and calling for emergency medical help *before* the person's heart stops beating — can save a life. Suspect a heart attack in someone who has any of the following symptoms:

■ chest pain or pressure that's severe, crushing (not sharp), and constant and lasts longer than several minutes. The pain, which may be mistaken for indigestion, isn't relieved by rest, changing position, or medicine. However, it may go away and come back.
■ chest discomfort that spreads to the arm, shoulder, neck, jaw, back, or pit of the stomach
■ profuse sweating
■ nausea and vomiting
■ extreme weakness
■ anxiety or fear
■ pale skin, possibly with blue fingernails and lips
■ extreme shortness of breath or rapid breathing
■ fast, slow, or irregular pulse.

Also, be aware that it's natural for someone with chest pain to deny that anything is wrong.

What should you do?

WHEN SECONDS COUNT

If someone who has recently complained of chest pain loses consciousness, call for immediate medical help. Then feel for a pulse and look, listen, and feel for breathing. If pulse and breathing are absent, start CPR, if you know how. *(See Performing CPR on an adult,* page 579, *Performing CPR on a child,* page 585, or *Performing CPR on an infant,* page 590.)

 Never delay getting help for someone with chest pain.

If the person is conscious and has chest pain, call for medical help immediately and describe the symptoms. If telephone service isn't available, go directly to the nearest hospital emergency department. (See *Alone with chest pain: What should you do?*)

Make the person comfortable
Next, place the person in a comfortable sitting or semisitting position. Use a pillow to prop up the person's head if that position is more comfortable.

 Don't let the person lie flat because this could make breathing more difficult.

Loosen any tight clothing, particularly neckties or other garments that constrict the neck. Keep the person warm by draping a blanket or coat around him or her.

Find out if the person has had chest pain before and uses a drug to relieve it. If the person has been taking nitroglycerin for chest pain, help him or her take it now.

Be sure not to let the person take someone else's nitroglycerin.

Don't give the person anything to eat or drink.

Never let the person talk you out of calling for help. Denial is normal, but it may prove fatal.

How is chest pain treated?
Diagnostic tests are performed to find out if the person is having a heart attack or is suffering from another disorder that mimics a heart attack.

If a heart attack is strongly suspected or confirmed, the person usually receives oxygen, and an electrocardiogram is taken to detect irregular heartbeats. An intravenous line is inserted so drugs can be given into a vein.

If irregular heartbeats occur, the doctor may prescribe a drug called an antiarrhythmic to steady the heartbeat. Some people also need to have a temporary pacemaker inserted in the chest.

Anyone who experiences chest pain must call the doctor promptly to investigate the cause.

Treating other causes

If the person is diagnosed with chest inflammation or infection, the doctor prescribes drugs and other therapies to relieve pain, reduce inflammation, and restore normal lung function.

For information on treatment of other conditions that can cause chest pain, see other sections of this book. For instance:

■ for treatment of pneumothorax, see "Chest injuries," page 123
■ for treatment of heart attack, see "Heart attack," page 283
■ for treatment of pulmonary embolism, see "Calf pain," page 119
■ for treatment of difficulty breathing or shortness of breath, see "Shortness of breath," page 456.

What else should you know?

Remember — not all chest pain signals a heart attack. But anyone who experiences chest pain must call the doctor promptly to investigate the cause.

CHILDBIRTH

If you're not far from a hospital, you may be able to make it there in time for delivery if the woman's contractions are more than 2 to 3 minutes apart.

Emergency childbirth takes place when a woman has little warning that she's about to give birth. Some births can take place within 2 hours after labor begins, so a woman may find herself about to give birth far from her doctor or midwife or a hospital.

What are the symptoms?

If you're not far from a hospital, you may be able to make it there in time for delivery if:

■ the woman's contractions are more than 2 to 3 minutes apart
■ the amount of the baby's head that's showing is smaller than a silver dollar
■ the woman doesn't feel the urge to bear down.

On the other hand, you should prepare for emergency childbirth if:

■ contractions are 2 to 3 minutes apart

■ the woman feels the urge to bear down or have a bowel movement
■ the amount of the baby's head that's showing is about the size of a silver dollar, meaning that the baby is "crowning." (See *Is the baby about to be born?* page 136.)

What should you do?

Call for emergency medical assistance, or at least try to get a doctor or 911 operator to assist you over the telephone.

Above all, don't panic — most childbirths are normal and natural. As you perform each of the steps below, calmly explain to the woman and any family or friends with her what you're doing. If you're the father and you've had childbirth preparation, you'll be somewhat ready. If you're assisting the family and the father is present, encourage him to help the woman with her breathing.

Prepare for delivery

■ Place clean sheets on the bed. (Birth is very messy.) If time permits, lay a shower curtain or rubber sheet under the fresh sheets. If you can't get the woman to a bed, place fresh newspapers or clean clothes under her hips.
■ Have the woman lie on her back with knees bent and feet flat on the floor or bed. Or, the father may sit behind her and support her in a semisitting position.
■ Then have her drop her knees wide apart. If she's on a bed, position her so you have room to work at the bottom of the bed.

If she prefers to squat or sit at the edge of a chair, don't argue with her. Gravity will aid the delivery. Just be prepared to catch the baby so it won't hit the floor.
■ Wash your hands thoroughly with soap and running water. (See *Understanding your priorities,* page 137.) Then sterilize a pair of scissors or a knife by immersing it in boiling water for at least 5 minutes. If boiling water isn't available, hold the scissors or knife over a flame for 30 seconds. You'll use the scissors later to cut the umbilical cord, so leave them in the water until you need them.
■ If you have someone to assist you, ask that person to gather the following equipment:
— something to wrap the baby in, such as a clean, soft blanket, towel, or sheet
— something to tie the umbilical cord with, such as a clean shoe lace, cord or string, or strips of cloth
— a bucket or container in case the woman needs to vomit

If you must assist with emergency childbirth, don't panic — most childbirths are normal and natural.

Is the baby about to be born?

If the baby's head is showing, as it is in this picture, birth is imminent. Don't move the mother. Prepare for emergency childbirth.

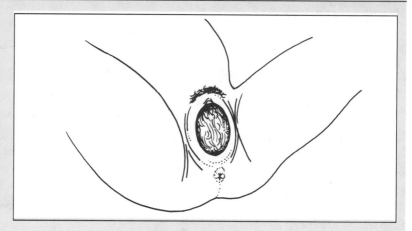

— a large bucket, container, or towel to hold the afterbirth (placenta) for later inspection by the doctor

— sanitary napkins, handkerchiefs, or clean folded cloths to place over the woman's vagina after she has delivered the baby and afterbirth

— disposable diapers or cloth diapers and safety pins.

■ Reassure everyone involved. Remember — most women don't plan on having their babies at the office or in the parking lot at the shopping mall.

Never try to delay the birth.

Don't deny that the birth is about to take place.

Never tell the woman to wait.

Avoid moving the woman if the baby's head is showing.

Never try to deliver a baby whose foot, arm, or shoulder appears first. This is difficult even for an experienced obstetrician. The baby and the mother could die.

Don't put your hands or any other object inside the vagina.

Be sure to not pull on the baby's head. Let the birth occur naturally.

Deliver the baby

■ As the baby's head emerges, take your dominant hand and extend it around the head with your fingers spread. Gently apply pressure to allow the head to emerge slowly, but don't use so much pressure that you slow the birth. Gentle pressure helps to prevent sudden expulsion of the head and shoulders, which could cause vaginal tearing. Also, the newborn is very slippery.

■ Press a folded towel or clean cloth against the baby's head. As the head emerges, check to see if the amniotic sac covering the head is intact. To keep the baby from breathing amniotic fluid, tear the membranes or break them with a fingernail. Note whether the fluid is clear or greenish brown so you can tell the doctor later.

■ If the umbilical cord is loosely wrapped around the baby's neck, gently lift it over the baby's head. (See *How to loosen the umbilical cord,* page 138.) If the cord is tight, tie a string around it tightly in two places, cut it between the ties, and release the cord before continuing.

■ Some babies emerge quickly, so be prepared to make a catch. Remember — babies are very slippery at birth.

Clear the baby's airway

■ You'll need to clear the baby's mouth and nose of mucus so he or she can breathe. After the baby's head has emerged, support the head between your hands and let it turn to the side. Don't pull. (See *Supporting the baby's head,* page 139.)

■ Stroke the baby's nose gently downward to help drain amniotic fluid and mucus. Stroke upward from the baby's neck to the chin.

■ Then sweep your fingers in the baby's mouth to clear away any mucus. Wipe any remaining mucus from the baby's face. While doing this, remember not to touch the mother's vagina.

■ Remove any remains of the amniotic sac at the base of the baby's neck.

Deliver the baby's shoulders

■ Depending on the baby's size, delivering the shoulders may be rapid or slow. You should deliver the shoulders with the next contraction. Tell the mother to breathe quickly four times — exhaling as if she's blowing out a candle — then to push hard.

■ Place a hand on either side of the baby's head for support and, as the contraction begins, exert gentle downward pressure to deliver the top shoulder.

Understanding your priorities

As you prepare to deliver the baby, keep the following priorities in mind.

Prevent infection in the mother and baby

You'll probably have just enough time to wash your hands. Make sure to put a clean towel under the mother during delivery.

Keep the delivery slow

Most babies are born head first without major difficulty. The most helpful thing you can do is urge the woman to pant and push slowly.

In a quiet, calm voice, tell her to "pant, pant, pant, as if you're blowing out candles." This will help avoid putting stress on the baby and prevent tearing as the woman's tissues stretch. (Torn skin requires stitching to prevent excessive bleeding.)

Protect the baby from cold

After delivery, dry the baby with a towel. Then wrap the newborn in a warm blanket, and lay him or her on the mother's stomach.

How to loosen the umbilical cord

If you see the umbilical cord wrapped around the baby's neck, gently lift it over the baby's head, as you see here.

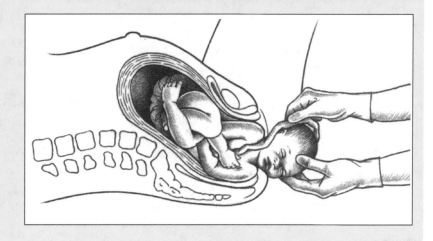

■ Then, at the next contraction, exert steady upward pressure to deliver the other shoulder. (See *Delivering the baby's shoulders,* page 140.)

> ⊗ Don't force the shoulder because this could damage the baby's spinal cord.

■ Tell the mother to push one more time when she feels the urge. Then the rest of the baby should emerge. The baby will be slippery, so cup one hand around the head and grasp the buttocks or feet as they emerge.

■ Supporting the baby with one arm, hold him or her securely with the head slightly downward to drain mucus from the mouth and nose. Gently rub the baby's back or soles until crying signals that the baby is breathing.

⊞ WHEN SECONDS COUNT

If the baby doesn't begin to breathe after birth, gently but firmly slap the soles of the feet or rub the baby's spine or breastbone. If the baby still doesn't start breathing, begin CPR at once, if you know how. (See *Performing CPR on an infant,* page 590.) Cover the baby's nose and mouth. Every 3 seconds, give a gentle puff — enough to cause a slight rise in the chest.

Supporting the baby's head

Using both hands, support the baby's head as it emerges from the birth canal.

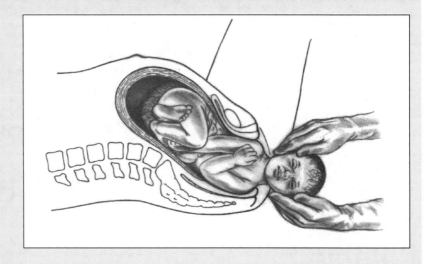

Care for the baby after birth

- Note the time of birth.
- Dry the baby and wrap him or her in a warm blanket. Place the baby on the mother's stomach.
- Encourage the mother to start breast-feeding right away if she wants to. Skin-to-skin contact will warm the baby.
- Cover the mother and baby with a warm blanket, but leave the mother's legs uncovered so you can deliver the placenta.

Cut the umbilical cord

If the ambulance has arrived, the mother and baby can be taken to the hospital with the umbilical cord still uncut, provided it's been tied or clamped. Place the baby on his or her side on the mother's stomach with the head down, facing the mother's feet. Keep the umbilical cord slack — don't stretch it taut.

If you can't get the mother and baby to a hospital, you'll have to cut the cord yourself. Here are the steps to take.

- If you haven't already boiled scissors, have someone do this now.
- Handling the cord gently, tie it at least 4 inches (10 centimeters) from the baby's navel (belly button), with two ties placed 2 inches

Delivering the baby's shoulders

To help deliver the *upper shoulder,* gently guide the baby's head downward.

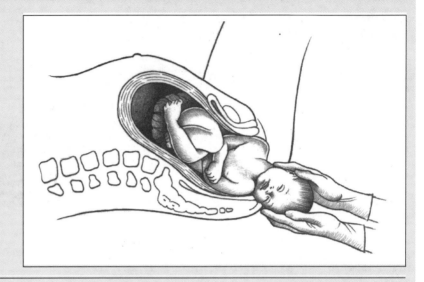

To help deliver the *lower shoulder,* guide the baby's head upward.

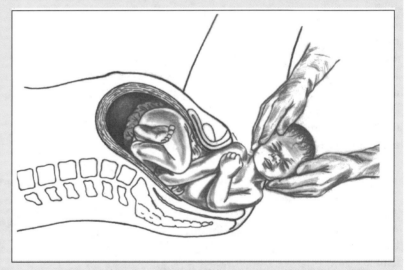

(5 centimeters) apart. Then, using the sterilized scissors, cut the cord between the two ties.

■ If the cut end attached to the baby is bleeding, tie the cord again next to the first tie. Don't remove the first tie. The baby's end of the cord shouldn't ooze.

Be sure not to pull on the umbilical cord; let it emerge naturally.

 Don't rush to cut the cord. And never cut it until it stops pulsating. The pulsations squeeze blood into the baby.

Deliver the placenta

The placenta is usually delivered within 5 to 20 minutes after the baby's birth. Here's how to deliver it:

■ When the placenta is about to be delivered, red blood will gush from the birth canal and the woman will feel a contraction. Encourage her to push the placenta out when she feels the contraction.

■ After the placenta emerges, place it in a container and send it to the hospital for examination. It's important for the doctor to see whether the placenta is in one piece. If the woman retains any pieces of the placenta, she may experience life-threatening bleeding.

Care for the mother after delivery

■ If everything appears normal after the placenta has been delivered, place a sanitary napkin or a clean, folded cloth against the woman's vagina to absorb the flow of blood. To help control bleeding, massage her uterus (the part of the abdomen below the navel). You'll recognize the uterus — it feels like a large, smooth ball. Massage every 5 minutes for 1 hour until it feels firm or until medical help arrives.

■ Give the mother something to drink — water, tea, coffee, or broth.

■ Keep her warm and comfortable. Congratulate her and all who helped in the delivery. Welcome the new baby.

 Don't give the mother alcoholic beverages.

 WHEN SECONDS COUNT

If vaginal bleeding is heavy or prolonged, seek medical help immediately. Heavy bleeding is life-threatening.

How is emergency childbirth treated?

At the hospital, the staff will care for both mother and baby.

Caring for the baby

The medical team clamps and cuts the umbilical cord using sterile equipment. Then they:

■ clean the baby

- weigh the baby
- assess the baby's breathing and other vital functions
- inspect for birth defects and possible injuries suffered during delivery
- put silver nitrate drops in the baby's eyes to prevent gonorrhea
- take footprints
- wrap the baby.

Caring for the mother
The doctor assesses the mother's general condition, then checks for tears in the vaginal area and for abnormally heavy vaginal bleeding.

What else should you know?
Even if the delivery goes smoothly, the mother and baby should get medical attention as soon as possible. Most serious problems associated with delivery occur within the first 24 hours.

> *Even if the delivery goes smoothly, the mother and baby should get medical attention as soon as possible. Most serious problems associated with delivery occur within the first 24 hours.*

CHOKING

About 3,000 Americans choke to death each year. Countless more have the frightening experience of a foreign substance "going down the wrong pipe." In fact, that's exactly what happens when someone chokes: Instead of the food or liquid going down the food tube, or esophagus, to the stomach, as it should, it goes down the windpipe to the lungs. (See *What happens when a person chokes.*)

Usually, having something go down the "wrong pipe" throws the person into a fit of coughing. The coughing gradually works the offending substance back up the windpipe so it can be spit out or swallowed the right way.

When coughing doesn't work
Sometimes, though, a piece of food gets stuck in the windpipe, leaving the person unable to breathe or to cough the food out. This is a medical emergency: The brain can't function without a steady sup-

ply of oxygen, so a person who can't breathe has only minutes to live. However, by acting quickly and appropriately, you can save a choking person's life.

What are the symptoms?

Coughing is the symptom most often associated with choking. Yet coughing doesn't necessarily signal that the person needs immediate help. Why? A person who can cough is able to breathe. Also, it's best to let the body remove a foreign substance on its own, if it can.

Universal choking signal

A much more ominous symptom of choking is when the person puts a hand to the throat and starts to turn blue. If the windpipe is completely blocked, the person won't be able to cough, speak, or breathe. Without assistance, the person will lose consciousness and die from lack of oxygen.

Important: If a person has symptoms of choking but *can* breathe, suspect a possible heart attack and get immediate help. (For more information, see "Heart attack," page 283.)

What should you do?

If the choking person can speak or cough, stay nearby, but let the person's cough reflex remove the foreign substance. (If you're alone and you start to choke, see *Clearing a blocked airway,* page 593.)

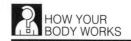 WHEN SECONDS COUNT

If the person can't breathe, you'll need to perform abdominal thrusts, also called the *Heimlich maneuver.* Stand behind and wrap your arms around the person's middle. Then make a tight fist with one hand and grasp it firmly with your other hand. (See *Positioning your hands for the Heimlich maneuver,* page 144.)

Then place your grasped fist, thumb inward, against the person's abdomen between the rib cage and navel. In one quick movement, press your clenched fists into the abdomen at an upward angle. Repeat the thrust as many times as it takes to clear the airway. (If the choking person is a child, see *Aiding a choking infant or child,* page 145.)

Don't tighten your arms around the person's middle when placing your fist between the rib cage and navel.

HOW YOUR BODY WORKS

What happens when a person chokes

Normally, when a person swallows, a flap of tissue called the *epiglottis* moves down to cover the opening of the windpipe.

Food's normal path

Food then goes down the esophagus to the stomach, and the epiglottis opens to restore breathing. This process explains why you can't breathe and swallow at the same time.

When food goes off-course

If something goes wrong and the epiglottis doesn't close properly, food may go down the windpipe instead of the esophagus. If the piece of food is big enough to block the windpipe, the person won't be able to breathe.

Positioning your hands for the Heimlich maneuver

To perform the Heimlich maneuver, stand behind the person and wrap your arms around the person's middle.

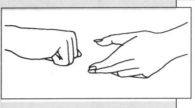

Make a fist
Make one hand into a tight fist, as shown in the small illustration. Then grasp the fist firmly with your other hand.

Press your fist into the abdomen
Next, place your fist against the person's abdomen as shown in the large illustration. In one quick movement, press your clenched fists into the abdomen at an upward angle. Repeat until the airway is clear.

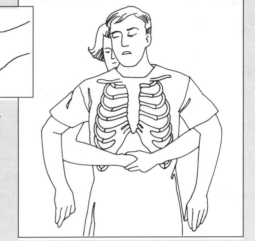

What to do if the person is lying down
If the person is lying down or unconscious, place him or her on the back and straddle the hips. Place the heel of one hand in the middle of the person's abdomen, halfway between the navel and rib cage. Then place your other hand on top of the first hand and interlace your fingers.

Lean forward and press with a quick, sharp upward thrust. Repeat up to five times.

How to remove a foreign object from the airway
If the person is lying down or unconscious, open the airway by using the *head-tilt, chin-lift maneuver.* Place one hand on the person's forehead and the fingers of your other hand on the bony portion of the lower jaw near the chin. Gently push the person's forehead back and pull upward on the chin. Keep the mouth partly open, making sure the teeth are almost touching.

Then perform five abdominal thrusts and check for breathing. If these methods fail, keep repeating the abdominal thrusts until the foreign object is expelled from the airway or help arrives.

If the object comes out of the mouth but the person still isn't breathing, the head and neck may be in the wrong position, allowing the tongue to block the airway. Reposition the person's head, if

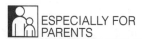
Aiding a choking infant or child

If you come upon a choking infant or child, call for emergency medical help right away. Then take the steps below.

For an infant

If the infant can breathe, cough, or cry, let him or her try to expel the object through the body's natural processes.

If the infant is having trouble breathing or coughing, place him or her facedown across your forearm or lap with the head facing downward. Using the heel of your hand, deliver five quick back blows between the shoulder blades, as you see here.

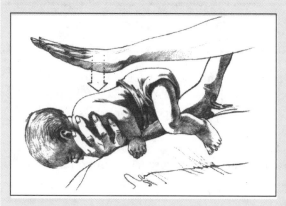

If the back blows don't dislodge the food or other object, turn the infant over and deliver five chest thrusts. To do this, place two fingers between the

infant's nipples and give quick, upward thrusts, as you see here.

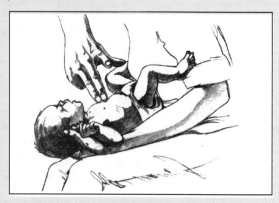

If the infant continues to choke, repeat the back blows and chest thrusts.

For a child

For a child up to age 8, use the same technique you'd use to perform the Heimlich maneuver on an adult. If the child continues to choke after the Heimlich maneuver, repeat the back blows and chest thrusts.

necessary, by putting your hand on the forehead and tilting the head backward.

How is choking treated?

The best treatment for choking is prevention. Some of the safety and etiquette rules our parents taught us serve as excellent guidelines for preventing choking:

■ Don't talk with your mouth full.

■ Chew your food well.
■ Don't put large pieces of food in your mouth.

What else should you know?

If the person who's choking is pregnant or obese, use *chest thrusts* instead of abdominal thrusts. To do this, stand behind the person with your arms wrapped around the front, under the person's armpits. Then place your clasped fists in the middle of the person's breastbone, and give four thrusts straight back toward you. Don't squeeze the person with your arms. (For more information on helping an obese or pregnant person who's choking, see *Clearing a blocked airway,* page 593.)

COLD EXPOSURE

Cold exposure, or hypothermia, occurs when a person's core (internal) body temperature drops below 95° F (35° C). The typical victim of cold exposure is a homeless person or a hiker caught in a sudden snowstorm.

Wind and wet weather increase the risk of cold exposure (See *Factors that speed heat loss.*) That's why it's so important to dress appropriately for outdoor activity.

Why it's life-threatening

Unlike frostbite, which affects only a specific body part, cold exposure affects the entire body. But both frostbite and cold exposure can quickly become life-threatening. If not treated promptly, cold exposure can cause severe infection, pneumonia, irregular heartbeats, and kidney failure.

Understanding the causes

Cold exposure can result from:
■ nearly drowning in cold water
■ prolonged exposure to cold temperatures
■ prolonged exposure to chilly weather (around 50° F [10° C]) if the person is also wet — for example, from being exposed to rain or fog for a long time

Cold exposure affects the entire body and can quickly become life-threatening. If not treated promptly, it can cause severe infection, pneumonia, irregular heartbeats, and kidney failure.

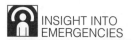
INSIGHT INTO
EMERGENCIES

Factors that speed heat loss

Of course, the body loses heat when it's cold outside. But two other factors increase the risk of cold exposure: wind and moisture.

What's the windchill factor?

Because wind causes the body to lose heat rapidly, weather forecasters talk about the windchill factor a lot. But do you know what windchill is?

A chilling combination

Windchill is a combination of the temperature and the wind speed. For instance, if the temperature is 10° F (–18° C) and the wind is blowing at 20 miles (32 kilometers) per hour, then the windchill factor is –25° F (–32° C). At this windchill, the skin can freeze within 1 minute of exposure.

That's why it always makes sense to listen to the weather forecast — including the windchill factor — when planning an outdoor activity. It could save your life.

How moisture comes into play

Keeping dry is equally important when you're out in cold weather. Moisture — whether it comes from rain, snow, or perspiration — cools your body by carrying heat away from it.

- transfusion of a large amount of cold blood or blood products
- drinking a large amount of cold fluids
- shock.

What are the symptoms?

Symptoms of cold exposure vary with the severity of the condition.

Symptoms of mild cold exposure

This condition is defined as a core body temperature below 96.8° F (36° C). Symptoms include:

- shivering
- increased pulse
- rapid breathing
- fine muscle tremors
- clumsiness
- apathy
- confusion
- slurred speech
- forgetfulness.

Symptoms of moderate cold exposure

In this state, the core body temperature measures 86° to 95° F (30° to 35° C). The person may have:

- violent shivering, followed by muscle rigidity

- memory loss
- bluish skin
- irregular heartbeats
- stupor
- disorientation
- decreased pulse
- slow breathing
- low blood pressure.

Symptoms of severe cold exposure
The person with this condition has a core body temperature below 86° F (30° C). Symptoms may include:
- further slowing of the pulse and breathing
- a further drop in blood pressure
- erratic heartbeat
- enlarged pupils
- stoppage of the heart
- lack of brain function.

What should you do?

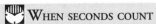 **WHEN SECONDS COUNT**

Check the person for a pulse and look, listen, and feel for breathing. If you're certain the person has no pulse and isn't breathing, start CPR, if you know how. (See *Performing CPR on an adult,* page 579, *Performing CPR on a child,* page 585, or *Performing CPR on an infant,* page 590.) Have someone call for emergency medical help at once.

Important: Before you stop CPR, be sure to rewarm the person to a core body temperature of at least 90° F (32° C), as measured rectally.

Perform CPR, if necessary. Gently move the person to a warm place and start rewarming.

Get the person out of the cold
If the person is breathing, gently move him or her to a warm place and start rewarming. Rewarming methods include:
- removing wet clothes
- drying the person and wrapping him or her in warm blankets
- offering warm, noncaffeinated beverages (if the person is conscious and can swallow).

 Don't warm the person too quickly.

Are you at high risk for cold exposure?

Knowing who is most at high risk for cold exposure can help you protect yourself and your family. The risk for serious injury from the cold increases with these factors.

Medical conditions
- Heart disease
- Malnutrition

Lifestyle habits
- Smoking
- Drug abuse
- Excessive alcohol intake

Other conditions
- Youth or old age
- Wet or inadequate clothing
- Fatigue
- Hunger
- Too little body fat (fat insulates a person against the cold)

Never use dry heat to warm the person because this can permanently damage body tissues.

Be sure not to let the person put his or her hands or feet on or near a radiator or hot stove.

Don't immerse the person's whole body in warm water. This could cause heart problems.

Never give alcohol or caffeine-containing drinks.

Don't let the person smoke. By impairing circulation, smoking slows the warming process.

What to do for minor cold exposure
Minor cold exposure can be treated at home. Cover the person with warmed blankets or towels or immerse him or her in warm water. Wrap a hot-water bottle in the blankets or towels before applying.

How is cold exposure treated?
In the hospital, the person may be warmed internally and externally, with constant monitoring of core body temperature. Rewarming methods include:
- giving heated intravenous fluids
- instilling warm fluids through a tube into the genitourinary tract
- instilling warm fluids through a tube inserted in the person's nose and stomach
- transfusing warmed blood products (hemodialysis)
- administering warmed, humidified oxygen.

What else should you know?

A condition called *rewarming shock* can occur if the outside of the person's body is rewarmed faster than the inside.

Also, be aware that some people are at greater risk for cold exposure. (See *Are you at high risk for cold exposure?* page 149.)

CONCUSSION

A concussion is a relatively minor brain injury. It typically comes from a direct blow to the head — for example, slipping on the ice and hitting your head on the sidewalk. The blow may cause the brain to rebound against the skull or drive the brain against the opposite side of the skull. (See *Brain shake-up*.)

For example, a head-on motor vehicle collision may cause an *acceleration-deceleration* injury: The person's head is hurled forward, then stops abruptly when it hits the windshield. But the brain keeps moving, slapping against the skull and then rebounding.

A concussion typically comes from a direct blow to the head. Most victims recover within 48 hours and don't suffer lasting damage.

Effects of repeated concussions

Most concussion victims recover within 48 hours and don't suffer lasting damage. However, repeated concussions take a cumulative toll on the brain.

What are the symptoms?

A person who has suffered a concussion may have:
- dizziness
- nausea and vomiting
- severe headache
- blurred or double vision
- confusion or disorientation
- inability to remember what happened just before or after the injury
- brief loss of consciousness.

What should you do?

Get the person to a doctor or hospital as soon as possible for evaluation.

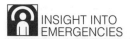
INSIGHT INTO
EMERGENCIES

Brain shake-up

A concussion "shakes up" the brain by driving it against the opposite side of the skull or by causing it to rebound against the skull.

BRAIN MOVEMENT DURING INJURY

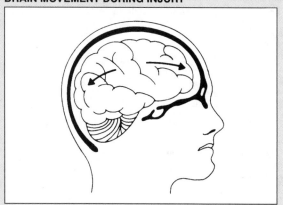

How is a concussion treated?

Treatment for a concussion may include bed rest, observation, and Tylenol (or another acetaminophen product) for headache. Usually, the person can recover at home, as long as someone observes him or her closely for at least 24 hours. (See *Caring for someone who has had a concussion,* page 152.)

What else should you know?

For up to 1 year after suffering a concussion, some people experience delayed symptoms, called *postconcussion syndrome.* Here's what to watch for:

- lack of usual energy
- occasional double vision
- dizziness, giddiness, or light-headedness
- memory loss
- emotional changes (such as feeling irritable or easily upset, especially in crowds)
- difficulty concentrating
- reduced sex drive
- easy intoxication by alcohol
- loss of inhibitions
- difficulty relating to others

Caring for someone who has had a concussion

A person who has been discharged from the hospital with a concussion needs to be observed closely for 1 or 2 days to detect any problems. If you'll be acting as caregiver, follow these guidelines.

Observe the person regularly
Awaken the person periodically the first night home and ask the following questions:
- What's your name?
- Where are you?
- Who am I?

If the person doesn't wake up or can't answer your questions, call for medical help right away.

Review the doctor's instructions
Read over and review with the person the doctor's discharge instructions for the first 48 hours. Usually, these instructions include the following:
- Take it easy and return gradually to usual activities.
- Avoid medicine stronger than Tylenol (or other acetaminophen products) for a headache. Don't take aspirin — it can worsen any internal bleeding caused by the injury. Try relieving a headache by lying down with your head raised slightly on pillows.
- Eat lightly, especially if nausea or vomiting occurs. (Occasional vomiting isn't unusual, but it should subside in a few days.)

Know when to get help
Call the doctor or get the person to the hospital at once if you notice:
- increasing irritability or personality changes
- increasing sluggishness
- confusion
- seizures
- persistent or severe headache that Tylenol doesn't relieve
- forceful or constant vomiting
- blurred vision
- abnormal eye movements
- staggering walk.

- noise intolerance.

These symptoms should subside over time. If they get worse, the person should consult the doctor.

CONFUSION

Confusion — the inability to think clearly — can vary from a mental muddling of people, places, time, and events to an alarming loss of contact with reality. Sudden confusion can affect anyone at any age, although we don't know for sure if it occurs in infants or very young children. (See *Helping a confused child.*)

Understanding the causes

Sudden confusion most commonly results from a head injury or lack of blood or oxygen supply to the brain, as occurs in a stroke.

Less often, sudden confusion stems from:

- progressive brain degeneration, such as Alzheimer's disease
- severe mental and emotional stress
- blood sugar that's too high or too low
- dehydration
- urinary tract infection (in older people).

What are the symptoms?

Sudden confusion may cause severe, unmistakable symptoms. These may include:

- lack of awareness of other people
- disorientation
- agitation
- hallucinations
- personality or mood changes — sudden depression, irritability, or even bizarre behavior.

Subtle clues

Sometimes sudden confusion causes more subtle symptoms. For instance, the person may:

- be less alert than before
- lack interest in usual pastimes
- neglect personal hygiene
- experience long- or short-term memory loss
- have difficulty concentrating on simple tasks
- have trouble thinking or speaking
- show unpredictable behavior (for example, suddenly becoming listless or, in contrast, overactive).

What should you do?

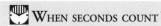 WHEN SECONDS COUNT

If the person has sudden, severe confusion — a condition called *delirium* — get medical help immediately. Also get immediate medical attention for someone who suddenly becomes confused after a head injury (even a minor one) or for a confused person who complains of dizziness, weakness, numbness, tingling, blurred vision, or difficulty speaking. These are symptoms of stroke.

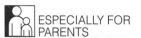 ESPECIALLY FOR PARENTS

Helping a confused child

Passing episodes of acute confusion, or delirium, are common in older children who have a fever. Read on for some tips on coping with a confused child.

Ensure safety

- If your child's bed has a side rail, attach it to the bed to prevent your child from falling out and getting injured.
- Walk with your child to the bathroom, and stay there until the child is finished.

Keep the child calm

- Try to keep your child calm and quiet.
- Don't leave the child alone.

Other tips

- If your child has a fever along with confusion, give Tylenol (or another acetaminophen product), not aspirin. But check with the doctor first.
- If your child's confusion doesn't disappear as his or her temperature decreases, call the doctor right away.

If stroke is the cause of confusion, the person needs surgery to improve blood flow to the brain.

What to do if the confusion is not severe

Try to keep the person quiet and calm while waiting for help. Urge him or her to rest without interruption, if possible. To help restore contact with reality, constantly tell the person where he or she is, what day it is, and who you are.

 Be sure not to leave a confused person alone.

 Don't give a confused person a sedative without consulting a doctor first. A sedative can worsen the confusion.

How is confusion treated?

Depending on the cause of confusion, the doctor may prescribe drugs to control symptoms. Some people may need surgery, drugs, or other methods to treat the underlying disorder.

If the person has had a stroke

A person whose confusion stems from a stroke may need surgery to improve blood flow to the brain. In an operation called an *endarterectomy,* the surgeon removes plaque (obstructing matter) from the inner walls of the affected artery. In a method called *microvascular bypass,* the surgeon joins a blood vessel outside the skull to one inside the skull.

Drugs useful for treating a person who's had a stroke include:
- Ticlid
- tissue plasminogen activator
- antiseizure medicines
- antibiotics
- stool softeners
- steroids
- pain relievers.

If the person has a brain tumor

If tests indicate a brain tumor, the person may need to undergo surgery. If the tumor is inoperable, the doctor may recommend some combination of radiation therapy, chemotherapy, and drug therapy.

Treating other conditions

If confusion stems from an imbalance of the body's fluids and salts, the doctor orders appropriate therapy to restore balance. If heatstroke, cold exposure, infection, or a head injury causes sudden confusion, the doctor orders appropriate treatments to correct these conditions.

What else should you know?

Sudden confusion sometimes comes from a high fever (over 104° F, or 40° C) or a brain infection, such as meningitis. Some people may become confused after drinking a large amount of alcohol or taking certain drugs, such as sedatives.

CONSTIPATION

If you're constipated, you pass your body's solid wastes, or feces, infrequently and with difficulty. Normally, muscle contractions in the digestive tract move feces through the intestines. During this motion, fluid is absorbed. But in someone who is constipated, intestinal motion decreases, more fluid is absorbed, and the wastes become harder and more solid.

Usually, constipation results from:
- not exercising enough
- not eating enough fiber
- not drinking enough liquids, especially water.

Constipation can also be caused by certain drugs, including codeine.

Life-threatening causes

Sometimes constipation signals a life-threatening condition, such as an intestinal obstruction. This serious disorder is most common in people who have just had abdominal surgery and in those with intestinal deformities at birth. Intestinal cancer is a major cause of large-intestine obstruction. Other serious medical conditions can also lead to constipation. (See *What causes constipation?* page 156.)

What are the symptoms?

Normal passage of stools varies greatly from one person to the next. Some people normally have one or two bowel movements a day, whereas others have a bowel movement every 2 to 3 days. How often you have a bowel movement depends on your:
- diet
- level of physical activity

Although constipation is usually no more than an annoyance, it sometimes signals a serious disorder.

What causes constipation?

Constipation most often comes from getting too little exercise or eating a low-fiber diet — not from a serious health problem. Both exercise and dietary fiber stimulate the natural wavelike contractions of the colon that trigger the urge to defecate.

Other common causes

Besides a low-fiber diet and too little exercise, common causes of constipation include:
- suppressing the urge to move the bowels — for example, because you're busy doing something else
- not drinking enough fluids
- overusing laxatives and enemas
- taking certain drugs and mineral supplements, such as narcotics, water pills (diuretics), iron, or calcium
- having hemorrhoids, which may cause you to avoid moving your bowels when they hurt or bleed.

More serious causes

Less often, constipation comes from a medical condition that should be investigated. These conditions include the following.

Digestive tract problems
- Inflammation of the appendix (appendicitis)
- Blockage of the intestine by a tumor, hernia, or hardened feces
- Pouches in the lining and wall of the intestine (diverticulosis)
- Tear or crack in the anus (anal fissure)

Other conditions
- Underactive thyroid gland
- Uterine cancer
- Spinal cord injury or disease

- amount of stress
- toilet habits
- overall health.

Symptoms of intestinal obstruction
Besides constipation, symptoms of *small-intestine obstruction* include:
- colicky pain
- nausea and vomiting
- a bulging abdomen
- intense thirst
- dry mouth
- aching
- general discomfort.

With *large-intestine obstruction,* constipation may be the only symptom for several days. Then abdominal pain may occur suddenly, with short spasms every few minutes. Other symptoms include:
- continuous pain and nausea
- visible bulges in the abdominal wall.

Adding high-fiber foods to your diet

High-fiber foods promote good digestion and may relieve constipation. Choose from the four main categories that follow:

High-fiber fruits
- Apples
- Apricots
- Avocados
- Cantaloupe
- Dates
- Figs
- Honeydew
- Oranges
- Peaches
- Pears
- Strawberries
- Watermelon

High-fiber vegetables
- Baked, green, or lima beans
- Bean sprouts
- Broccoli
- Brussels sprouts
- Cabbage
- Carrots
- Corn
- Peas
- Potatoes
- Squash
- Sweet potatoes
- Turnips

High-fiber nuts
- Almonds
- Peanuts
- Pecans

High-fiber whole-grain breads and cereals
- Bran cereal
- Oatmeal
- Puffed wheat
- Shredded wheat
- Whole wheat bread

What should you do?

If constipation isn't treated, it can lead to headache, appetite loss, and stomach discomfort. Most people can treat constipation with the following self-care steps:

- Drink at least eight glasses of water daily, especially if you're elderly. (Many older adults lose the sensation of being thirsty.)
- Eat high-fiber foods, such as grains, fruits, vegetables, and nuts. (See *Adding high-fiber foods to your diet.*)
- Avoid highly refined foods, such as white flour products.
- Stimulate your intestine by drinking hot or cold water — plain or with lemon — or prune juice before meals.
- Respond promptly when you get the urge to defecate.
- Establish a regular toilet time, such as after breakfast.
- Get some exercise every day.

The road to a lazy bowel

Taking laxatives too often can make your bowel "lazy." In this state of chronic constipation, called lazy bowel syndrome, the contractions that normally move wastes through the bowel may stop completely. To avoid this problem, consult the doctor if you find yourself taking laxatives regularly.

Other causes

Other conditions that can lead to lazy bowel syndrome include:

■ not eating enough dietary fiber
■ not drinking enough fluids, especially water
■ not getting enough exercise.

When should you turn to laxatives or enemas?

If self-treatment doesn't bring relief within a few days, try taking an over-the-counter laxative. Then, if you're still constipated, try giving yourself an enema.

> ⊠ Don't take laxatives more than once or twice a month without consulting your doctor. (See *The road to a lazy bowel.*)
>
> ⊠ Be sure not to use enemas regularly.

How is constipation treated?

Someone whose constipation doesn't improve after a week of self-treatment should call the doctor, who will evaluate for an underlying health problem.

Treating an intestinal obstruction

The person with this disorder must be hospitalized. Intravenous fluids are given to correct fluid and body salt imbalances. To relieve pressure in the abdomen, a tube is passed down the person's throat to bring up material trapped in the intestine; the person isn't allowed to eat or drink at this time. If this method doesn't work, intestinal surgery is necessary.

Treating constipation caused by drug therapy

If a person becomes constipated while taking a drug like codeine or an antihistamine, the doctor may be able to substitute another drug.

What else should you know?

If you're bottle-feeding an infant, be aware that cow's milk contains ingredients that can make your infant constipated or cause hard stools.

In older children, constipation usually results from drinking too much milk and consuming too little fiber. Other causes of constipation in older children include:

■ intestinal spasm
■ a blocked intestine
■ an underactive thyroid.

COUGHING UP BLOOD

Coughing is a normal body function. It helps to keep your lungs clear and removes germs and foreign objects from your airways.

But sometimes an illness or injury can cause a person to cough up phlegm (also called *sputum*) that's streaked or tinted with blood. An illness as minor as a cold can cause this. Why? When a person has a cold, coughing irritates and places stress on the tender, swollen mucous membranes of the respiratory tract.

The link with smoking
More often, though, coughing up blood signals a more serious problem — sometimes an emergency. Coughing up blood has been showing up more often among people with chronic bronchitis or lung cancer; both conditions are more prevalent in heavy smokers over age 40. (See *How lung disease causes coughing*, page 160.)

Understanding the causes
The most common causes of coughing up blood include:
- cancer of the lung or larynx (voice box)
- chronic inflammation of the air passages (chronic bronchitis)
- injury to the windpipe
- chronic abnormality of the walls of the airways (bronchiectasis)
- buildup of fluid in the lungs (pulmonary edema)
- tuberculosis, a contagious lung infection
- pneumonia, an acute lung inflammation
- a clot in one of the blood vessels in the lungs
- chest injury
- certain fungus infections of the lung
- diseases caused by inhaling lung irritants — silicosis and silo-filler's disease, for example. (See *Avoiding lung irritation,* page 161.)

What are the symptoms?
The color and nature of coughed-up blood vary with the underlying cause. Here are some examples:
- A chest injury may cause a person to cough up bright red blood, possibly in very large amounts.
- Tuberculosis leads to coughing up of bloody, pus-filled phlegm with a foul odor.
- Blood-streaked phlegm may be linked to lung cancer.

Sometimes an illness or injury can cause a person to cough up phlegm that's streaked or tinted with blood. An illness as minor as a cold or as serious as lung cancer can cause this.

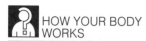

How lung disease causes coughing

Coughing, perhaps streaked with blood, may occur when an illness such as chronic bronchitis irritates or damages the airways and lungs.

Bronchitis and coughing
In chronic bronchitis, the mucous membrane that lines the small airways in the lungs becomes swollen and irritated. This narrows the airways, makes breathing difficult, and causes coughing.

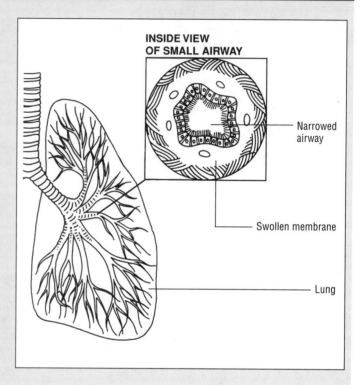

INSIDE VIEW OF SMALL AIRWAY

Narrowed airway

Swollen membrane

Lung

■ Pink, frothy phlegm typically comes from fluid build-up in the lungs.

Other symptoms to watch for
Someone who's coughing up blood also may have shortness of breath, fever, and chest pain.

What should you do?
If the person has never coughed up blood before, seek medical attention right away. Be sure to give the doctor a detailed description of the blood. Also mention whether the person:
■ has had a recent medical or dental procedure that could affect the mouth, throat, or lungs
■ has had pneumonia or another illness

- has recently suffered a chest injury
- smokes cigarettes and, if so, how many a day and for how long
- has associated symptoms, such as nausea, vomiting, fever, trouble swallowing, shortness of breath, or pain in the neck, chest, or abdomen
- takes drugs that could interfere with bleeding, such as aspirin or blood thinners.

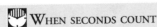 ## WHEN SECONDS COUNT

If the person is coughing up a lot of blood, get emergency help immediately. Forceful coughing up of a great deal of blood could mean internal bleeding from a recent chest injury. This is a dire emergency.

How is coughing up blood treated?

Depending on how much blood the person is coughing up, the medical team may insert a tube in the windpipe to keep it open and use a suction device to remove the blood. They usually place an intravenous line to give fluids, drugs, and blood and start administering oxygen. The medical team monitors the person for symptoms of shock and collects blood repeatedly to measure levels of various gases.

Emergency bronchoscopy

The person may have to undergo an emergency bronchoscopy. In this procedure, the doctor inserts a thin, flexible tube called a bronchoscope into the air passages and lungs to see where the bleeding is coming from and help determine how to stop it.

Less urgent treatments

If the situation is less urgent, the medical team positions the person comfortably sitting up or lying on the affected side. This makes it harder for blood to enter the other lung or impede breathing. The person also undergoes a series of X-rays and other diagnostic tests to help determine the cause of the bleeding.

Drug therapy

The person may receive antibiotics and drugs to stop the urge to cough. But the doctor probably won't prescribe a sedative or tranquilizer because these drugs depress the urge to breathe.

What else should you know?

Don't confuse blood that has been coughed up with blood that has

 PREVENTION TIPS

Avoiding lung irritation

The best way to avoid coughing up blood is to keep your lungs free from irritation. Here are some suggestions.

Stay away from irritants
- Don't smoke. If you do smoke and you're over age 40, be sure to have a chest X-ray every year.
- Don't spend much time in heavily polluted areas.
- Wear a protective mask if you work with or near irritants.

Prevent blood clots
If you're bedridden for any length of time, perform the leg exercises recommended by the doctor, and get out of bed and take walks as often as possible. This will help prevent blood clots in your legs and lungs.

Take prompt action
If you do cough up blood, call the doctor right away.

been regurgitated. Blood that is coughed up comes from the respiratory tract. Because it's mixed with air, it usually appears as bright red phlegm.

Blood that is regurgitated comes from the digestive tract. It may be bright red, or it may not be blood exactly, but a material that looks like coffee grounds. The coffee-ground appearance means it has been held in the stomach and partially digested. Often the person who vomits blood also complains of stomach upset.

COUGHING UP PHLEGM

Many people who cough up phlegm minimize or overlook the problem or accept it as normal.

Coughing up phlegm, or sputum — a mixture of mucus and saliva — results from a productive cough. By bringing mucus from the lungs to the mouth, coughing is the body's way of getting rid of secretions that have built up in the lungs. Smoking is a major cause of coughing up phlegm. (See *What causes a productive cough?*)

An often-overlooked problem
Many people who cough up phlegm minimize or overlook the problem or accept it as normal. They may not seek medical attention until they develop a related health problem, such as shortness of breath, coughing up blood, chest pain, weight loss, or recurrent respiratory infections.

What are the symptoms?
Productive coughing can occur as a single cough or as forceful, noisy coughing. The color, consistency, and odor of the phlegm are important clues to the person's condition. So is the sound of the cough.

What phlegm color and consistency signify
■ Clear, thin, watery phlegm usually comes from a cold or other upper respiratory tract infection, asthma, an allergy, or exposure to irritants (such as cigarette smoke).
■ Thick greenish or yellow phlegm may signal a sinus infection, bronchitis, or pneumonia.

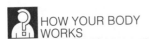

HOW YOUR BODY
WORKS

What causes a productive cough?

Dozens of disorders can make a person cough up phlegm, but smoking is the number one reason. Why? Smoking makes the airways produce more mucus, which in turn creates more phlegm that must be cleared. Smoking also paralyzes tiny hairs in the respiratory tract that normally help move phlegm out of the airways.

The conditions below also can cause a productive cough.

Asthma

This condition often starts with a dry cough and mild wheezing, then progresses to severe wheezing and a productive cough. The person may produce thick mucus secretions.

Chronic bronchitis

In this condition, chronically blocked breathing passages cause a dry cough that later produces phlegm. The phlegm may contain pus.

Common cold

A person with a cold may cough up phlegm made up of mucus or a mixture of mucus and pus.

Exposure to irritants

A person who inhales particles from paint, dust, or other substances may have extra airway mucus. The mucus trickles down the throat, irritating the airways enough to cause coughing. This problem is especially common in people with chronic sinus infections or allergies.

Lung cancer

An early symptom of this disease is a chronic cough that produces a small amount of blood-streaked phlegm. The phlegm may contain pus or a mixture of mucus and pus.

Pneumonia

This disorder may cause a dry cough that becomes productive. Phlegm color varies with the bacteria present.

Tuberculosis

A person with this disease may cough up a small or large amount of phlegm. The phlegm may contain mucus, blood, or pus.

■ Brown or reddish phlegm usually contains blood. It may result from injury caused by coughing or from a condition like pneumonia, tuberculosis, severe lung irritation, or even lung cancer.

What the odor signifies
The odor of the phlegm can be revealing too. Foul-smelling phlegm could mean bronchitis, lung abscess, or another infection, such as tuberculosis.

What certain coughing sounds indicate
A hacking cough means the voicebox is involved, whereas a brassy cough means a major airway is affected.

How to do deep-breathing exercises

If you have a productive cough, special breathing exercises can expand and clear your lungs. This will help you avoid getting pneumonia or other respiratory infections. To learn how to do deep-breathing exercises, follow these instructions.

Prepare for deep breathing
Position yourself comfortably on your back. Then put one hand on your chest and the other hand over your upper abdomen at the base of your breastbone.

Bend your knees slightly and support them with a small pillow. Try to relax. *Note:* If you've just had surgery on your chest or abdomen, keep that area still by hugging a pillow.

Inhale deeply
Exhale normally, and then close your mouth and inhale deeply through your nose. As you do this, concentrate on feeling your abdomen rise, *without expanding your chest*. If the hand on your abdomen rises as you inhale, you're breathing correctly.

You should be using your diaphragm and abdominal muscles — not just your chest muscles — to breathe.

Next, hold your breath and slowly count to five.

Exhale through pursed lips
Purse your lips as though you're whispering, and exhale completely through your mouth without puffing out your cheeks.

Use your abdominal muscles to squeeze all the air out as your ribs sink down and in. Exhaling should take twice as long as inhaling.

Repeat the exercise
Rest for a few seconds. Then continue the exercise until you've done it correctly five times. Gradually increase the number of repetitions until you can do the exercise 10 times.

Perform deep breathing often
Once you've learned the exercise, you can do it while sitting, standing, or lying in bed. Try to deep-breathe every 1 to 2 hours while you're awake.

Other symptoms to watch for
Depending on the medical condition that's causing the cough, the person may have other symptoms too. For example, *pneumonia* can cause:

- shaking chills
- high fever
- muscle pain
- headache
- chest pain
- a fast pulse
- rapid breathing
- sweating.

  Tuberculosis causes:
- a general feeling of illness
- chest pain
- night sweats
- shortness of breath.

How to do coughing exercises

Like deep-breathing exercises, coughing exercises can help clear lung secretions and prevent respiratory infections. Read what follows to learn the proper techniques.

Prepare for coughing
Sit on the edge of the bed with your body leaning slightly forward. If your feet don't touch the floor, rest them on a stool. If you feel weak, rest your arms on a bedside table with a pillow on it.

Breathe and exhale through pursed lips
To stimulate your cough reflex, breathe deeply and exhale while pursing your lips. Make sure you exhale completely through your mouth without puffing out your cheeks. Using your abdominal muscles, squeeze out all the air.

Cough vigorously
Now inhale again, hold your breath, and cough twice vigorously while concentrating on forcing all the air out of your chest. If you can't cough effectively, cough three times gently instead of twice vigorously.

Repeat the exercises
Rest for a moment, then do the exercises at least five times. Repeat them at least once every 2 hours.

What should you do?

In someone who doesn't normally have a cough, persistent coughing up of phlegm is a danger sign — one that could indicate a life-threatening disorder. The person should see a doctor quickly, especially if the phlegm is bloody, pus-filled, yellow, greenish, or rust-colored.

Also seek medical attention quickly if the person becomes restless or confused or starts to have shallow, irregular, rapid, or slow breathing. These symptoms could indicate acute breathing distress.

Self-care

If the doctor rules out a serious underlying disorder, the person can try doing deep-breathing and coughing exercises to help clear the lungs. (See *How to do deep-breathing exercises,* and *How to do coughing exercises.*) Other self-care treatments include the following:

■ Drink plenty of fluids to thin lung secretions and increase their flow. However, if you've had fluid in your lungs (pulmonary edema), check with your doctor first.

■ Use a room humidifier to add moisture to the air. This will help to ease inflamed airways and loosen dried secretions.

■ Rest frequently.

■ Avoid respiratory irritants — especially cigarette smoke.

■ Sit or stand upright when coughing to increase lung expansion.

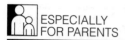

What to do if your child coughs up phlegm

Because children have narrow airways, a child who has been coughing up phlegm can quickly develop a blocked airway and have trouble breathing if the phlegm accumulates. That's why you should consult a doctor if your child develops a productive cough.

Possible causes
Conditions that can cause a child to cough up phlegm include:
- asthma, a chronic lung disease that leads to recurrent attacks of troubled breathing
- bronchitis, a chronic blockage of the breathing passages
- acute bronchiolitis, a virus of the lower respiratory tract seen mainly in infants ages 2 to 12 months
- cystic fibrosis, a chronic disease that affects many of the body's organs

- whooping cough (pertussis), a highly contagious respiratory infection that causes sudden attacks of high-pitched whooping sounds as the child breathes.

How to help clear up the cough
To clear phlegm from your child's breathing passages, the doctor may prescribe an expectorant. Be sure to use this drug exactly as directed. Don't give any other drugs — for example, cough suppressants such as Robitussin DM — without the doctor's approval. Suppressing a cough could worsen your child's condition.

Humidify the air
To soothe your child's inflamed airways and prevent lung secretions from drying up, ask the doctor about using a room humidifier.

Don't encourage the person to suppress a productive cough. Doing so may interfere with lung function or increase the risk of respiratory infection. (See *What to do if your child coughs up phlegm.*)

How is coughing up phlegm treated?
The doctor may prescribe drugs to dissolve the phlegm (called mucolytics), to help clear phlegm from the lungs (called expectorants), and to open the airways (called bronchodilators). To treat an underlying bacterial infection, the doctor prescribes antibiotics.

What else should you know?
To help avoid spreading the infection, the person should:
- cover the mouth and nose with a tissue when coughing
- always dispose of tissues in a trash can with a lid
- wash the hands after touching used tissues.

CRUSH INJURIES

Crush injuries occur when a person's arm or leg is pressed or squeezed by a heavy object, such as rollers in an industrial machine. If the rollers are reversed, the limb may suffer a second compression.

Bone, muscle, and nerve damage
Crush injuries are serious because they can:
- break bones into small pieces
- cause extensive damage to muscle and tissue
- injure nerves
- impair blood circulation.
    Sometimes the damage is so severe that the person eventually loses the limb.

What are the symptoms?
A person with a crush injury may show no obvious damage or may have the following symptoms:
- extreme pain
- inability to move the injured limb
- considerable swelling at the injury site
- an obvious wound
- blood-filled, swollen areas (hematomas)
- large bruised or torn areas with bleeding, cuts, and purplish or red skin patches.

What should you do?

WHEN SECONDS COUNT

Call for emergency medical help immediately. Splint the injured limb in the position in which you found it; don't try to straighten it first. The splint supports and immobilizes injured tissues and helps prevent further damage to muscles, nerves, and blood vessels. (For information on how to make a splint, see *How to splint a broken bone or dislocated joint,* page 596.) After splinting the limb, elevate it above the level of the person's heart. Try to keep the person calm and quiet until help arrives.

> *Crush injuries can break bones into small pieces, cause extensive damage to muscle and tissue, injure nerves, and impair blood circulation. Sometimes the damage is so severe that the person eventually loses the limb.*

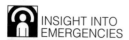

INSIGHT INTO
EMERGENCIES

What happens in crush syndrome

A severe crush injury may lead to crush syndrome. A person with this complication suffers:

■ massive bleeding
■ destruction of muscle and bone tissue
■ fluid loss.

A perilous chain of events
Crush syndrome may result in shock, kidney failure, coma, and, possibly, death. This flowchart shows how a crush injury can lead to crush syndrome.

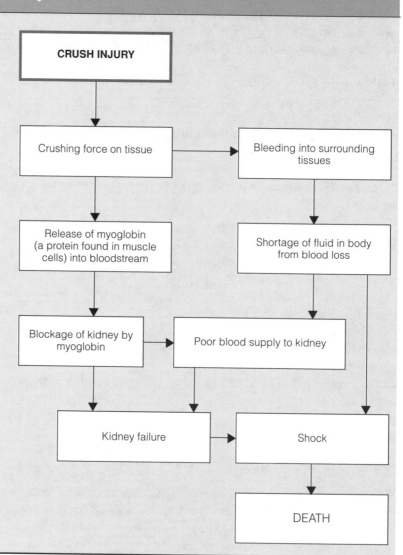

CRUSH INJURY

Crushing force on tissue

Bleeding into surrounding tissues

Release of myoglobin (a protein found in muscle cells) into bloodstream

Shortage of fluid in body from blood loss

Blockage of kidney by myoglobin

Poor blood supply to kidney

Kidney failure

Shock

DEATH

How are crush injuries treated?

Emergency medical personnel check the person's pulses beyond the injured area to make sure the blood is circulating properly. They also try to find out the extent of damage to muscles, tissue, and nerves.

Understanding compartment syndrome

When a person suffers a serious injury, such as a broken or crushed leg or a bad burn, the tissue around the injury can become quite swollen. Usually, the swelling gradually subsides. But in some people, the swelling becomes so severe that the swollen tissue cuts off blood flow and presses on nerves around the injured area. This condition is called compartment syndrome.

A threat to the limb

This syndrome may arise right after an injury occurs or may be delayed for a few days. Either way, the person needs immediate medical treatment to restore blood flow and nerve function to the affected area. Otherwise, muscle and nerve damage may become so severe that the leg develops gangrene and must be amputated.

How to recognize symptoms

Suspect compartment syndrome if the person's injured leg becomes extremely painful — well out of proportion to the extent of the injury. The pain probably won't subside no matter how the person holds the leg. Don't expect it to respond to pain-relieving drugs either.

Stay alert for numbness and tingling

Also, the leg or the space between the toes may feel numb. The person may feel a tingling or pins-and-needles sensation in the leg. If these symptoms occur or if the leg becomes extremely painful, call the doctor immediately or take the person to an emergency facility.

What treatment to expect

The doctor removes any tight dressings or cuts off the cast, if the person has one. The leg is elevated, ice packs are placed on it, and the person receives a pain reliever.

Relieving pressure

The doctor also may perform a minor operation called *fasciotomy* to relieve pressure in the leg. Afterward, the medical staff checks to make sure the swelling is under control and blood flow is returning to normal.

Evaluating and treating the injury

At the hospital, the doctor orders X-rays to evaluate the damage and check for broken bones. If the person has an open wound, it's cleaned with mild antiseptic soap, rinsed with warm sterile water, and wrapped in a bulky dressing. The injured limb is kept elevated and immobilized to control swelling. The person may receive a tetanus shot to help prevent infection and pain relievers to reduce pain.

Other treatments

The person also may receive:
- antibiotics to prevent infection
- other drugs
- intravenous fluids to ward off shock, kidney problems, and *crush syndrome* — a dire complication of severe crush injury (see *What happens in crush syndrome*)
- surgery, if needed, to remove dead tissue.

Fat embolism syndrome can occur 1 to 3 days after a crush injury. Unless detected and treated quickly, it can cause severe breathing difficulty and death.

What else should you know?

Crush syndrome isn't the only serious complication of crush injury. *Fat embolism syndrome* can occur 1 to 3 days after the injury. Unless detected and treated quickly, it can cause acute breathing distress and death. Symptoms of fat embolism syndrome include:

- fever
- weak, spastic, rigid muscles
- chest pain during inhalation
- changes in mental status
- wheezing
- gradually increasing pulse and breathing rates
- tiny purple or red spots on the torso, eyes, and roof of the mouth and in the armpits.

Other complications

After a crush injury, the person may go into shock or suffer *compartment syndrome* from swelling of the injured part. For more information, see *Understanding compartment syndrome,* page 169.

CUTS (LACERATIONS)

Cuts occur when a sharp object penetrates the skin or, less often, when a blunt object strikes a severe blow to the body. *Lacerations* are deep cuts that may extend far into the skin layers and into fat and muscle. The edges of the wound may be rough or jagged. If foreign matter has been rubbed or pressed into the wound, the wound is likely to become infected.

How the body reacts

Just after the skin is torn, more blood flows to the area, and it becomes inflamed. The blood brings white blood cells and other elements of the immune system to the injured area to help fight infection. After a few days, a scab forms to protect the injury as it heals.

What are the symptoms?

A cut usually causes an obvious wound or break in the skin. Other

symptoms of a cut or laceration include:
- bleeding
- bruising
- swelling.

What should you do?

Usually, bleeding from a small cut stops on its own. If it doesn't, take the following steps.

Apply direct pressure
- Put on disposable latex gloves to guard against blood-borne diseases. If gloves aren't available, use a waterproof material, such as a plastic bag, plastic wrap, or several layers of gauze pads.
- Remove or cut any clothing covering the wound so you can see where the blood is coming from.
- Make a compress using gauze or the cleanest material available. Press the compress firmly against the wound with your fingers or palm. Usually, this stops the bleeding by allowing normal blood clotting to occur.
- If the bleeding doesn't stop after you've applied direct pressure for 10 minutes, the pressure may be too light or applied in the wrong area. Press harder over a wider area for another 10 minutes.

�֍ Never apply direct pressure to a cut over the eye or to a wound with an object still impaled in it. Instead, cover the wound with a loose dressing.

✖ Don't remove the original dressing if it becomes blood-soaked. Just place another dressing over it and keep applying pressure until the bleeding stops.

Elevate the limb
If the cut is in an arm or a leg, raise the injured limb above the level of the person's heart while you apply pressure.

Use indirect pressure
If the cut continues to bleed, apply pressure at a *pressure point* while still keeping direct pressure on the cut. (But don't do this unless you've been trained in pressure point technique.) The combination of direct and indirect pressure should slow the blood flow. (See *Using pressure points to stop bleeding,* page 76.)

If the bleeding doesn't stop after you've applied direct pressure for 10 minutes, press harder over a wider area for another 10 minutes.

Dress the wound

■ Once the bleeding has stopped, apply a bandage over the cut. To do this, place the center of a gauze strip or other long, thin material (like cloth strips) directly over the compress. Then wrap both ends of the gauze around the wound and tie a knot over the compress.

■ When the bleeding is under control, keep the injured limb elevated.

> ✪ Be sure not to apply the bandage too tightly, or it could cut off the circulation. Apply it just tightly enough to stop the bleeding. To make sure it's not too tight, check for a pulse at a point below the bandage. If you don't detect a pulse, loosen the bandage.
>
> ✪ Don't use a tourniquet except as a last resort. A tourniquet can injure blood vessels and nerves — and even lead to loss of an arm or a leg.

Don't use a tourniquet except as a last resort. A tourniquet can injure blood vessels and nerves and lead to loss of an arm or a leg.

If the person has hemophilia

Get the person to the nearest hospital emergency department immediately. Hemophilia impairs blood clotting. Without special measures, a person with hemophilia may bleed to death from even the slightest cut.

How are cuts and lacerations treated?

In the doctor's office or hospital, direct or indirect pressure is applied to the wound if it's still bleeding. If the cut is in an arm or a leg, the limb is kept elevated. The doctor gives a tetanus shot if the person hasn't had one in the past 7 to 10 years.

A person who has suffered a severe laceration may need surgery to repair the wound and any related damage.

What else should you know?

A small amount of blood can look like heavy bleeding — especially if the cut is on the person's face, scalp, or hand. So even if you see what looks like a lot of blood, stay calm — the wound may be minor. Getting upset will only make the person panic.

DELIRIUM

Delirium is a form of severe confusion that strikes suddenly and requires immediate medical attention. It's caused by some condition that impairs the brain regions that control higher functions, such as comprehension, abstract thinking, judgment, reasoning, attention, and memory.

A treatable cause
Unlike dementia, which causes confusion by chronically disrupting brain cells, delirium results from a treatable condition. (See *What causes delirium?* page 174.) However, a person can suffer from delirium and dementia at the same time. (See *Is it delirium or dementia?* page 175.)

What are the symptoms?
Typically, symptoms of delirium arise over hours or days and fluctuate as the day progresses. The person shows a diminished attention span and disorganized thinking, plus at least two of the following symptoms:
- decreased level of consciousness
- problems in perception, such as misinterpretations, illusions, or hallucinations
- disrupted sleep-wake cycle with inability to sleep at night or drowsiness during the day
- enhanced or diminished ability to perform skills that involve both mental and muscle activity
- disorientation to time, place, or person
- loss of short- or long-term memory.

What should you do?
Get medical help at once if a person suddenly shows symptoms of severe delirium. Make a special effort to communicate with the person. Address him or her by name and identify yourself. Speak calmly in a normal tone of voice, using simple words and sentences.

Unlike dementia, delirium results from a treatable condition. However, a person can suffer from delirium and dementia at the same time.

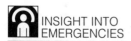

What causes delirium?

Delirium may result from many conditions, such as those listed below. Most of these conditions are treatable.

Body temperature changes
- Abnormally low temperature (hypothermia)
- Fever

Heart and blood vessel problems
- Heart attack
- Irregular heartbeats
- Stroke
- Heart failure

Nervous system problems
- Nervous system infection or inflammation
- Head injury
- Seizures

Drugs and other substances
- Alcohol
- Amphetamines
- Antiarrhythmics (drugs used to steady the heartbeat)
- Antidepressants (drugs used to treat depression, including MAO inhibitors)
- Antihistamines
- Antiseizure drugs
- Barbiturates (like some sleeping pills and antiseizure drugs)
- Beta blockers (drugs used to treat high blood pressure or angina)
- Cocaine

- Digitalis glycosides (drugs used to treat heart attack, heart failure, and irregular heartbeats)
- Lithobid (used to treat bipolar mood disorder)
- Opium-like drugs
- Penicillins
- Phenothiazines (used for anxiety, nausea, vomiting, or psychosis)
- Steroids (used to treat severe inflammation and other problems)
- Water pills (diuretics)

Imbalances in the body's salts
- Too much calcium
- Too much or too little magnesium
- Too much or too little sodium

Other causes
- Imbalance in the body's acids and bases
- Disorders of the adrenal, parathyroid, pituitary, or thyroid gland
- Infection
- Kidney failure
- Liver failure
- Low blood sugar
- Oxygen shortage in the blood — for example, from anemia
- Poisoning from cyanide, heavy metals
- Vitamin deficiencies — folic acid, niacin, thiamine

Stay nonthreatening

Try to look nonthreatening. Move slowly, and stand directly in the person's line of vision. Maintain eye contact. Ask one question at a time and give the person time to answer. Be aware of your own emotional responses to the person.

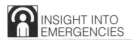

INSIGHT INTO
EMERGENCIES

Is it delirium or dementia?

Although delirium and dementia share such symptoms as agitation, confusion, and restlessness, the two conditions have different causes. There are other important differences too. Read on for details.

When to suspect delirium

Delirium strikes suddenly, progresses rapidly, and lasts 1 month or less. It can affect any age-group. Typical symptoms include hallucinations, illusions, and lack of inhibitions.

Conditions that can cause delirium

Usually, delirium results from a treatable condition, such as:

- infection
- oxygen shortage
- imbalance of the body's acids and bases
- depression
- injury
- drug or alcohol toxicity
- drug side effects
- drug interactions.

When to suspect dementia

Dementia comes on gradually and typically affects people age 65 and older. Although sometimes dementia can be halted or corrected, its normal course is progressive and long-term. Symptoms include impaired judgment and resistance to change.

Conditions that can cause dementia

Some of the conditions that cause dementia are treatable — Parkinson's disease, brain tumor, and heart attack, for instance. But more often the underlying cause is an irreversible disorder like Alzheimer's disease, Huntington's disease, or AIDS.

❌ Don't overreact to the person's condition. Doing so could cause anxiety.

Keep the environment calm and safe

If necessary, use fewer lights for a more relaxing atmosphere. Keep drapes open to let in natural light and help orient the person to the time of day.

Make sure the environment is safe, with enough light so the person won't trip or bump into objects. If the person has impaired judgment, don't leave him or her alone.

❌ Be sure not to provide too much or too little stimulation. Doing so could make the delirium worse.

How is delirium treated?

Depending on the cause of the delirium, the doctor may order drugs to control symptoms or treat an underlying disorder, such as depression. Drugs called neuroleptics can help change the mood and thoughts of a person with an altered perception of reality. Antianxiety drugs are tranquilizers that ease anxiety and tension. Drugs called beta blockers may help treat agitation and anxiety when other medicines don't work. (Drugs won't be given if the person is in a coma or in shock or has unstable vital signs.)

Treating drug or alcohol abuse

If delirium results from drug or alcohol abuse, the doctor recommends a detoxification program. The doctor may prescribe drugs to make withdrawal symptoms less severe.

What else should you know?

If you're caring for a delirious person at home, try to set a predictable routine. For instance, schedule activities like eating, dressing, and bathing at the same time each day so the person knows what to expect and when.

Using comfort measures like repositioning and massage can help reduce the person's agitation. First determine what makes the person agitated, then try to alleviate the cause. For example, a person who is in pain or needs to go to the bathroom may become restless.

DEPRESSION

People with a family history of depression are three times more likely to experience depression than those without such a history.

Most people experience occasional, brief feelings of sadness or dejection. But when these emotions become more intense and last longer than usual, the person may be suffering from depression. In severe depression, feelings of sadness and dejection are especially pronounced.

Risk factors

Although depression can occur at any age, the first symptoms commonly appear between ages 20 and 24. People with a family history of depression are three times more likely to experience depression than those without such a history. Other risk factors include:

■ low family income

- unemployment
- obesity
- lack of confidence.

Risk groups for severe depression include:
- married women
- children
- teenagers
- older adults
- members of dysfunctional families
- bereaved people
- caregivers of people with chronic disorders
- hospital patients
- people with certain medical conditions — heart attack, cancer, AIDS, dementia, or schizophrenia, for instance.

What are the symptoms?

A severely depressed person may have a sullen expression and look older than his or her stated age. Other symptoms may include:
- poor hygiene
- an unkempt appearance
- slouching
- a slow, shuffling gait
- significant weight loss or gain over a short period
- trouble thinking clearly or communicating with others
- reduced ability to see, hear, taste, feel, or perceive things accurately.

What should you do?

Get help from a mental health professional if a severely depressed person is suicidal or shows five or more of the following symptoms for 2 weeks or longer:
- depressed mood most of the time
- apathy or indifference
- significant weight loss or gain due to a change in appetite
- difficulty sleeping, or sleeping too much
- agitation
- fatigue or loss of energy
- low self-esteem, feelings of worthlessness, or excessive or inappropriate guilt
- feelings of hopelessness or helplessness
- diminished ability to think

A severely depressed person may have a sullen expression and look older than his or her stated age. Other symptoms may include poor hygiene and an unkempt appearance.

Shock therapy: Return of a controversial treatment

You've probably heard of electroconvulsive therapy, also called ECT or shock therapy. Once widely used to treat severe depression, this controversial treatment fell out of favor a few decades ago but has made a recent comeback.

Who can benefit?

Shock therapy is known to help certain depressed people, especially those who have tried various antidepressant drugs unsuccessfully and elderly people who can't tolerate these drugs.

A jolt to the brain

In shock therapy, an electric current is passed through the person's brain. Doctors don't know how shock therapy works against depression, but they do know that it causes loss of consciousness and induces a series of seizures lasting about 10 seconds. On awakening, the person has no memory of the shock.

Most people require 8 to 12 treatments. Some may need monthly treatments to prevent depression from recurring.

What are the side effects?

Possible side effects of shock therapy include:

- confusion
- headache
- short-term memory loss.

- recurrent thoughts of death
- suicidal thoughts or a suicide plan. (See "Suicide potential," page 502.)

Promote self-esteem

If you're living with a severely depressed person, try to help him or her set realistic goals. To promote feelings of self-worth, encourage the person to assert opinions and make decisions. Also encourage open expression of feelings, including anger, which often underlies depression.

Provide outlets for anger

To help the person overcome feelings of helplessness, plan physical activities that provide a controlled outlet for anger and at which the person can succeed. Focus on past and present experiences in which the person was successful. Make sure the person gets enough rest and nourishment, and keep the surroundings calm and relaxing.

How is depression treated?

Treatment for severe depression depends on how marked it is and what is causing it. If the depression stems from a physical disorder, treating that disorder may ease the depression. If the cause of depression isn't apparent, a trained professional may be able to help the person identify what triggers the depressive moods and then develop effective coping strategies.

Special therapies

For some people, drug therapy, behavioral therapy, or cognitive therapy can also play important roles in overcoming depression. When other treatments fail, some severely depressed people may benefit from electroconvulsive therapy. (See *Shock therapy: Return of a controversial treatment.*)

What else should you know?

Depression can be classified as follows:

■ *Mild depression.* The person seems quiet, withdrawn, and melancholy until he or she gradually accepts reality.

■ *Major depression.* The person is depressed or takes no pleasure in daily activities over a 2-week period. He or she can't concentrate or make decisions.

■ *Melancholia.* The person may feel apathetic and seem unable to get pleasure from any activity. These symptoms are more or less constant over a prolonged period.

■ *Manic-depressive illness.* In this condition, also called bipolar disorder, the person's mood swings abruptly from depression to elation (mania), or the person has prolonged episodes of either mood.

■ *Seasonal affective disorder.* The person regularly becomes depressed and reclusive during the fall and winter.

DIABETIC COMA

Diabetic coma is a blood sugar crisis. An acute complication of diabetes mellitus, it occurs when the body has too much sugar (glucose) and not enough of the hormone insulin (made by the pancreas).

Risk factors

The typical victim of this life-threatening emergency is a diabetic person who:

■ hasn't taken the correct dosage of insulin or antidiabetic drug

■ has consumed more sugar than he or she is supposed to

A blood sugar crisis, diabetic coma is an acute complication of diabetes. It occurs when the body has too much sugar and not enough insulin.

- gets an illness that affects the body's insulin production
- loses a lot of fluid, such as through vomiting. (See *Ways to prevent diabetic coma.*)

Don't confuse diabetic coma, which takes a few days to develop, with insulin shock, which can come on suddenly if the blood sugar level is too low. For information on insulin shock, read "Insulin shock," page 324.

> *Diabetic coma comes on slowly. A relative or friend may notice that the person has become confused or disoriented. Sometimes this behavior is mistaken for drunkenness.*

What are the symptoms?

Diabetic coma comes on slowly. A relative or friend may notice that the person has become confused or disoriented. Sometimes this behavior is mistaken for drunkenness.

Other symptoms of diabetic coma include:
- drowsiness
- extreme thirst
- rapid, labored breathing
- warm, dry skin
- sunken eyes
- weak, rapid pulse
- frequent urination
- nausea and vomiting
- fruity or sickly sweet breath odor
- abdominal pain
- eventual loss of consciousness or coma.

To help detect these symptoms early, relatives and friends of a person with diabetes should learn how to recognize the symptoms of both high and low blood sugar.

What should you do?

 WHEN SECONDS COUNT

If the person is unconscious, call for emergency medical help at once. Check for a pulse and look, listen, and feel for breathing. If a pulse and breathing are absent, start CPR, if you know how. (See *Performing CPR on an adult,* page 579, *Performing CPR on a child,* page 585, or *Performing CPR on an infant,* page 590.) If the person has a pulse and is breathing, keep the airway open, place the person on the left side, and watch for vomiting.

Never try to give an unconscious person anything to eat or drink.

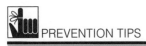

Ways to prevent diabetic coma

Good health habits can help prevent diabetic coma and other complications of diabetes. Make the following habits a way of life.

Manage minor illnesses properly

The flu, a cold, or an upset stomach can cause your body to release certain hormones that increase your blood sugar level. To make matters worse, illness often affects your appetite, causing you to eat less than usual.

Consult your doctor

When you get sick, be sure to take insulin, if prescribed. But consult your doctor — he or she may want to adjust your insulin dose. Also, drink more fluids and check your blood sugar level more often than usual. Call the doctor if your blood sugar level steadily rises.

Alter your diet

If illness causes you to eat less, spread half your daily carbohydrate allowance over 24 hours. If you can't eat solid foods, consume foods with more simple sugars than you're normally allowed — for instance, gelatin, custard, and nondiet soft drinks.

Check your blood sugar level

Even when you're not sick, be sure to follow your doctor's advice on how often to check your blood sugar level. For reliable results, use good technique and accurate timing. Make sure you know what your blood sugar level *should* be as well as what to do if the level is too high.

Test your urine

The doctor may want you to test your urine daily for substances called ketone bodies. If these bodies are present, it means that your diabetes isn't well controlled.

The doctor may also check your urine routinely for protein, which can signal kidney disease related to diabetes. Don't delay telling the doctor if you have symptoms of a urinary tract infection: burning, painful or difficult urination, and blood or pus in the urine.

Keep your heart healthy

Because diabetes raises your risk of heart disease, take care of your heart by following these American Heart Association guidelines:
- Maintain a normal weight.
- Get regular exercise, following your doctor's recommendations.
- Eat a low-fat, high-fiber diet, as your doctor prescribes, to help control your blood pressure and cholesterol level.

Treat your skin with care

Bathe daily with warm water and a mild soap, and apply a lanolin-based lotion afterward to prevent dryness. Pat your skin thoroughly dry, taking extra care between your toes and in other areas where skin surfaces touch.

Avoid skin irritation

Breaks in your skin can put you at risk for infection. So check your skin daily for cuts and irritated areas, and see your doctor if necessary. Also, be sure to wear cotton underwear so moisture can evaporate and help prevent skin breakdown.

Take care of your feet

Diabetes can reduce blood supply to your feet. So normally minor foot injuries, such as a blister, can lead to dangerous infection. To prevent foot problems, wash your feet daily in warm soapy water. Check water temperature with a thermometer before putting your feet in — diabetes reduces sensation in your feet.

(continued)

PREVENTION TIPS

Ways to prevent diabetic coma *(continued)*

Keep your feet dry
After washing your feet, dry them thoroughly, especially between the toes. Then apply lotion immediately to prevent evaporating water from drying your skin. Avoid walking barefoot.

Get your eyes checked
Have your eyes examined by an eye doctor at least once a year. He or she may detect diabetes-related damage (which can cause blindness) before symptoms appear.

Have regular checkups
See your doctor regularly so he or she can detect early symptoms of complications and start treatment promptly.

What to do if the person is conscious

If someone who is a known diabetic shows symptoms of diabetic coma, give a food or beverage that contains sugar, such as fruit juice, candy, a soft drink, or table sugar. (Giving sugar won't cause added harm — and it could save the person's life if he or she is in insulin shock rather than diabetic coma.)

Also give a beverage. If the person doesn't feel better in 15 minutes, call for emergency medical help.

Be sure not to give a diet soda or other diet drink because it doesn't have the sugar the person needs.

How is diabetic coma treated?

The person receives intravenous fluids, intravenous insulin, and, possibly, sodium bicarbonate to correct a condition called acidosis. Antibiotics may be given to treat an infection.

Other treatments

Most people also need supplements of potassium and, possibly, other body salts (called electrolytes). That's because diabetic coma disturbs the body's salt balance.

What else should you know?

Researchers are working on new treatments to help people with diabetes better monitor and control the disease. This in turn can help them to prevent diabetic coma and other complications. Here are some examples of recent advances.

Glycemic index

This form of diet therapy links changes in blood sugar levels with specific foods. It also identifies low-fat, starchy foods that people with diabetes can eat to boost their carbohydrate intake without triggering high blood sugar. With this therapy, the person measures the blood sugar level after every meal and snack.

Implantable probes and pumps

These devices permit more precise blood sugar control by monitoring blood sugar levels and automatically delivering the correct insulin dose.

Sandimmune therapy

This drug is a promising treatment for people with insulin-dependent (type I) diabetes. It aims to interfere with the conditions that stop the pancreas from making enough insulin.

DIARRHEA

Diarrhea is the frequent passage of loose or liquid stools. Typically, it occurs when some condition causes the muscles of the digestive tract to contract too rapidly. (See *How diarrhea occurs,* page 184.)

Most of us experience diarrhea at one time or another. Sometimes the trigger is simple stress or nervousness. Other times diarrhea serves as a defense mechanism by which the body attempts to remove something it's not used to. For example, if you've been limiting your dietary fat intake for a while and then suddenly eat a high-fat meal, your body may respond by eliminating the fats quickly through loose stools.

Understanding the causes

Besides stress and unfamiliar foods, diarrhea also may result from:
- intestinal flu
- caffeine, spicy foods, or foods that can irritate the intestine, like cabbage or sauerkraut

Sometimes diarrhea comes from simple stress. Other times it serves as a defense mechanism by which the body tries to remove something it's not used to.

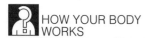

HOW YOUR BODY WORKS

How diarrhea occurs

Normally, a series of wavelike muscle contractions forces food through the digestive tract.

Fast contractions

If these contractions become too rapid, the large intestine can't absorb as much fluid from foods as it should. This leads to diarrhea.

DIGESTIVE TRACT

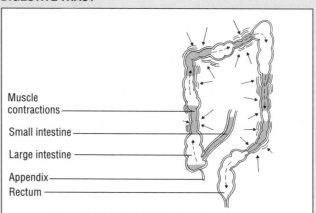

Muscle contractions

Small intestine

Large intestine

Appendix

Rectum

■ food poisoning, usually from *Salmonella* or *Staphylococcus* bacteria (see "Food poisoning," page 238)

■ acute intestinal infection caused by bacteria, viruses, or other organisms

■ irritable bowel syndrome

■ long-term inflammation of the layers of the colon (chronic ulcerative colitis)

■ growths on the inner surface of the intestinal tract (polyps)

■ cancer of the rectum or colon

■ lactose intolerance caused by shortage of the enzyme lactase, which the body needs to digest the sugar in milk; undigested milk sugar (lactose) ferments and causes gas, cramps, and diarrhea

■ certain drugs. (See *Is your medicine giving you diarrhea?* page 186.)

What are the symptoms?

Diarrhea can be acute or chronic; the frequency of loose or liquid stools can vary from one person to the next or from one day to the next. The stools may be bloody or contain mucus or pus — or both.

Along with diarrhea, the person often has abdominal pain or cramping, nausea, vomiting, fatigue, and appetite loss. The nature of the stools and the presence of other symptoms vary with the cause of diarrhea.

Symptoms of acute intestinal infection
The person usually has:
- extremely watery diarrhea of sudden onset
- increased stool odor
- a painful and tender abdomen
- nausea
- fever
- chills
- weakness
- a poor appetite
- weight loss.

Symptoms of cancer of the large intestine
Symptoms of this disease include:
- bloody diarrhea alternating with pencil-thin stools
- abdominal pain
- appetite loss
- weight loss
- weakness
- depression.

Symptoms of irritable bowel syndrome
In this condition, diarrhea may alternate with constipation or normal bowel function. The person may also have:
- a painful, tender, or bloated abdomen
- stomach upset
- nausea.

Symptoms of ulcerative colitis
This disease causes:
- recurrent bloody diarrhea that contains pus or mucus
- cramping pain in the lower abdomen
- a slight fever
- appetite loss
- occasional nausea and vomiting.

The person with cancer of the large intestine may have bloody diarrhea alternating with pencil-thin stools.

Is your medicine giving you diarrhea?

Diarrhea can be a side effect of many drugs. For instance, it can come from taking an antibiotic (an infection-fighting drug). Antibiotics that can cause diarrhea include:

- Ceftin
- Cleocin
- Keflex
- Keflin
- Omnipen
- Rocephin
- tetracycline.

Other drugs that can cause diarrhea

Also watch out for these other drugs:

- antacids that contain magnesium, such as Di-Gel and Maalox
- birth control pills
- Cardioquin, a drug used to steady the heartbeat (can cause diarrhea when taken in high doses)
- colchicine, a medicine used to treat gout
- Dantrium, a muscle relaxant
- Edecrine, a water pill (diuretic)

- estrogens
- Inderal, a drug used to treat high blood pressure and certain heart conditions
- Ismelin, a drug used to control high blood pressure
- laxatives (can cause diarrhea when used excessively)
- Lanoxin, a drug used to steady the heartbeat (can cause diarrhea when taken in high doses)
- Mexate, a drug used to treat cancer, arthritis, and some other conditions
- Ponstel, a nonsteroidal anti-inflammatory drug used to relieve pain, ease inflammation, and reduce fever
- vitamin C (can cause diarrhea when taken in high doses).

Important precaution

If you get diarrhea while using a drug, check with your doctor before taking diarrhea medicine. Such medicine may make your diarrhea worse or make it last longer.

What should you do?

If the diarrhea is severe or prolonged, check the person for symptoms of shock, such as:

- fast pulse
- dizziness or light-headedness (especially when rising from a sitting to a standing position)
- cool, pale, sweaty skin.

If any of these symptoms are present, call for medical help immediately. Then raise the person's legs about 8 to 12 inches until help arrives.

Self-treatment

In an otherwise healthy person, diarrhea typically clears up within a few days or even sooner. Using simple self-care measures may help it go away.

Drinking a lot of fluids, for instance, is crucial. Until the stools are normal again, the person should sip 8 to 10 large glasses of water (or other clear fluid) every day. Instruct the person to avoid beverages like colas, coffee, milk, fruit juices, and alcohol. Also, caution the person not to gulp fluids. Gulping can trigger cramps by over-stimulating the digestive tract.

Encourage the person to eat regularly but to avoid foods that are spicy, fried, or high in fat until the diarrhea goes away. You may want to recommend the BRAT diet — bananas, rice, applesauce, and toast. These foods often ease diarrhea because they're binding.

If diarrhea persists after a day or two of high fluid intake and the BRAT diet, the person may consider taking an over-the-counter diarrhea medicine like Kaopectate.

When to consult the doctor
Call the doctor if:
- diarrhea lasts more than 24 hours
- stools contain bright red or darkened blood or appear black (which signals the presence of blood)
- stools are bulky and greasy
- you suspect food poisoning.

How is diarrhea treated?
Severe or prolonged diarrhea can interfere with the body's fluid and salt balance. This could trigger life-threatening complications like irregular heartbeats, dehydration, and shock. The person with severe diarrhea may even need to be hospitalized to find out the cause of the problem. He or she also needs intravenous fluids to fight off the dehydration that comes from excessive fluid loss — especially if the person is unable to eat or drink anything. The doctor may also order medicine to decrease intestinal contractions.

What else should you know?
Call the doctor promptly if your infant develops diarrhea. Why? Diarrhea can be life-threatening in a young child, causing severe dehydration from rapid loss of a great deal of body fluid. This condition poses the risk of seizures and other serious problems. Be sure to get medical attention quickly for a child under age 3 who has diarrhea for more than a day or who has bloody stools.

Severe or prolonged diarrhea can interfere with the body's fluid and salt balance. This could trigger life-threatening complications like irregular heartbeats, dehydration, and shock.

DISLOCATIONS

A dislocation is the displacement of a part of the body from its normal position — especially a bone from its normal connection with a joint. In this injury, the ends of the bone are no longer held together by the shiny, white fibrous bands called *ligaments*. In fact, the injury may stretch the ligaments or even tear them loose. (See *What happens in a dislocation*.) Dislocations often accompany fractures and sometimes cause fragments of broken bone to become lodged between joint surfaces.

The most vulnerable joints
The joints most commonly dislocated are the freely movable ones:
- shoulders
- elbows
- wrists
- fingers
- toes
- hips
- knees
- ankles
- lower jaw.

Understanding the causes
A dislocation may be present at birth (as in congenital dislocation of the hip), or it may follow injury or disease of surrounding joint tissues. Injuries that can lead to dislocations include:
- sharp twisting or straining
- sudden muscle contractions
- force applied at or near the joint
- a fall in which the force stresses a joint — for example, a fall on the shoulder, hand, or elbow can dislocate the shoulder. (See *Advice for the dislocation-prone,* page 190.)

What are the symptoms?
A dislocation typically causes symptoms of joint injury, such as:
- a popping sound heard or felt at the time of injury
- swelling
- tenderness
- severe pain

In a dislocation, the ends of the bone are no longer held together by the ligaments. The injury may stretch the ligaments or even tear them loose.

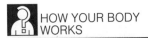 HOW YOUR BODY WORKS

What happens in a dislocation

When the bones in a joint are dislocated, they move out of their normal alignment. The near illustration shows the normal position of the three bones that meet at the elbow. The far illustration shows how the bones are no longer aligned because the elbow is dislocated.

NORMAL ELBOW JOINT

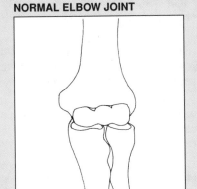

DISLOCATED ELBOW JOINT

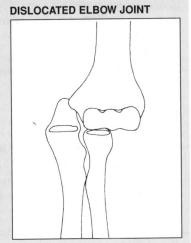

- bruising
- deformity
- inability to move the injured part
- decreased sensation (if nerves have been damaged)
- pale skin
- tingling sensations
- a weak pulse (if the dislocated bone is pressing on an artery)
- coolness of the skin below the injury site.

  Other symptoms vary with the specific dislocation.

Symptoms of a dislocated wrist

This injury causes:
- tenderness
- pain
- swelling.

Symptoms of a dislocated finger

The person with this injury may have:
- pain

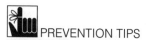 PREVENTION TIPS

Advice for the dislocation-prone

Dislocations typically result from an injury, such as a fall on the shoulder or an outstretched arm.

A family matter?
Some people seem to be genetically predisposed to frequent dislocations. For instance, members of the same family may have noticed a tendency for their shoulders to "pop" or "go out of joint."

Strengthen your muscles and ligaments
If dislocations run in your family, you can help prevent these injuries by avoiding high-risk activities. If this isn't possible, consider weight training to strengthen your muscles and ligaments. A physi-cal therapist or trainer can advise you on the correct weight-training techniques.

Dress for the occasion
Another must: Wear layers of clothing to help cushion falls — even if you're not planning to engage in sports.

And speaking of sports, be aware that contact sports — especially football — account for many dislocations. Other risky sports include downhill skiing, hockey, volleyball, rugby, soccer, lacrosse, and rollerblading. Before participating in *any* sport, put on all the protective gear you can, including elbow and knee pads.

- swelling
- a crooked joint that can't be bent
- a shortened finger.

Symptoms of a dislocated shoulder
This injury may cause:
- tenderness or pain
- one shoulder that looks different from the other
- tendency to hold the elbow 1" or 2" from the body
- inability to touch the elbow to the side of the body.

Symptoms of a dislocated hip
This injury can result from a fall onto the foot or knee or a direct blow to the thigh. Symptoms include:
- intense pain
- shortening of the leg with the foot turned out or in
- pain
- swelling.

Symptoms of a dislocated jaw
The person may have:
- difficulty speaking

- pain
- inability to close the mouth
- a rigid jaw.

What should you do?

 WHEN SECONDS COUNT

If the person has been in a serious accident and is unresponsive, check for an open airway, feel for a pulse, and look, listen, and feel for breathing. If you can't feel a pulse, severe internal bleeding may have caused the person to go into shock; send someone to call for emergency medical help. If the person isn't breathing and has no pulse, start CPR, if you know how. (See *Performing CPR on an adult,* page 579, *Performing CPR on a child,* page 585, or *Performing CPR on an infant,* page 590.)

Apply a splint and use ice
Next, immobilize the injured part by applying a splint. (See *How to splint a broken bone or dislocated joint,* page 596.)

To control swelling and reduce pain, apply ice or a cold pack. But first, wrap the ice in a towel or cloth so it doesn't directly touch the skin.

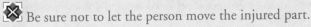 Don't try to place the injured part in its normal position before splinting. Splint it in the position in which you found it.

Be sure not to let the person move the injured part.

Avoid moving someone who has an injured hip. And don't try to transport him or her to the hospital yourself. Wait for professional rescuers to arrive.

Seek assistance
Get medical help as soon as possible. If treatment is delayed, the ligaments may start to get used to the new, wrong position. This will make it harder for the doctor to correct the dislocation.

You shouldn't try to treat a dislocation yourself because you could seriously damage blood vessels and ligaments. However, several types of dislocation may yield to self-treatment. For instance, a person with a dislocated jaw may be able to fix the problem by yawning. (Ironically, yawning *causes* most jaw dislocations.) Also, some people who repeatedly dislocate their shoulders have learned how to pop

Get medical help as soon as possible. A delay in treatment can cause difficulty correcting the dislocation.

their shoulders back into place. However, despite these exceptions, *it's always best to get prompt medical treatment for a dislocation.*

How are dislocations treated?

The sooner the displaced parts are restored to their normal position, the sooner they can start to heal — and the less damage they'll inflict on soft tissue, nerves, and blood vessels. Preferably, a procedure called *reduction* should take place before swelling and muscle spasms make repositioning difficult.

Reducing the injury

Reduction can be done in several ways. In *closed reduction*, the doctor manually manipulates the injured part without making an incision. The person receives a general anesthetic (or a local anesthetic and sedatives). An intravenous medicine like morphine is given to control pain and an intravenous sedative like Versed is given to control muscle spasms and ease muscle stretching during traction.

Some injuries require *open reduction*. In this operation, the surgeon makes an incision into the injury site and then wires the joint and repairs damaged ligaments.

Immobilizing the joint

After reduction, the doctor applies a splint, cast, or traction to immobilize the joint. Usually, a dislocated finger or toe is immobilized for 2 weeks to allow time for surrounding ligaments to heal. A hip is immobilized for 6 to 8 weeks; other dislocated joints are immobilized for 3 to 6 weeks.

What else should you know?

After treatment, the person should report numbness, pain, or coldness in the arm, leg, hand, foot, fingers, or toes below the cast or splint. These symptoms may mean the dressing is too tight and the injured area isn't getting enough circulation. The person should also report pain or pressure inside or outside the cast or bandage.

After the cast or splint is removed, the person may gradually return to normal activities.

> *After the displaced parts are restored to their normal position, a splint, cast, or traction is used to immobilize the joint.*

DIZZINESS

Dizziness is the sensation that the room — or the world — is spinning. This sensation can come from many conditions, including:
- ear infection
- other types of infection
- Ménière's disease, a dysfunction of the inner ear
- inflammation of inner ear structures, such as the labyrinth (labyrinthitis) or the mastoid process (a bone located behind and below the ear)
- low blood pressure.

What are the symptoms?
The person may complain of a spinning, whirling, off-balance feeling. Some people describe dizziness as light-headedness, "wooziness," confusion, or a feeling of being about to faint or "black out." Fainting — a temporary loss of consciousness — may signal a more serious condition. (See "Fainting," page 231.) Depending on what is causing the dizziness, the person may have other symptoms too, as described below.

Symptoms of inner ear infection
The person may have hearing loss and severe vertigo with movement of the head. That's because the inner ear controls both hearing and balance. (See *Dizziness and the inner ear,* page 194.)

Symptoms of mastoid inflammation (mastoiditis)
The person with this condition may have:
- dull ache and tenderness below and behind the ear
- slight fever
- swelling and blockage of the external ear canal
- thick, pus-filled ear discharge
- hearing loss.

Symptoms of labyrinthitis
This viral infection of the inner ear produces severe dizziness, which may incapacitate the person for 3 to 5 days. Other symptoms include:
- vertigo beginning gradually and peaking within 48 hours
- loss of balance and falling in the direction of the affected ear

Dizziness can result from such conditions as an ear infection, dysfunction or inflammation of the inner ear, and low blood pressure.

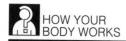
HOW YOUR
BODY WORKS

Dizziness and the inner ear

The inner ear houses the body's center of balance. That's why an inner ear disorder is often the cause of dizziness.

How the ear works
Sound waves enter the ear canal and strike the eardrum, making it vibrate and creating pressure on the ossicles (three small bones in the middle ear). The ossicles, in turn, vibrate, transmitting sound waves to the inner ear.

The labyrinth within the ear
The inner ear — tiny enough to fit inside a marble — contains two structures: the cochlea and the semicircular canals. Together, these structures form the *labyrinth,* named for its complicated twists and turns. The snail-shaped cochlea converts sound waves into nerve impulses, which travel to the brain.

How the ear canals monitor balance
The loop-shaped semicircular canals detect changes in balance and body orientation. Changes in the amount of fluid in these canals can throw off a person's sense of balance.

What happens when fluid pressure rises
Increasing fluid pressure within the labyrinth can make a person lose the sense of balance. In Ménière's disease, for example, the result is hearing loss, dizziness, and ringing in the ears.

What happens when fluid thickens
If fluid in the labyrinth thickens, as may occur with infection or severe dehydration, the fluid moves slowly and can't keep up with the person's movement.

- jerking movements of the eyes toward the unaffected ear
- nausea and vomiting
- giddiness
- drainage of pus from the ear (with severe bacterial infection).

Symptoms of Ménière's disease
The person with this condition may have:
- severe vertigo
- hearing loss
- tinnitus (ringing in the ears).

   Sudden, violent attacks of Ménière's disease last from 10 minutes to several hours. During such an attack, the person may also experience:
- severe nausea
- vomiting
- sweating
- giddiness
- involuntary movements of the eyeball.

What should you do?

Most conditions that lead to dizziness aren't strictly medical emergencies. But the person may need prompt treatment to avoid serious complications.

Keep the person safe and comfortable

If you're with someone who becomes extremely dizzy, help the person to lie down. Check for a pulse and look, listen, and feel for breathing. Loosen any tight clothing.

If you think the person is about to faint, try to prevent a fall. Elevate the person's legs 8 to 12 inches. Stay with the person until he or she is fully conscious.

If the person is at home and you know the cause of the dizziness (for example, because a child has a middle ear infection), help the person get into bed. Provide reassurance and comfort. If you're not sure what is causing the dizziness, call the doctor.

> Never offer anything to eat or drink if the person feels faint or nauseated.
>
> Don't let a dizzy person move about if nausea is present. Instead, have the person lie down until the spinning sensation goes away.

If you think the person is about to faint, try to prevent a fall. Elevate the person's legs 8 to 12 inches.

How is dizziness treated?

If the dizziness is caused by an underlying infection, the doctor prescribes antibiotics. Other treatments are used for other underlying conditions.

Treating labyrinthitis

Treatment includes bed rest with the person's head immobilized between pillows. Usually, the doctor prescribes Antivert, an antivertigo drug, and antibiotics if the person has a bacterial infection. To combat dehydration from vomiting, the person is encouraged to drink plenty of fluids after the nausea goes away. For severe nausea and vomiting, hospitalization and intravenous fluids may be necessary.

Treating mastoiditis

Typically, the person receives intravenous antibiotics to treat the infection. If bone damage is minimal, the doctor may perform *myringotomy*. In this procedure, the eardrum is punctured to drain pus-filled fluid and a specimen of the drainage is collected. The specimen is then tested to see which type of bacteria is causing the infection; this in turn helps the doctor decide which drugs to administer.

Some people with mastoiditis need surgery. A *simple mastoidectomy* may be done if the person has recurrent or persistent infection or develops complications within the skull. In this procedure, the surgeon removes the diseased mastoid bone. Then the affected area is cleaned and a drain is inserted. Afterward, the person must take antibiotics for several weeks.

Surgery for Ménière's disease can permanently relieve symptoms, but causes irreversible hearing loss.

Treating a middle ear infection
Early and vigorous treatment can prevent complications like labyrinthitis and mastoiditis. Antibiotics may be prescribed. To relieve pain, the doctor prescribes a mild pain reliever, such as aspirin or Tylenol (or another acetaminophen product), or heat applications to the external ear. Rarely, the person must be hospitalized.

Treating Ménière's disease
Various drugs may be used to treat this disease. For an acute attack, Dramamine, Antivert, or Valium may be effective.

What else should you know?
Sometimes the doctor recommends surgery for a person with Ménière's disease. The surgery destroys the affected labyrinth, which permanently relieves the symptoms, but causes irreversible hearing loss. Usually, surgery is done only if the disease:
- persists after 2 years of treatment
- causes incapacitating vertigo
- resists medical management.

DOUBLE VISION

Double vision refers to seeing two images of an object at the same time. This happens when the eye muscles fail to function together as a team. (See *Understanding how your eyes move*.)

Double vision may be present at birth in a child who has crossed eyes, or *strabismus*. It can also result from a problem with nerves in the brain or in the eyes themselves.

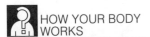

HOW YOUR BODY
WORKS

Understanding how your eyes move

Try as you might, you simply can't will your eyes to move in different directions independent of one another. If you could, you'd have double vision. Read what follows to understand how the eye muscles move.

The shifting functions of eye muscles

Six muscles control how each eyeball moves. Each one has a main function and several minor functions. Which function a muscle performs depends on which other muscles it's working with at a given time.

EYE MUSCLES

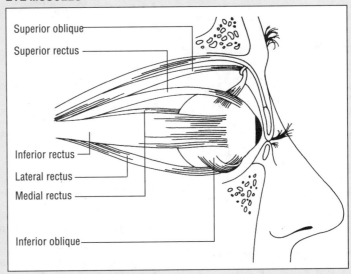

Superior oblique
Superior rectus
Inferior rectus
Lateral rectus
Medial rectus
Inferior oblique

How the eyes move in the same direction

Normally, the muscles of both eyes work together as a team to keep the eyeballs moving in the same direction at the same time.

A group effort

Groups of eye muscles work together to:
- move the eyeballs up and down
- turn the eyeballs from side to side
- rotate the eyeballs in a circle.

Double vision and stroke

Sometimes double vision signals a potentially serious condition. For instance, it may be a symptom of a "little stroke" — a brief episode of decreased blood supply to the brain. (See "Stroke," page 494.) Double vision can precede a major stroke by weeks or months. Treating the person in time can prevent the little stroke from turning into a disabling one.

Understanding other causes

Besides stroke, common causes of double vision include:
- fatigue, which can cause the eye muscles to become too tired to work together properly
- a type of migraine called *ophthalmoplegic migraine*

- alcohol intoxication
- head injury
- nervous system disorders, such as myasthenia gravis and multiple sclerosis.

What are the symptoms?

A person with double vision sees two images of the same object at the same time.

What should you do?

Report any episode of double vision to the doctor at once. Until the person gets to the doctor's office, patching one eye can relieve double vision. Although this will reduce depth perception, at least the person will see the correct number of objects.

How is double vision treated?

In children, crossed eyes can be corrected by surgery. For double vision resulting from other conditions, treatment varies with the underlying cause. For instance, if fatigue is the cause of double vision, getting rest may cure the problem. If migraine is the culprit, the person should be sure to take prescribed drugs or follow the doctor's advice for relieving symptoms.

What else should you know?

Less common causes of double vision include:
- botulism, an often fatal form of food poisoning
- infection
- brain tumor
- a broken bone near the eye
- an overactive thyroid, which causes bulging eyeballs.

> *Report any episode of double vision to the doctor at once. Until the person gets to the doctor's office, you can relieve double vision by patching one eye.*

DRUG OVERDOSE

Abuse of prescription or "street" drugs may lead to an overdose — a medical emergency. A wide range of drugs are abused in any number of settings — from elementary school children sniffing inhalants to middle-aged professionals snorting cocaine. (See *When to suspect your kids are abusing drugs or alcohol,* page 200.)

The drugs that people may abuse and overdose on are mainly those that affect the central nervous system by either stimulating or depressing it. These drugs can be classified by type:

- depressants
- stimulants
- hallucinogens.

Depressants

These include narcotics, sedatives, cannabis drugs, and depressant tranquilizers. Examples of depressants are:

- opium
- heroin
- morphine
- codeine
- "downers"
- phenobarbital
- hashish
- marijuana.

(Alcohol is also a depressant, but isn't covered here. See "Alcohol intoxication," page 20.)

Stimulants

Examples of stimulants are:

- cocaine
- crack cocaine
- "ice" (crystal meth)
- "speed"
- "uppers"
- "pep pills"
- "bennies"
- "whites"
- "dexies"
- glue
- lighter fluid
- paints and lacquers and their thinners (gasoline, kerosene, nail polish and remover).

Hallucinogens

Also called psychedelic drugs, hallucinogens alter a person's perception of reality by changing brain chemistry. They include:

- LSD ("acid")

The drugs that people overdose on are mainly those that affect the central nervous system. They include depressants, stimulants, and hallucinogens.

When to suspect your kids are abusing drugs or alcohol

How can you tell if your children are abusing drugs or alcohol? It's not always easy; normal teenage mood swings can mimic the dramatic behavior changes that drug abuse can cause.

Unfortunately, by the time drug-related behavior changes are apparent, the child may already have a severe problem. If you can intervene early — with firmness but not anger — you have a better chance of stopping the problem long before a drug overdose can occur.

Has your child's behavior changed?

Look for a *pattern* of change. For example, is your child sluggish or sleeping more than usual? Has he or she suddenly stopped paying attention to personal hygiene? Such behavior may signal drug abuse, or it may mean the child is depressed.

Show concern, not criticism

If you notice behavior changes, show your concern without criticizing. One way to do this is to use "I" statements. For example, "I've noticed you're not eating much lately. I'm concerned that you're losing weight."

Encourage your child to express feelings

Try to get your child to express feelings. If he or she tends to give one-word answers, ask open-ended questions instead of those that call for a yes or no answer. For example, ask "What's going on?" instead of "Are you OK?" Allow silence, and your child may open up.

Is your child hanging out with a different crowd?

You may become alarmed if your child has a new group of friends and seems disgusted with all the old ones — especially if the new friends dress or wear their hair in unconventional ways.

Don't let appearances deceive you

Switching old friends for new, seemingly "wilder" ones could mean drug abuse. But don't automatically assume that drug abuse goes along with new friends and a new hairstyle. And remember that a clean-scrubbed appearance can be deceiving too: Many teenagers who dress like model children have drug problems.

Has your child had a sudden weight loss?

Weight loss can be a warning sign of drug use, or it can be a symptom of an eating disorder. Is your child also moody or easily agitated? If so, take him or her to a medical professional before the situation gets worse.

- PCP ("angel dust")
- mescaline (peyote buttons)
- psilocybin mushrooms ("shrooms").

What are the symptoms?

A drug overdose may cause vomiting, breathing difficulty, and loss of consciousness. Other symptoms vary with the type of drug taken.

Symptoms of depressant overdose

Because depressant drugs depress the central nervous system, most symptoms reflect slowness — chiefly of thought and reaction time.

Look for:
- drunken behavior
- slurred speech
- sleep, possibly leading to coma
- shallow breathing
- slow pulse
- low body temperature
- heavy sweating
- very relaxed muscles
- tiny (pinpoint) pupils.

Symptoms of stimulant overdose

Stimulants cause symptoms of overstimulation, such as:
- overactivity
- aggressive behavior
- confusion
- disorganization
- mindless repetition of an act
- irritability
- anxiety
- suspiciousness or paranoia
- hallucinations
- exaggerated perception of personal abilities (such as delusions of grandeur).

Symptoms of hallucinogen overdose

Suspect hallucinogen use in a person with:
- delusions (misinterpretation of sounds, movements, or objects)
- hallucinations or visions (seeing things or hearing sounds that have no factual basis)
- fast pulse
- increased blood pressure
- enlarged pupils
- reddened face
- lack of emotional control (periods of inappropriate laughing or crying)
- depression (appearing sad or moving or talking slowly)
- panic, fear, tension
- varying changes in the level of consciousness
- disorientation
- poor memory of recent events.

A person who experiences delusions, hallucinations, or visions may be using hallucinogens. Other symptoms of hallucinogen use are enlarged pupils and poor emotional control.

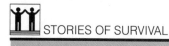

"It was so *not* cool when you took all those sleeping pills!"

"You really want to hear about this, Trish? Are you sure? OK.

"Well, you really scared me when you called. I mean, I was like, 'What?' And you go, 'I took some pills.'

"Some pills! I knew you were depressed about Kevin, but I didn't think you'd try something like that.

"So I go whipping over to your house in my mom's car, which by the way I wasn't supposed to use, but when I told her why I used it, she goes 'OK,' so I didn't get in trouble or anything."

Really out of it

"So I go flying into the house and find you passed out on the couch with an empty bottle of your mom's sleeping pills on the floor. You were like really out of it, OK?

"I ran into the kitchen to get some coffee, because that's what they always do on TV, but then I remember, 'Duuuh, your mom doesn't drink coffee.'

"So I just grab some cold water in a glass and toss it in your face. But you didn't wake up, so I knew something really bad was going on."

I lost it

"So I call 911 and tell them, 'Get over here! My best friend took a whole bunch of sleeping pills and now she won't wake up!' And they go, 'Is she breathing?' and I go, 'Yeah, but not very much.' And they go, 'Is she vomiting?' and I go, 'No.'

"Then they ask me a whole bunch of questions about what kind of pills you took and do I know how long you've been out of it — stuff like that. I mean, I like lost it. It was so *not* fun.

"The EMTs got there in about a second, which was totally cool. They took you to the hospital and pumped your stomach. Then they sent you to the psych unit, which I guess you already know 'cause you're still here."

Any cute doctors here?

"So anyway, I came by because I want you to know we're all thinking about you and we want you to get better — even Jill, who by the way says she doesn't want anything to do with Kevin, he's such a loser.

"So now that you're feeling better, do they, like, have any cute doctors here?"

AfterWords

Trish's friend was obviously concerned about Trish's well-being. But she probably could have handled the situation better.

For instance, she might have skipped trying to find coffee and called 911 as soon as she realized her friend was "really out of it." And she might have checked Trish's airway to make sure it was clear and turned her onto her side to prevent any vomit from blocking her airway.

When the going gets tough, take a deep breath

She also might have taken a deep breath to calm herself. By concentrating on staying calm, she might have been better able to assess the situation and respond appropriately.

What should you do?

 WHEN SECONDS COUNT

If you suspect a person is experiencing a drug overdose, call for medical help immediately. (See *"It was so not cool when you took all those sleeping pills!"*) Check the person for an open airway, feel for a pulse, and look, listen, and feel for breathing. If the airway is obstructed and the person has no pulse and isn't breathing, start CPR at once, if you know how. (See *Performing CPR on an adult,* page 579, *Performing CPR on a child,* page 585, or *Performing CPR on an infant,* page 590.)

Never leave the person alone; drug abuse impairs judgment.

Don't induce vomiting if the person is sleepy or can't be aroused.

If you suspect a person is experiencing a drug overdose, call for medical help immediately. If the person has no pulse and isn't breathing, start CPR at once.

How is drug overdose treated?

If the person has trouble breathing, the emergency medical team gives oxygen through a tube, by mask, or by mechanical ventilation. The person is hooked up to a heart monitor to check heart function. If the person is violent, he or she may be restrained. (See *Understanding drug overdose,* pages 204 to 206.)

Other treatments

Depending on which drug the person took and when, the doctor may induce vomiting if the person is awake. Sometimes the stomach is pumped or the person receives activated charcoal to help absorb the drug, along with a cathartic to help speed elimination of the charcoal through the digestive tract.

In some people, a drug overdose causes the body temperature to decrease or increase. To treat a low body temperature, the person may be covered with extra blankets or a hyperthermia mattress. To treat a fever, the person may receive a drug like aspirin and be placed on a hypothermia mattress.

What else should you know?

After the crisis passes, the doctor will probably recommend drug counseling to prevent future overdoses.

(Text continues on page 207.)

Understanding drug overdose

Symptoms of drug overdose vary with the drug the person has taken. Read this chart to learn about overdose symptoms of a wide range of drugs and what type of treatment the person needs.

DRUG	SYMPTOMS OF OVERDOSE	POSSIBLE TREATMENTS
Amphetamines ■ Amphetamine (Benzedrine) ■ Methamphetamine (Methadrin) — "speed," "meth," "crystal," "ice" ■ Dexedrine — "dexies," "hearts," "oranges"	■ Large pupils ■ Changes in mental status, from confusion to paranoia or coma ■ Hallucinations ■ Tremors ■ Seizures ■ Exhaustion ■ Dry mouth ■ Shallow breathing ■ Fast pulse ■ Fever ■ Dizziness ■ Sweating	■ Activated charcoal to absorb drug ■ Forced vomiting ■ Pumping of stomach ■ Checking of pulse for irregular heartbeats ■ Restraints ■ Suicide watch ■ Barbiturates to control seizures ■ CPR
Barbiturate sedative-hypnotics ■ Barbiturates — "downers," "sleepers," "barbs" ■ Amytal sodium — "blue angels," "blue devils," "blue birds" ■ Luminal — "phennies," "purple hearts," "goofballs" ■ Seconal — "reds," "red devils," "seccy"	■ Unusual pupil reaction to light ■ Wandering eye movements ■ Decreased mental status, from confusion to coma ■ Limp muscles ■ Fever or low body temperature ■ Slow breathing ■ Bluish skin ■ Dizziness or weakness ■ Blisters or skin lesions	■ Forced vomiting ■ Activated charcoal to absorb drug ■ Pumping of stomach ■ Intravenous fluids to raise blood pressure ■ Cooling or warming with hyperthermia or hypothermia blanket ■ CPR

Understanding drug overdose *(continued)*

DRUG	SYMPTOMS OF OVERDOSE	POSSIBLE TREATMENTS
Cocaine ■ Cocaine, or "coke" ■ "Free base" ■ Crack	■ Large pupils ■ Confusion ■ Increased excitability ■ Hallucinations ■ Muscle spasms ■ Seizures ■ Coma ■ Rapid, shallow breathing or no breathing ■ Pale or bluish skin ■ Rapid pulse ■ Fever ■ Nausea and vomiting ■ Abdominal pain ■ Irritation or tearing of lining of nose ■ Mouth sores	■ Activated charcoal to absorb drug ■ Laxative to induce bowel evacuation ■ Pumping of stomach ■ Tepid sponge bath plus aspirin or Tylenol to reduce fever ■ Valium to control seizures ■ Checking of heart rate and rhythm (cocaine overdose can cause heart attack) ■ CPR
Hallucinogens ■ LSD — "acid," "hawk," "sunshine" ■ Mescaline (peyote) — "mes," "cactus," "big chief" ■ Psylocybin — "shrooms"	■ Large pupils ■ Agitation, anxiety ■ Hyperactivity ■ Flashbacks ■ Hallucinations ■ Fast pulse ■ Fever	■ Reorientation to time, place, and person ■ Forced vomiting ■ Activated charcoal, with laxative to induce bowel evacuation ■ Pumping of stomach ■ Valium to control seizures ■ CPR

(continued)

Understanding drug overdose *(continued)*

DRUG	SYMPTOMS OF OVERDOSE	POSSIBLE TREATMENTS
Hallucinogens *(continued)* ■ PCP — "angel dust," "peace pill," "hog"	■ Blank staring ■ Wandering eye movements ■ Memory loss ■ Recurrent coma ■ Hyperactivity ■ Seizures ■ Clumsy walk ■ Rigid muscles ■ Drooling ■ Fever ■ Severe rise in blood pressure ■ Heart attack	■ Forced vomiting ■ Activated charcoal given repeatedly to absorb drug ■ Pumping of stomach ■ Valium to control agitation or psychotic behavior ■ CPR
Narcotics ■ Heroin — "smack," "H," "junk," "snow" ■ morphine — "mort," "monkey," "M," "Miss Emma" ■ Dilaudid — "D," "lords"	■ Small pupils ■ No awareness of surroundings (will respond if you keep talking to person or slapping person) ■ Seizures ■ Low body temperature ■ Dizziness or weakness ■ Slow pulse (less than 60 beats per minute) ■ Itching, hives, or flushed skin	■ Narcan (drug used to counteract nervous system depression) ■ Warming, such as with extra blankets or hyperthermia blanket ■ Oxygen by tube, mask, or mechanical ventilator ■ Checking of heart rate and rhythm ■ CPR
Sedatives or tranquilizers (antianxiety drugs) ■ Valium ■ Librium ■ Quaaludes — "ludes"	■ Confusion ■ Stupor ■ Slow reflexes ■ Seizures ■ Coma ■ Dizziness or weakness	■ Forced vomiting ■ Activated charcoal, with laxative to induce bowel evacuation ■ Pumping of stomach ■ Intravenous fluids to raise blood pressure ■ Monitoring of vital signs ■ CPR

EAR INFECTION

Ear infection is a painful inflammation or infection of the internal, middle, or external ear. A common affliction of childhood, it can interfere with daily activities and sometimes causes hearing loss.

Some ear infections are mild and temporary. Others can be debilitating. (See *Guarding against ear infections,* page 208.)

Understanding the causes
An ear infection can result from:
- allergy
- bacteria
- fungi
- viruses
- injury.

Types of ear infections
External ear infection (which doctors call otitis externa) affects the ear's outer structure — the earlobe and ear canal. Swimmer's ear is a common form of external ear infection. Occurring mainly in the summer, it is caused by infection transmitted in the water of a swimming pool. Swimmer's ear may be acute or chronic. With treatment, the infection usually subsides in 7 days.

Middle ear infection (otitis media) is an infection of the tympanic cavity — the small cavity in the temporal bone that includes tiny bones called ossicles (the malleus, incus, and stapes). Like an external ear infection, a middle ear infection may be acute or chronic. The acute form is common in children, especially in winter, when cold viruses make the upper respiratory tract vulnerable to bacterial infection. Doctors sometimes classify middle ear infection as pus-producing (suppurative) or secretion-producing (secretory).

Inner ear infection (otitis interna) is also called labyrinthitis. This inflammation affects the labyrinthine canals of the inner ear. (For more information, see "Dizziness," page 193.)

Swimmer's ear is a common form of external ear infection. Occurring mainly in the summer, it is caused by infection transmitted in the water of a swimming pool.

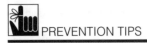
PREVENTION TIPS

Guarding against ear infections

To reduce your chance of getting recurrent ear infections, follow these suggestions.

Avoid swimmer's ear
Swimmer's ear tends to recur. But you can lower your risk of getting future infections by taking the following steps.

Keep water out of your ears
- Use lamb's wool earplugs coated with Vaseline when showering or washing your hair.
- When swimming, wear earplugs or keep your head above water.

Avoid other risk factors
- Don't swim in contaminated water.

- Avoid cleaning your ear canal with a cotton-tipped swab, bobby pin, finger, or other foreign object.
- Be sure not to expose your ear to dust, hair spray, or other hair care products or irritants.
- Don't wear earphones, earplugs, or earmuffs for prolonged periods. These items trap moisture in the ear canal, creating a perfect growing environment for germs.

Keep the eustachian tube working properly
Using a method called *Valsalva's maneuver* can help you avoid middle ear infection. To perform the maneuver, inhale deeply, hold your nose for at least 10 seconds, and then exhale forcefully. This action creates pressure in your eustachian tubes. Perform Valsalva's maneuver several times a day.

What are the symptoms?
Symptoms vary with the type of ear infection.

Symptoms of external ear infection
The person may have:
- fever
- itching
- moderate to severe pain
- foul-smelling discharge
- pain on clenching the teeth, opening the mouth, chewing, or touching the external part of the ear
- a red, swollen, moist, pus-filled earlobe
- partial hearing loss if the ear canal becomes swollen or filled with pus.

Symptoms of middle ear infection
Symptoms depend on the form of the infection. Acute pus-produc-

ing infection may produce no symptoms — or many. For instance, the person may have:

- severe, deep, throbbing pain
- runny nose
- sneezing
- cough
- mild to high fever
- nausea
- dizziness
- hearing loss (usually mild)
- a bulging eardrum, which may rupture and cause swelling and drainage of pus in the ear canal.

Acute secretion-producing infection can cause:

- a sensation of fullness in the ear
- popping, crackling, or clicking sounds on swallowing or moving the jaw
- echo heard when speaking
- a vague feeling of top-heaviness
- severe hearing loss.

What should you do?

Call the doctor promptly to report symptoms of an ear infection. Once the condition is diagnosed, the person should follow the doctor's instructions on taking drugs and practicing self-care.

Many parents have been awakened in the middle of the night by a child crying from the pain of an ear infection. For advice on dealing with this problem, see *Coping with your child's ear infection,* page 210.

How is an ear infection treated?

For *external ear infection,* the ear is cleaned. The doctor prescribes antibiotic eardrops and may prescribe aspirin or acetaminophen (Tylenol or Tylenol with codeine) to relieve pain. (See *Giving eardrops,* page 212.) If the person has a persistent fever, the doctor may prescribe an oral antibiotic too.

The person with an acute *middle ear infection* typically receives an antibiotic like Omnipen or Amoxil. A person who is allergic to penicillin derivatives may take Ceclor instead. Aspirin or acetaminophen is used to reduce pain and fever.

For swimmer's ear, antibiotic eardrops may be prescribed. If the condition becomes chronic, the ear is thoroughly cleaned and wet

Call the doctor promptly to report symptoms of an ear infection. Once the condition is diagnosed, the person should follow the doctor's instructions on taking drugs and practicing self-care.

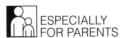

Coping with your child's ear infection

Some young children have as many as six colds over the course of the winter. Each of these upper respiratory infections gives bacteria the chance to take hold and cause an ear infection.

Know the consequences
Middle ear infection can lead to rupture of the eardrum. That's one reason it's so important to get prompt treatment if your child has symptoms of ear infection.

Expect symptoms to vary
Keep in mind that two children, even in the same family, may show different symptoms of an ear infection. Your daughter, for instance, may run a high fever, while your son complains of pain or shows no symptoms.

Try not to get frustrated, though. You'll soon recognize each child's particular combination of symptoms.

Speed your child's recovery
If your child has been diagnosed with an ear infection, applying heat to the ear can help relieve pain. Use a heating pad or hot, damp towels. For other ways to speed your child's recovery and prevent the infection from coming back, read the following advice.

Use drugs properly
■ If the doctor prescribes antibiotics, discuss matching the drug form to your child's age. For instance, an infant or a toddler should probably take a liquid antibiotic. Elementary school age children may be ready for a chewable form, whereas older children may be able to swallow pills.

■ To prevent hearing loss, ensure that your child finishes the full course of antibiotics.

■ If the doctor prescribes decongestants, make sure you understand — and follow — the instructions for instilling them.

Other instructions
■ Take your child back to the doctor for a follow-up visit, usually scheduled 2 to 4 weeks after the first visit. Some children need a second course of antibiotics to clear up the ear infection.

■ If your child has an acute secretory middle ear infection, watch for and immediately report pain or fever. These symptoms may signal an additional infection (called a *secondary infection*).

■ If your child has a ruptured eardrum, don't let the ear get wet.

■ If your child suffers a temporary hearing loss from a middle ear infection, know that the hearing should return to normal once the infection clears up or the eustachian tube blockage is relieved.

Prevent ear infection in an infant
■ Don't breast-feed your infant while lying down.

■ Never let your infant drink from a propped-up bottle. When an infant swallows while lying down, discharge from the nose can drain into the eustachian tubes, setting the stage for middle ear infection.

Coping with ear tubes
If your child has been taking antibiotics for 1 to 3 months without improved hearing or has had frequent ear infections, the doctor may recommend that ear tubes, called tympanostomy tubes, be inserted into the ear. The tubes won't prevent ear infection, but they will ease drainage from the ear canal.

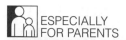

Coping with your child's ear infection *(continued)*

Check for drainage
If the ear tubes are functioning normally, you'll see drainage from the outer ear canal. If they're clogged, your child may show symptoms of ear infection — fever, pain, irritability, restlessness, and tugging at the ear. Call the doctor if these symptoms occur.

Prevent complications
To help prevent complications after tube insertion, remind your child not to blow his or her nose until the ear has healed. Also, don't let your child get the ear wet when bathing.

soaks applied to oozing or affected skin. The doctor may prescribe an exfoliative ointment for a chronic fungal infection.

Surgery
If the person has a severe, painful bulging of the eardrum, the doctor may recommend *myringotomy*. In this operation, performed in the doctor's office, the doctor cuts into the eardrum and gently suctions fluid or pus from the middle ear to relieve pressure. The person remains awake during the procedure.

Ear tubes
For someone with recurrent ear infections, the doctor may recommend insertion of ear tubes, called *tympanostomy tubes*. The tubes help to drain the ear canal. They fall out on their own after 9 to 12 months.

What else should you know?
A person with a blocked eustachian tube may develop a secretion-producing middle ear infection. Why? The blockage causes negative pressure to build up in the middle ear, allowing fluid from blood vessels to enter.

When pressure isn't equalized
Such fluid entry may result from a viral infection or an allergy. Or it may stem from inability to equalize pressures between the environment and the middle ear. In a person with an upper respiratory infection, this may happen during rapid descent in an airplane. It may also occur in a scuba diver who rapidly rises to the water surface.

Giving eardrops

The structure of a child's ear is different from that of an adult's — so different that you give eardrops to a child differently than you give them to yourself or to another adult.

Understanding the anatomy
The difference lies in both the eardrum and the ear canal. In a child, the eardrum slants horizontally and the entire external ear canal slants upward. This means you must hold the child's earlobe down and back to give eardrops.

In the adult, the eardrum is more vertical and the ear canal eases upward. So to instill eardrops, you hold the adult's earlobe up and back.

Here are step-by-step instructions to follow when giving eardrops.

Giving eardrops to an adult
■ Shake the bottle if directed. Then open it and fill the dropper.
■ Tilt the person's head so the affected ear is facing up. Then gently pull the top of the ear *up and back* to straighten the ear canal as shown in the illustration below.

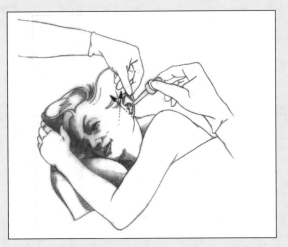

■ Position the dropper above the ear but not touching it. Then release the prescribed number of drops.
■ Have the person lie on the side with the affected ear facing up for 10 minutes.
■ Repeat the procedure for the other ear if the doctor has told you to.

Giving eardrops to a child
■ Lay the child on the side so the affected ear is facing up.
■ Gently pull the ear *down and back* to straighten the ear canal as shown in the illustration below. Then slowly release the prescribed number of drops.
■ Repeat the procedure for the other ear if the doctor has told you to.

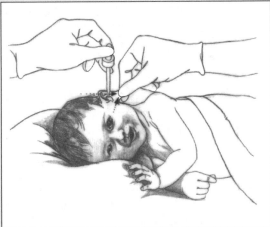

ELBOW INJURIES

The elbow — where three main arm bones, major nerves, and major arteries converge — is vulnerable to several kinds of injuries. Called *overuse injuries,* they come from the repetitive motions we make when engaging in many sports and daily activities. For instance, repetitive motion can cause *golfer's elbow* or *tennis elbow.* Both injuries also go by the name *tendinitis.*

Golfer's elbow
This injury is an inflammation or a tear in the tendon that attaches the muscles on the *inside* of the forearm to the bony protrusion on the *inside* of the elbow, called the *medial epicondyle.* Seen in both golfers and tennis players, golfer's elbow can come from:
■ an improper downward stroke in golf
■ hitting the ground when swinging the golf club
■ an improperly executed forehand stroke in tennis
■ underdeveloped flexor (bending) muscles in the arm.

Tennis elbow
The opposite of golfer's elbow, tennis elbow is an inflammation or a tear in the tendon that connects the muscles on the *outside* of the forearm to the bony protrusion on the *outer* part of the elbow, called the *lateral* epicondyle. (See *The elbow's parts,* page 214.)
    Causes of tennis elbow include:
■ a poorly executed backhand tennis stroke
■ improper tennis equipment, such as loose strings, a too-stiff or too-heavy racquet, or a grip that's too small or too large
■ snapping the wrist on the tennis serve
■ underdeveloped extensor muscles — the ones you use when you reach out your arm.

What are the symptoms?
Golfer's elbow causes pain on the inside of the elbow. Often intense, the pain can limit movement. The person may feel the pain when carrying heavy objects or lifting boxes as well as when doing the activity that originally caused the injury.
    Tennis elbow, in contrast, causes pain on the outside of the elbow. As with golfer's elbow, the pain may be severe enough to limit movement. It may occur during such activities as turning a doorknob, shaking hands, or picking up a piece of paper.

Golfer's elbow causes pain on the inside of the elbow. Tennis elbow causes pain on the outside of the elbow. Pain from either injury may be severe enough to limit movement.

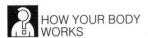

HOW YOUR BODY
WORKS

The elbow's parts

The elbow, a hinge (swinging) joint, is the place where three arm bones — the ulna, radius, and humerus — meet. White, shiny, flexible bands of fibrous tissue called *ligaments* connect the three bones here. *Tendons,* which are also made of fibrous tissue, join the muscles to the bones. *Epicondyles* are the bony protrusions on the inside and outside of the elbow.

An inside look

The top illustration on the right shows one type of movement that may injure the inner elbow, along with a close-up of inner elbow structures. The bottom illustration on the right shows one type of movement that may injure the outer elbow, along with a close-up of outer elbow structures.

INNER ELBOW

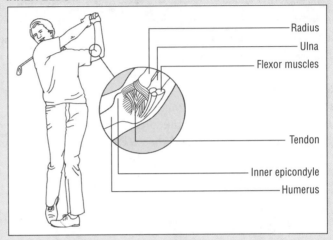

OUTER ELBOW

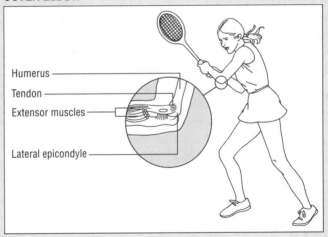

What should you do?

If the person can't bend or straighten the elbow without pain or can't extend the arm forward, have him or her stop the activity that's causing the pain. Place an ice pack on the elbow to help stop internal bleeding and reduce pain and swelling. Then consult the doctor.

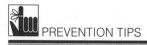
PREVENTION TIPS

How to avoid more elbow trouble

If you've had one bout of golfer's or tennis elbow, you may be afraid to go back to the activity that brought on the injury. But keep this in mind: Even though these injuries recur in some people, your fate needn't be a lifetime of arm pain. Here are some self-care measures that may help you avoid recurrences.

Ease into activity slowly
■ Give yourself plenty of time to heal. Don't engage in the activity that caused the pain until your symptoms go away.
■ Once the pain is gone, resume the activity *gradually,* in limited workouts. For example, start with a few minutes of swinging a tennis racquet or golf club and working with light weights.

Strengthen your arms
■ Ask the doctor or a physical therapist about exercises to help strengthen the muscles, ligaments, and tendons of your hand, wrist, and forearm.
■ Ask your golf or tennis pro for advice on proper technique and equipment.

Wear protective gear
Wear a tennis strap or band just below your elbow. The strap reduces pain by constricting your arm muscles and taking pressure off the areas where they attach to the elbow.

How are elbow injuries treated?

The doctor may recommend aspirin, Motrin or Advil (ibuprofen), or another mild pain reliever to reduce pain and swelling. If the pain is severe, the doctor may suggest a low-dose injection of cortisone or another steroid-like drug to reduce inflammation.

Never give aspirin to a child under age 16 who also has a cold, flu symptoms, or chickenpox. Doing so may cause Reye's syndrome, a life-threatening condition that affects the brain.

Other treatments

Other treatments for golfer's elbow and tennis elbow include:
■ using an ice pack at least once a day for the first 2 to 4 days, then switching to a heating pad
■ resting the arm for 4 to 8 weeks (see *How to avoid more elbow trouble*)
■ avoiding (at least until the pain goes away) the activities that bring on symptoms

■ doing exercises for the hand, wrist, and forearm to strengthen arm muscles, ligaments, and tendons.

Don't apply heat to the elbow until swelling has subsided. Warming an area that's still swollen may increase the swelling.

Surgery

Some people eventually may need surgery to release tension on the tendon. In this operation, the surgeon detaches the tendon from the bone.

What else should you know?

You don't have to be a golfer or tennis player to get golfer's elbow or tennis elbow. You can get *golfer's elbow* from:

■ archery
■ bowling
■ table tennis
■ rowing
■ racquetball
■ waterskiing
■ weight lifting.

You can get *tennis elbow* from:

■ archery
■ golf
■ bowling
■ fly fishing
■ table tennis
■ racquetball
■ skiing.

Not just for athletes

In fact, you don't have to engage in *any* sport to get these injuries. Golfer's elbow and tennis elbow can come from doing construction work and other forms of repetitive manual labor — say, painting, gardening, mopping floors, or moving furniture.

Even "couch potatoes" can get tennis elbow if they write a lot. Over time, writing can strain an elbow tendon.

ERECTION THAT IS PAINFUL

A painful, persistent erection of the penis not associated with sexual arousal is both frightening and puzzling. The man may be too embarrassed to seek medical help and may try to treat himself through sexual activity.

However, this condition is a medical emergency. In fact, without swift treatment, irreversible complications may occur. Fortunately, this type of erection, which doctors call *priapism*, is relatively rare. (See *What causes a painful erection?*)

What are the symptoms?

The problem may start during sleep and may seem to be a normal erection, but it may last for several hours or days. Besides the prolonged and painful erection, the man typically has constant, dull aching in the penis. Other symptoms may include:

- difficulty urinating
- urine retention
- extreme anxiety.

What should you do?

Call the doctor at once. Apply an ice pack to the penis.

How is it treated?

The man usually is hospitalized. To ease his discomfort, he may receive a pain reliever. To drain retained urine, a urinary catheter may be inserted. In some cases, the drug epinephrine is given.

If these measures don't help the erection subside, the man may need surgery or aspiration (withdrawal of blood by a suction device). Both of these procedures aim to remove blood from the corpora cavernosa — the cylindrical mass of spongelike tissue inside the penis that fills with blood and causes the penis to become erect.

Determining the cause

The doctor also examines the man's urologic system to find out the cause of his condition. Treating the cause, such as sickle cell anemia or leukemia, is important. A man with sickle cell anemia, for example, may receive intravenous fluids. A man with leukemia may receive a chemotherapeutic drug to reduce the number of white blood cells in his circulation; this relieves the erection.

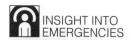

INSIGHT INTO EMERGENCIES

What causes a painful erection?

A painful, prolonged erection of the penis occurs when veins in the erectile portion of the penis, called the corpora cavernosa, fail to drain correctly. The tissues of the penis then become swollen and congested with blood. In about half the cases, the doctor can't determine the cause of the abnormal erection.

Tracking the cause

In the other half of the men who get this condition, the problem results from one of the following conditions:
- a blood disorder, such as acute leukemia, sickle cell anemia, or sickle cell trait
- a tumor in the penis
- injury to the penis
- spinal cord injury
- infection of the urinary tract (rare).

Drug culprits

Certain drugs can cause a painful erection too. They include:
- Desyrel, an antidepressant
- Thorazine, used to treat mental illness
- Alazine Tabs and Minipress, drugs used to control high blood pressure.

What else should you know?

Without prompt treatment, a painful, prolonged erection can cut off blood flow to the penis and cause a blood clot in this organ. If the shortage of blood flow is prolonged, gangrene of the penis may develop.

EYE INFECTION

An eye infection occurs when a germ that can cause disease — like a bacterium, virus, or fungus — gets into the eye or related tissues. (See *The eye's parts*.)

Types of eye infections

An eye infection may take one of the following forms:

■ *blepharitis*, a common inflammation of the eyelid edges

■ *chalazion*, an infection of a deep gland in the eyelid. The gland may grow large enough to press on the eyeball.

■ *pinkeye* (conjunctivitis), an infection of the conjunctiva — the membrane that lines the eyelids and covers the exposed surface of the eyeball. It's usually caused by bacteria, allergies, fungi, or chemicals; when caused by bacteria, it's highly contagious.

■ *stye*, a red, swollen abscess caused by inflammation of the glands at the rim of the eyelid

■ *uveitis*, an inflammation of a structure called the uveal tract (see *Three types of uveitis,* page 220). Uveitis is a serious condition that occasionally causes partial loss of vision.

What are the symptoms?

Symptoms depend on the type of infection.

Symptoms of blepharitis

The person with this infection may have:

■ burning and itching of the eye

■ a foreign-body sensation in the eye

> *An eye infection occurs when a disease-causing germ gets into the eye or related tissues. Types of eye infections include blepharitis, chalazion, pinkeye, stye, and uveitis.*

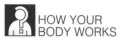

HOW YOUR
BODY WORKS

The eye's parts

The eyes are complex organs with many parts. Each part has a different job to do.

Sclera
This is the eye's dense, fibrous, outer protective coat. The sclera is often called the white of the eye.

Cornea
The curved, transparent part of the eye, the cornea is continuous with the sclera. Made up of five layers, it covers the iris and the pupil. The cornea's job is to let light into the inside of the eye.

Iris
This is the colored part of the eye. The iris regulates the amount of light entering the eye.

Pupil
This is the round opening that light rays pass through. It is surrounded by the iris.

Lens
The completely transparent part of the eye, the lens is located behind the iris. It changes shape to focus clear images of objects on the retina.

Ciliary body
This is the thickened part of the eye's vascular coat. It controls the thickness of the lens and, along with the iris, regulates the light focused through the lens onto the retina.

Retina
The eye's lining, the retina receives light rays from all other parts of the eye and receives the image of objects through the lens.

Choroid
This thin membrane covers the rear five-sixths of the eye between the retina and sclera. It contains many small arteries and veins.

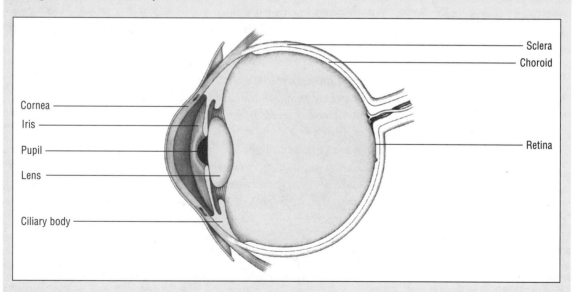

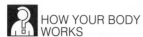

Three types of uveitis

In uveitis, all or part of the *uveal tract* of one eye becomes inflamed.

Structures of the uveal tract
The uveal tract consists of:
- the iris — the portion that gives the eye its color, such as blue, brown, or hazel
- the choroid — a thin membrane covering the rear part of the eye behind the retina
- related tissues in the eye.

Where inflammation can strike
- *Anterior uveitis* affects either the iris alone or both the iris and the ciliary body (a thickened part of the choroid).
- *Posterior uveitis* affects the choroid alone or both the choroid and the retina — the part of the eye that receives impulses and sends them to the brain.
- *Panuveitis* affects the entire uveal tract.

- greasy or flaky scales on the eyelashes
- loss of eyelashes
- ulcers on the eyelid edges
- nits (louse eggs) on the eyelashes, if blepharitis is caused by lice
- sticky, crusted eyelids on waking up in the morning
- frequent blinking or rubbing of the eyes, caused by constant irritation.

Symptoms of chalazion
The person with this eye condition may have a painless, hard swelling of the eyelid.

Symptoms of pinkeye
This eye infection may cause:
- a pink tinge to the eyes
- increased tearing
- eye itching or burning
- eye pain
- light sensitivity (if the cornea is also inflamed)
- eye discharge, which is sticky and profuse with bacterial pinkeye and less abundant with viral pinkeye.

Symptoms of a stye
A stye commonly leads to:
- redness, swelling, and pain in the eye
- discharge of pus from the eye
- a red, swollen, tender abscess at the edge of the eyelid, with an eyelash pointing outward from its center.

Symptoms of uveitis
The person may have such symptoms as:
- moderate to severe pain in one eye
- increased tearing
- eye sensitivity to light
- a small pupil that doesn't react to changes in the amount of light
- blurred or decreased vision
- seeing floating spots, if the disease is in the back portion of the uveal tract.

What should you do?
The actions you should take vary with the type of eye infection.

How to administer eye medicines

To clear up an eye infection, the doctor will probably prescribe eye medicines, such as eyedrops or ointment.

How to instill eyedrops

To instill eyedrops, gently pull the person's lower eyelid down until you can see the space between the lid and the eyeball. Then tell the person to look up and away. Squeeze the prescribed number of drops into this space without letting the applicator touch the eye, as shown in the illustration below. Next, let go of the eyelid and tell the person to blink. This will spread the drops throughout the eye.

INSTILLING EYEDROPS

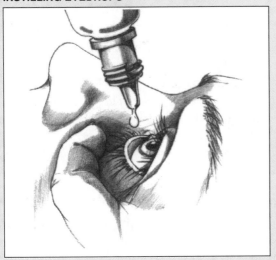

How to apply an eye ointment

To apply an eye ointment, gently pull the person's lower eyelid down until you can see the space between the lid and the eyeball. Then squeeze a thin strip of the ointment into this space, as shown in the illustration below. Start at the inner fold and move toward the outer fold of the eye. Don't let the tube touch the eye. Now, let go of the eyelid. Tell the person to close the eyes and roll the eye around to spread the ointment. Expect the person's vision to be blurry for a few minutes.

APPLYING EYE OINTMENT

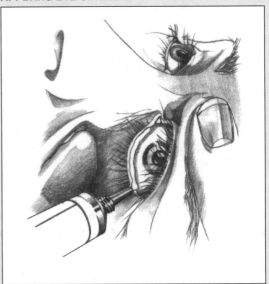

With any eye infection, don't let the person touch or rub the eyes with the fingers. Doing so can cause more germs to get into the eye, complicating the infection. Touching the eye can also pass the infection on to other people.

What to do for blepharitis

Have the person wash the eyelashes daily with a mild shampoo on a damp applicator stick or a washcloth to remove scales. Make sure

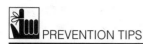

PREVENTION TIPS

Avoiding complications of blepharitis

To prevent blepharitis from getting worse, read over these suggestions.

Use warm compresses
Apply warm compresses to your eyelids. To do this, fill a clean bowl with warm water. Then place a clean cloth in the water and wring it out.

Next, hold the cloth against your closed eyelid — but be careful not to burn your skin. Hold the compress over your eyelid until it cools. Repeat this procedure for 15 minutes.

Remove eyelid scales
Every day remove the scales from the edges of your eyelid. To do this, use an applicator stick or a clean washcloth.

the person frequently shampoos the scalp and eyebrows. Thorough hand washing before and after touching the eye is important.

What to do for a chalazion
Apply warm compresses to the person's outer eyelid a few times a day. If the bump remains for more than a few days or if it comes back after clearing up, get medical attention.

 Avoid trying to pop the swollen area.

What to do for pinkeye
Consult the doctor. For temporary pain relief, put an ice cube in a plastic bag and hold the bag over the eyelid. Wash your hands before and after any contact with the infected eye, and tell the person with pinkeye to do the same. Also wash any cloths or towels that have touched the infected eye.

What to do for uveitis
Call the doctor right away if the person has symptoms of uveitis. This emergency condition puts the person's eyesight at risk.

How is an eye infection treated?
All eye infections require a doctor's care. The goal is to treat the cause of the infection. To do this, the doctor usually prescribes antibiotic eyedrops. (See *How to administer eye medicines,* page 221.) Often the person is instructed to apply warm compresses to the eye every few hours.

Treating blepharitis
If blepharitis is caused by seborrhea (overproduction of the natural lubricant called sebum), the person must shampoo daily to remove scales from the eyelid rims, scalp, and eyebrows. For blepharitis caused by lice, the nits are removed or an insecticide ointment is applied. The doctor may also recommend putting warm compresses on the eye. (See *Avoiding complications of blepharitis.*)

Treating a chalazion
If the chalazion doesn't get better after treatment with drugs and compresses, the doctor may recommend injection of steroids or even surgery.

Treating uveitis
The person may need a cycloplegic, a type of drug that paralyzes certain eye muscles. The doctor may also prescribe a steroid drug applied directly to the eye. For severe uveitis, treatment includes taking steroids orally. Other treatments for uveitis include rest and wearing dark glasses to ease discomfort from light sensitivity.

What else should you know?
Some eye infections, such as blepharitis and stye, may come back after they clear up and then become chronic. Uveitis also has a tendency to recur.

Watch for symptoms
That's why someone who has recovered from an eye infection should watch for eye symptoms — including eye pain, increased tearing, light sensitivity, and decreased vision — and seek treatment immediately.

EYE INJURIES

Eye injuries are caused by a penetrating object or a blow from a blunt object. In a penetrating injury, an object becomes impaled in the eye. In a blunt injury, the eye suffers a direct blow — for example, from a fist or a moving ball.

A serious injury may even knock the person's eye out of the socket, causing an *eye avulsion*. Or it may separate the layers of the retina, causing *retinal detachment*.

What are the symptoms?
Symptoms vary with the type of injury.

Symptoms of a penetrating injury
This injury may cause:
- eye pain
- visible bleeding within the eye
- increased tearing

Eye injuries are caused by a penetrating object or a blow from a blunt object. A serious injury may knock the person's eye out of the socket or separate the layers of the retina.

- decreased vision
- a visible eye wound
- a torn eyelid.

Symptoms of a blunt injury
This injury may result in:
- eye pain
- visible bleeding within the eye
- a reddish tint or drifting spots (floaters) seen before the eyes.

What should you do?
Always assume any eye injury poses a danger to the person's vision. Specific steps to take depend on the type of injury.

What to do for a penetrating injury
Call for medical help immediately. Then cover both eyes with a gauze dressing or similar material. This will prevent further damage that can occur if the injured eye moves in unison with the unharmed eye.

> Never remove — or move — any object that's impaled in the eye. Only a doctor should do this.
>
> Don't flush the eye with water or apply pressure to the eye.

Next, place a paper cup or cone over the object that's stuck in the eye. Place a bandage over the cup and dressing to hold them in place. Make sure the bandage covers both eyes. (See *Protecting an injured eye.*)

> Don't let the object touch the top or sides of the cup.

Tell the person to lie on his or her back. Then immobilize the head by using large pads or sandbags. Instruct the person not to touch the dressing or the impaled object.

> Be sure not to leave the person alone if both eyes are bandaged. Providing reassurance and staying in constant physical contact can help prevent the person from panicking.

What to do for a blunt injury
Call for medical help. Then apply cold compresses or an ice pack to the injured eye. This will decrease pain and swelling. Leave the cold treatment on for about 15 minutes. Keep the person lying down with the eye closed.

Protecting an injured eye

To prevent the impaled object from being driven deeper into the eye, cut a paper cup, as shown by the dotted line in this illustration. Then place the end of the cup (or cardboard folded into a cone) over the impaled object and tape it to the person's face as shown here.

Margin of safety
Don't let the impaled object touch the top or side of the cup. If the object is longer than the cup, make a hole in the bottom of the cup.

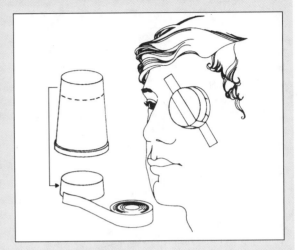

What to do for an eye avulsion

If the person's eye has been knocked out of the socket, get medical help immediately. Cover the injured eye loosely with a moist sterile dressing and a protective cup. Cover the unharmed eye with a bandage or patch.

 Don't try to put the eye back into the socket.

 Never apply pressure to the eye.

How are eye injuries treated?

Treatment varies with the type of injury.

Treating a penetrating eye injury

If necessary, the person has X-rays, a computed tomography scan (commonly called a CAT scan), or ultrasound to locate the penetrating object. Then an ophthalmologist removes the object during surgery and repairs the eye and any related injuries. Afterward, the person wears an eye shield. The doctor usually prescribes the following drugs:

- antibiotics to prevent infection
- steroids to decrease swelling and inflammation
- analgesics to relieve pain.

(Text continues on page 228.)

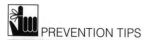

Safeguarding your eyes

More eye injuries occur in the home than anywhere else. Of course, eye injuries can also occur at work or during recreational activities.

Some of the activities that can injure your eyes are so obvious that they're easy to avoid — playing with fireworks or guns, for instance. Others, such as playing tennis, may seem harmless.

Recognize obvious threats

Take special precautions to avoid eye injuries, such as cuts, burns, scratches, and punctures. Stay away from:

- rifles and other firearms, unless you've been trained to use them
- fireworks and firecrackers
- dangerous sports equipment, such as air rifles, bows and arrows, swords, wrist rockets, and slingshots
- flying objects
- spatter from frying foods
- sharp or protruding objects
- chemical sprays
- dangerous liquids, including cleaning fluids and detergents, battery acids, painting supplies, and hot liquids
- high-speed tools, such as drills, chain saws, chisels, solderers, sanders, polishers, and lawn and farm equipment

Watch for environmental hazards

Be aware of the threat from automobile exhaust, tobacco smoke, and other pollutants.

Store objects safely

Any pointed object — especially one that sticks out at eye level — poses a danger to your eyes. Be wary of knives, scissors, pencils, cooking forks, workbench tools, countertops, table corners, and even tree branches.

Keep pointed objects away from children

Pointed objects are especially risky for young children. Keep them out of children's reach, and remove any objects that stick out at a child's eye level.

Celebrate with care

In the exuberance of toasting the future, assure yourself and your friends of being able to see in the new year. Popping champagne corks have destroyed many special occasions.

Point champagne bottles away from people

Before opening your bottle of bubbly, wrap the cork end in a towel. Don't bend over the cork or point it toward anyone — not even yourself.

Use contact lenses safely

If you wear contact lenses, follow the eye doctor's directions for wearing and caring for them.

Don't wear contact lenses to bed unless they're extended-wear lenses. Also remove contact lenses before swimming. After getting out of the water, rinse your eyes with fresh water or saline solution before putting the lenses back in.

Keep smoke out of your eyes

Don't smoke while wearing contact lenses. Smoking hampers the normal exchange of oxygen and carbon dioxide on the surface of your eyes.

Protect your eyes during sports

You need as much — if not more — eye protection if you're active in sports as you do at home or at work. Eye injuries are becoming much more common as more people engage in athletic activities. Using safety gear specially designed for your activity can protect your eyes from such hazards as:

- fast-moving balls

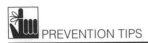

PREVENTION TIPS

Safeguarding your eyes *(continued)*

- branches
- trees
- blows to the head
- excessive exposure to sunlight.

The most dangerous games

Squash and racquetball account for many sports-related eye injuries. The small balls used in these sports can ricochet straight into unprotected eyes. Even tennis players with vigorous net games flirt with disaster if they don't wear safety goggles.

But the "gentlemanly" sport of badminton results in eye injuries that are more serious than most. An unprotected eye that's hit with a badminton bird has about a 10% chance of never seeing again.

Wear masks, eye guards, and goggles

To avoid sports-related eye injuries, always protect your eyes. Sporting goods stores offer:

- catcher's and goalie's masks
- batting helmets with eye guards
- racquetball and squash goggles
- elastic eyeglass guards for people who wear eyeglasses
- headgear for boxers and wrestlers
- face masks for football players
- goggles for tennis, skiing, and swimming.

Take care around your car

Wear protective goggles when working on your car — especially while doing auto body work. Before opening the hood of your car, put out all cigarettes and matches. Why? Battery acid can explode. Also, never light a match to look at a dead battery at night.

Look before you jump-start

When jump-starting your car, make sure the two cars and the jumper cables aren't in contact with each other. And never attach a booster cable to the negative terminal of a dead battery.

Always use protective eyewear

Wear protective glasses or goggles during activities in which a foreign object can easily enter your eyes, such as chipping paint, painting a ceiling, clearing brush, and sandblasting.

Get safety glasses

You can obtain safety eyeglasses from your optician, who will make sure they fit you correctly. Safety lenses won't break, are much thicker than normal lenses, and provide excellent protection from flying particles. They can be modified with side shields for more protection.

If you wear corrective lenses, an optician and many hardware stores can grind safety glasses to your prescription. However, they will be expensive and may not be necessary unless you have some specific occupational need for them.

Look into safety goggles

If you work around flying particles, harsh sprays, or fumes, consider getting safety-thickness goggles. They offer front and side protection. Most can be worn over your own eyeglasses or contact lenses. They're available at many hardware stores or through the yellow pages under "Safety Equipment and Clothing" or similar headings.

Treating a blunt eye injury

The person is kept on bed rest and receives various drugs to help the eye recover. The drugs paralyze certain eye movements, halt bleeding inside the eye, and reduce pressure within the eye.

If internal eye bleeding is extensive, the person may need surgery. Afterward, the person wears an eye shield, takes antibiotics to help prevent infection, and takes pain relievers to reduce pain.

What else should you know?

Many common activities done at work or at home can cause eye injuries. Most people don't realize that some of these activities can be dangerous. For advice on how to avoid these injuries, see *Safeguarding your eyes*, pages 226 and 227.

EYE PAIN

The degree of eye pain doesn't always indicate how severe the problem is. The eyes are so sensitive that any injury or irritation may cause pain out of proportion to the extent of the damage.

Because the eyes are fragile, complex organs, sudden pain in or around the eye is always a cause for concern. Possible causes of sudden eye pain include such serious conditions as glaucoma and eye infection.

Acute closed-angle glaucoma

This condition, which can lead to blindness within days, causes severe eye pain as pressure within the eye rises dangerously high. (See *What happens in closed-angle glaucoma?*)

What are the symptoms?

Eye pain may be sharp, aching, throbbing, burning, or stabbing. But remember — the degree of eye pain doesn't always indicate how severe the problem is. The eyes are so sensitive that any injury or irritation may cause pain out of proportion to the extent of the damage. Even a hairline scratch on the cornea — the clear covering on the front of the eyeball — can cause extreme pain and damage.

The nature of the pain and the accompanying symptoms vary with the underlying condition.

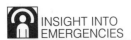

What happens in closed-angle glaucoma?

In a normal eye, fluid travels from the back chamber through a meshwork of tissue. Eventually, it reaches the *canal of Schlemm*, an outflow channel in the front chamber. The fluid then travels from the canal of Schlemm into the venous (vein) circulation.

The starved optic nerve

If the iris — the colored part of the eye — comes in contact with the meshwork, it blocks the fluid. This blockage increases fluid pressure within the eye. As a result, the optic nerve doesn't receive its blood supply. Blindness may result if the blockage isn't repaired.

When fluid forces the iris into the angle

In acute closed-angle glaucoma, normal drainage may be blocked by a sudden rise in fluid pressure that pushes the iris into the angle of the eye, where the iris joins the cornea. Thickening or bulging of the iris can also increase eye pressure.

Detecting glaucoma early

Acute closed-angle glaucoma can cause blindness in the affected eye in 3 to 5 days. Fortunately, early treatment can preserve vision. That's why it's so important to get medical help immediately if you experience these symptoms:

- blurred vision
- pressure over the eye
- seeing halos around lights.

Get yearly screenings

If you're over age 35, have yearly glaucoma screenings. This is especially important if glaucoma runs in your family.

Symptoms of acute closed-angle glaucoma

The pain, which may be severe, may start in one eye and spread to other parts of the head. The person may also have:

- pressure over the eye
- blurred or decreased vision
- unusual light sensitivity
- nausea and vomiting
- halos seen around lights
- a slightly enlarged pupil.

Symptoms of an eye infection

An infection that involves the inside of the eye may cause sudden, intense eye pain. The eyes may be reddened and unusually sensitive to light.

What should you do?

Call the doctor immediately if the person has moderate to severe eye pain or, if necessary, take the person to the nearest hospital emergency department. If the person has sudden eye pain along with visible eye damage, a change in vision, or light sensitivity, get him or her to an emergency department immediately.

How is eye pain treated?

The doctor tries to find the cause of the sudden eye pain. For instance, to see if the pain stems from a corneal injury, the doctor does a simple, painless test: After wetting the tip of a strip containing fluorescein dye, the doctor touches it to the lower part of the eye. As the person blinks, the dye flows over the surface of the eyeball and stains the edges of a corneal scratch or ulcer. Using a special lamp called a slit lamp, the doctor can easily see the problem.

Also, an antibiotic ointment is applied to the eye to help prevent infection. The person may need to wear a patch for 12 to 24 hours to prevent rubbing and blinking.

Treating closed-angle glaucoma

The person with closed-angle glaucoma receives drugs to reduce pressure within the eye. Some of these drugs are applied directly to the eye. Others may be given intravenously.

Other treatments for glaucoma may include pain relievers to ease pain and antinausea drugs to control nausea and vomiting. If the internal eye pressure doesn't drop to an acceptable level within a few hours, surgery may be necessary.

What else should you know?

Eye pain may also result from less serious conditions. The most common causes of sudden eye pain are:

- eye injury (most often abrasion of the cornea) from a sharp object, such as a fingernail or pencil
- eye dryness and irritation from such things as exposure to the wind or sun and swimming in chlorinated or salt water
- a cold or congested sinuses
- contact lenses that don't fit properly or aren't well lubricated
- wearing hard or non-extended-wear lenses to bed
- eyestrain
- internal (and invisible) eye injury from such things as being hit by a ball or someone's elbow.

The person with closed-angle glaucoma receives drugs to reduce pressure within the eye. If the pressure doesn't drop within a few hours, surgery may be necessary.

FAINTING

Fainting is a sudden, brief loss of consciousness. It happens when the brain doesn't get enough blood and oxygen. (See *What makes a person faint?* page 232.)

A fainting spell may last from several seconds to a few minutes. Typically, the person regains consciousness without treatment shortly after fainting.

What are the symptoms?
The person may feel weak, dizzy, or light-headed and the skin may become pale, cool, and moist. Other symptoms may include:
- nausea
- blurred vision or seeing spots
- a weak, rapid pulse
- shallow breathing.

These symptoms may precede fainting, or they may occur as the person faints.

What should you do?
Whether the person has already fainted or merely complains of feeling light-headed, you can take steps to avoid injury.

What to do if the person has already fainted
- Make sure the airway is open. Check for a pulse and look, listen, and feel for breathing. If pulse and breathing are absent, perform CPR if you know how. (See *Performing CPR on an adult,* page 579, *Performing CPR on a child,* page 585, or *Performing CPR on an infant,* page 590.)
- If the person has a clear airway and a pulse and is breathing, lay the person down and raise the legs 8 to 12 inches, unless you suspect a head injury.
- Look for a medical identification necklace or bracelet. It may indicate a medical condition that could be responsible for the fainting spell.

Check for medical identification. It may indicate a medical condition that could be responsible for the fainting spell.

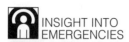

INSIGHT INTO
EMERGENCIES

What makes a person faint?

Fainting is caused by an interruption of the blood supply to the brain.

Typical causes

Usually, fainting comes from a condition that isn't serious, such as:

- emotional distress — for example, from the sight of blood
- strong emotions like joy or fear
- standing too long without moving
- exhaustion
- hunger
- severe pain
- a hot, stuffy environment — especially one filled with cigarette smoke.

More serious causes

Some causes of fainting require a doctor's care. They include:

- irregular heartbeats — especially if the person has a history of heart disease, palpitations, or chest pain
- seizures (also called convulsions or epilepsy)
- use of certain drugs, like those prescribed to control high blood pressure
- low blood sugar — especially in someone with diabetes.

- Loosen any tight clothing, such as a belt or collar.
- Place a wet cloth on the person's forehead, or gently bathe the face with cool water.
- If the person vomits, place him or her on the side. Or turn the head to the side to prevent the person from choking on vomited matter.
- If the person is unconscious for more than a few minutes, suspect a more serious problem and get medical help at once.

Don't slap the person or pour water in the person's face.

Avoid giving smelling salts or ammonia.

Be sure not to give the person anything to drink or eat until he or she recovers.

How to help prevent fainting

- If someone complains of feeling faint or light-headed, first try to stop him or her from falling.
- Then have the person lie down and raise his or her legs 8 to 12 inches. Or instruct the person to sit down and then slowly bend the body forward until the head is between the legs.
- Calm the person.
- Loosen any tight clothing, especially around the neck.
- Place a wet cloth on the person's forehead.
- Move harmful objects out of the way in case the person does faint.

How is fainting treated?

The medical team monitors the person's pulse, breathing, blood pressure, and temperature. Intravenous fluids are given if the person has symptoms of dehydration. To check for a heart problem (which can cause fainting), an electrocardiogram and other heart tests may be done. Also, blood is collected to measure the levels of body salts; an imbalance in these salts can be corrected by giving certain drugs.

Evaluating for other causes

If the doctor suspects that fainting has resulted from taking a drug, the person's drug use is reviewed and, if necessary, adjusted. Some people may need to be evaluated for anxiety too.

What else should you know?

Fainting calls for medical attention if the person:

- faints for no apparent reason
- faints while sitting or lying down
- doesn't recover within 5 minutes
- has a history of fainting spells
- is over age 40.

FEVER

A fever is a body temperature that's above normal. What's normal? That varies from one person to the next. For this reason, the definition of fever varies among individuals — and among doctors. Some doctors consider anything above 99° F (37.2° C) a fever. Others push the lower range of fever up to 101° F (38.3° C).

Message from the body

However it's defined in terms of degrees, fever is a common symptom and the body's way of saying that something is wrong. A fever can come from hundreds of illnesses.

Usually, a fever means the body is fighting an infection. Why? Most disease-causing germs can't reproduce at temperatures much above normal. During an infection, chemicals released into the bloodstream tell the brain to boost the body's temperature so that germs will stop reproducing. Sometimes, though, a fever isn't caused by an infection but by a drug, an injury, or an immunization.

How serious is it?

The most important features of a fever are its severity and its duration. Most fevers are mild and last a short time. What's more, a slight rise or fall in body temperature is rarely significant. But a steep increase — say, to 104° F (40 °C) or higher — may signal a serious condition.

What are the symptoms?

Fever seldom occurs alone. A fever usually causes a feeling of being overheated and generally ill.

The person's other symptoms can help reveal what's causing the

A fever is a common symptom and the body's way of saying that something is wrong. It can come from hundreds of illnesses.

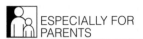

ESPECIALLY FOR
PARENTS

Coping with your child's fever

A high fever in a child can be frightening. But following these suggestions can help you stay calm and collected.

Take the right temperature
If your child is too young to hold an oral thermometer in the mouth, take the temperature *rectally,* using a rectal thermometer. If your child is older, take the temperature *orally* with an oral thermometer.

A child with a rectal temperature of 101.5° F (38.6° C) or higher probably has a fever. But keep in mind that some children can have high fevers without having a serious illness. For example, a minor infection can produce a very high temperature in a young child.

Why rectal temperature is the most accurate
Rectal temperature represents the body's "core" temperature and isn't affected by external environmental conditions, such as rapid breathing and poor positioning of the thermometer in the mouth.

Take the right actions
If your child has a fever, take the following steps to help him or her recover more quickly.
- Give your child plenty of fluids.
- Encourage your child to eat often, but give smaller portions. Don't give your child fried foods, milk, or dairy products.
- Have the child rest — preferably in bed.

Seek medical attention
- Consult the doctor if your child's temperature is over 101° F (38.3° C) — especially if the child doesn't look or feel well.
- Get immediate medical attention if your child has a fever of 101.5° F (38.8 °C) or higher.

How to ease a high fever
To reduce a high fever, the doctor may recommend tepid sponge baths. To give this type of bath, sponge the child with warm water and let the skin air-dry. (But don't let your child become chilled; shivering can increase the body temperature.)

Check the rectal temperature every 30 minutes. Keep giving sponge baths until the temperature drops below 102° F (38.9° C).

Important warnings
- *Never* give aspirin to a feverish child under age 16 who also has a cold, flu symptoms, or chickenpox. Giving aspirin to such a child may cause Reye's syndrome, a life-threatening condition that affects the brain. Instead, give Tylenol (or another acetaminophen product).
- Make sure not to give more of the drug or give it more often than the doctor or package instructions direct.
- If your child is under age 1 year, check with the doctor before giving *any* medicine.

fever. For instance:
- an infection may cause a cough, a sore throat, or an earache
- an inflammation causes redness or swelling of the inflamed area.

Symptoms in a child
Children can have fevers — even very high ones — without being

seriously ill or appearing uncomfortable. But this doesn't mean you should ignore a fever in a child. (See *Coping with your child's fever.*)

What should you do?

To know for sure whether a fever is present, you must measure the person's temperature. A slight to moderate fever may be best left untreated because it aids healing. Urge the person to drink plenty of fluids.

Other ways to ease discomfort from a fever include:
- taking a tepid bath
- removing excessive clothing
- reducing room temperature
- taking certain drugs to bring the temperature down.

Give fever-reducing drugs

Taking aspirin, Tylenol (or another acetaminophen product), or an ibuprofen product (such as Motrin) can reduce a fever. Make sure the person takes only as much of the drug as the doctor directs or the package instructions specify.

When to call the doctor

Sometimes a fever signals a dangerous condition. Here's when to call the doctor:
- The fever occurs for no obvious reason.
- The fever occurs in someone with a serious chronic disease, such as respiratory disease or heart disease.
- The fever occurs in an infant less than age 1 year.
- The fever lasts longer than 5 days (3 days for a child).
- The fever comes back after going away with treatment.
- The person also has extreme thirst, dry mouth, a light-headed feeling, less elastic skin than normal, dark urine, or decreased urination.
- The fever suddenly rises from slight (99° F [37.2°C]) to high (104° F [40° C]) — especially in an infant. If you can't reach the doctor, take the infant to the nearest hospital emergency department.

When to get immediate medical help

Call the doctor immediately if the person's fever is accompanied by:
- a rash
- a severe headache
- a stiff neck
- confusion or irritability

Sometimes a fever signals a dangerous condition. Call the doctor if the fever occurs for no obvious reason, if it occurs in an infant less than age 1 year, or if it lasts longer than 5 days (3 days for a child).

- abdominal pain
- severe back pain
- coughing up of brown or green sputum
- painful urination.

These symptoms may signal meningitis, pneumonia, or another serious disease.

How is fever treated?

For a high fever, rapid cooling measures are used, such as:
- tepid sponge baths
- a special blanket called a hypothermia blanket
- intravenous fluids
- Tylenol (or another form of acetaminophen).

The doctor may also order a spinal tap (removal of a fluid sample from the lower spine) and other diagnostic tests to find out what's causing the fever.

What else should you know?

Adults normally have an average body temperature of 98.6°F (37° C). But body temperature commonly rises and falls slightly throughout the day.

Also, some people normally have temperatures slightly above or below 98.6° F. For others, 97.4° F (36.3° C) or 100° F (37.7° C) is a normal temperature.

Adults normally have an average body temperature of 98.6° F (37° C). But some people normally have t emperatures slightly above or below 98.6° F.

FISHHOOK INJURIES

A fishhook getting caught in a person's body is a fairly common injury. If the hook penetrates deeply, the barb may become impaled in the skin.

What are the symptoms?

This injury is unmistakable. If the hook penetrates the skin, the wound may bleed slightly.

Removing a fishhook

To remove a fishhook that's embedded beyond the barb, push the hook through the skin until you can see the tip of the barb.

Cut the hook
Next, cut the hook at the barb or shank, and carefully remove the part of the hook that's still in the skin.

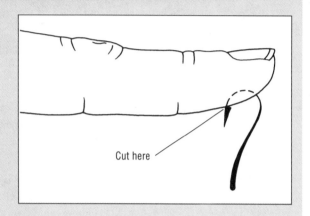

Cut here

What should you do?
If just the point of the hook — not the barb — is caught in the person's skin, gently pull backward on the hook and then remove it.

What to do if the barb is deeply embedded
Preferably, a doctor should remove the fishhook if the barb is deeply embedded. But if a doctor isn't available, follow these steps.
■ Carefully push the hook through the skin until the barb comes out.
■ Cut the hook at its shank or at the barb, using clippers or pliers. (See *Removing a fishhook.*)
■ Remove the part of the barb that's still in the skin.
■ Wash the wound with soap and water and cover it with a bandage.
■ Get medical help as soon as possible to help prevent infection.

Don't try to remove a fishhook that's caught in a person's eye or face. Instead, get medical help immediately.

How are fishhook injuries treated?
The doctor removes the hook if it's still embedded. Usually, the person gets a tetanus shot and, possibly, antibiotics to reduce the risk of infection.

What else should you know?

You can avoid fishhook injuries by following some basic safety rules. For instance, don't put your hand in a tackle box without looking first. Also, don't cast while another person is behind you.

FOOD POISONING

Botulism is the most serious type of food poisoning. Eating even a small amount of tainted food can be fatal.

Food poisoning is a catchall term for what happens when we eat food that's spoiled, tainted, or contaminated. In most cases, bacteria are what make food go bad.

You've probably heard of some of the most common food poisoning culprits — the bacteria *Salmonella, Staphylococcus,* and *E. coli.* But occasionally, the culprit is not bacteria but an amoeba, a protozoa, a parasite, a virus, or a plant toxin.

Botulism

Botulism, which can cause paralysis, is the most serious type of food poisoning. Eating even a small amount of tainted food can be fatal. Of those who do eat such food, one in four dies, usually of respiratory failure during the first week of the illness. Symptoms typically appear 12 to 36 hours after the person eats the tainted food. (See *What happens in botulism?*)

Salmonella

Eating fresh or raw foods contaminated by *Salmonella* — the leading cause of food poisoning in the United States — results in an illness called salmonellosis. Frequently implicated foods include:
- uncooked eggs
- milk
- raw meats
- undercooked poultry
- raw fish.

Although salmonellosis is seldom fatal and usually clears up in a few days, it can be serious in infants, young children, the elderly, and the chronically ill. Symptoms usually appear within 6 to 24 hours. (See *Turn up the heat on bacteria,* page 240.)

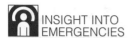
INSIGHT INTO
EMERGENCIES

What happens in botulism?

Botulism occurs when a spore-forming bacterium called *Clostridium botulinum* releases one of the world's most potent toxins into a person's body.

How the bacterium enters the body
Typically, the bacterium enters the body when the person eats improperly canned or preserved food. The spores, found in the soil and in certain foods, such as honey, can cause botulism by contaminating deep wounds or by being eaten.

Toxic reaction
After a person ingests *C. botulinum,* the digestive tract absorbs the toxin. Then the toxin interrupts the chemical reactions needed for muscles and nerves to function properly.

The result: progressive paralysis of the muscles and respiratory system, along with a host of digestive symptoms. Only with prompt medical treatment can the person avoid stoppage of breathing and death.

No chance for immunity
Ironically, the botulism toxin is an antigen to which the body — in theory — could become immune. Unfortunately, the body can't develop immunity because the lethal dose is smaller than the amount required for the body to produce antibodies.

E. coli

Some strains of *E. coli* are normally present in the digestive tract. But other strains of this bacterium are toxic and can be ingested by drinking or eating contaminated water or food — especially undercooked hamburger meat.

A small percentage of people with *E. coli* food poisoning develop a potentially fatal complication called hemolytic-uremic syndrome. Children under age 5 and elderly people are most susceptible.

Staphylococcus aureus

When you hear on the evening news that a number of people who attended the same picnic got sick, chances are they ate food contaminated by a toxic strain of *Staphylococcus aureus.* The second most common type of food poisoning in the United States, this illness typically comes from eating food that hasn't been properly refrigerated. The foods most commonly contaminated are:

- meat
- poultry
- eggs
- milk
- cream-filled bakery goods
- salads with a mayonnaise base (tuna, potato, and macaroni salads, for example).

Turn up the heat on bacteria

Most cases of food poisoning result from contamination by bacteria. You can help make bacteria harmless by storing foods at cold enough temperatures and by cooking them at hot enough temperatures. The illustration at right shows these critical levels.

When in doubt, take the temperature

Don't guess what a food's temperature is. Use a meat or candy thermometer to make sure foods reach 165° F.

FOOD TEMPERATURE: SAFE OR DANGEROUS

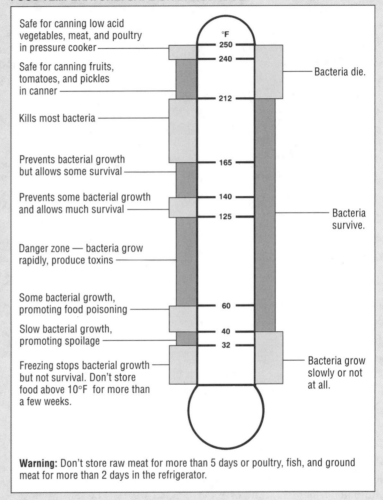

Safe for canning low acid vegetables, meat, and poultry in pressure cooker — 250, 240

Safe for canning fruits, tomatoes, and pickles in canner — 212

Kills most bacteria

Bacteria die.

Prevents bacterial growth but allows some survival — 165

Prevents some bacterial growth and allows much survival — 140, 125

Bacteria survive.

Danger zone — bacteria grow rapidly, produce toxins

Some bacterial growth, promoting food poisoning — 60

Slow bacterial growth, promoting spoilage — 40, 32

Freezing stops bacterial growth but not survival. Don't store food above 10°F for more than a few weeks.

Bacteria grow slowly or not at all.

Warning: Don't store raw meat for more than 5 days or poultry, fish, and ground meat for more than 2 days in the refrigerator.

Symptoms usually occur 1 to 6 hours after ingestion and subside in about 18 hours. Most healthy adults recover completely in 1 to 3 days.

Ciguatera poisoning

Once rare, ciguatera is now a common type of fish poisoning in the United States. It comes from eating warm-water fresh fish like grouper and red snapper.

The poison stems from toxins produced by the tiny marine protozoa responsible for the discolored seawater called "red tide." These organisms live on dead coral reefs, where they're eaten by snails (cigua) and fish.

In the past, ciguatera poisoning was restricted to the warmer oceans, mainly the Caribbean basin and the Hawaiian islands. But the disease is spreading as fish shipments span the world.

Ciguatera contamination has no telltale taste or smell. The toxin isn't destroyed by freezing or cooking.

Most symptoms resolve on their own within hours or days. But some nervous system problems, such as numbness and tingling in the arms or legs, may linger for 6 months.

What are the symptoms?
Symptoms vary with the type of food poisoning.

Most symptoms of ciguatera resolve on their own within hours or days. But numbness and tingling in the arms or legs may linger for 6 months.

Symptoms of botulism or salmonellosis
The person usually has some of the following symptoms:
- nausea and vomiting
- diarrhea or constipation
- abdominal cramps and tenderness
- fever or chills
- below-normal body temperature
- weakness
- lack of energy
- dizziness
- headache
- blurred vision
- dry, sore throat with hoarseness
- impaired speech
- shortness of breath
- partial or complete paralysis of the arms, legs, or torso
- worsening muscle failure
- vertigo.

Symptoms of *E. coli* poisoning
This condition may cause:
- watery or bloody diarrhea
- severe abdominal cramps
- slight fever.

Symptoms of *Staph* poisoning
The person typically has:
- abdominal cramps

- nausea
- vomiting
- diarrhea.

Symptoms of ciguatera poisoning
Strangely, ice may feel hot to the person with this type of poisoning. Other symptoms include:
- numbness and tingling around the mouth and other areas
- nausea
- vomiting
- diarrhea.

Call for emergency medical help at once if the person has severe symptoms or experiences blurred vision, paralysis, or muscle problems.

What should you do?

If the person's symptoms are severe or involve the nervous system (blurred vision, paralysis, or muscle problems), call for emergency medical help at once. If the person must be taken to the hospital, send some of the suspected food along, if possible.

What to do if symptoms aren't severe
If the person is able to drink, give clear fluids, such as broth, ginger ale, fruit juice, or lemonade. This will help replace fluids lost through vomiting and diarrhea.

❖ Don't give milk or dairy products to a person whose stomach is upset.

Be sure to ask the doctor which symptoms to stay alert for; some may indicate that the person needs further medical care. To ease anal irritation from diarrhea, the person can apply soft pads soaked in witch hazel to the rectal area.

To avoid future bouts of food poisoning, make sure you know how to prepare and cook foods properly. (See *How to avoid food poisoning.*)

How is food poisoning treated?

In the hospital, the person usually receives intravenous fluids to replace lost fluids. If he or she seems to be in relatively stable condition, the medical team then focuses on finding out what caused the illness. For instance, they ask the person about foods he or she has eaten within the past few days and obtain fresh specimens of stool and urine, a blood sample and, if possible, samples of suspected foods to test for contamination.

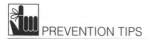

How to avoid food poisoning

An almost sure way to avoid food poisoning is to prepare and cook foods properly. Read what follows to learn more.

Put cleanliness first
- Always wash your hands with warm water and soap before preparing food — especially after using the bathroom.
- Wash your hands, the countertop, all dishes, and all utensils before and after handling raw meats, poultry, and eggs.
- Never put cooked meats back onto the plate that carried them when they were raw unless you wash it first.
- Clean utensils thoroughly.
- Every once in a while, run your kitchen sponge or washcloth through the dishwasher or heat it in the microwave until it steams.

Store foods properly
- Refrigerate perishable foods, such as milk, mayonnaise, potato salad, and cream-filled pastry.
- Thaw frozen foods in the refrigerator, not at room temperature.
- Serve foods immediately after cooking them. Refrigerate leftovers promptly so they'll cool rapidly.

Stay away from risky foods
- Don't eat raw eggs, rare meats, or bloody poultry.
- Don't eat home-preserved foods if the container bulges or the seal isn't intact when you open it.
- When visiting a foreign country, don't drink the local water or eat raw fruits or vegetables unless you're sure they're safe.

Treating botulism
Botulism can be deceiving because progressive symptoms may develop over several days. If the doctor suspects botulism but the person doesn't have severe symptoms, the doctor may send him or her home with instructions to return to the hospital right away if neurologic symptoms, such as weakness, blurred vision, or slurred speech, develop.

The person with severe symptoms receives an antitoxin plus other drugs to help the antitoxin work. (The antitoxin is made from horse serum, so the doctor will need to know if the person has any allergies.) With an infant or a person who has botulism wound contamination, the doctor may give penicillin too.

The medical team pays close attention to the person's breathing and administers oxygen, if needed. (Rarely, the person requires mechanical ventilation.) Reflexes and muscle movement are checked regularly.

Treating salmonellosis
Salmonellosis typically clears up on its own in 2 to 4 days, so treat-

ment aims at helping the person feel better, not curing the illness. Therapy often includes intravenous fluids and body salts.

What else should you know?

Eating wild mushrooms can cause an illness similar to bacterial food poisoning. The person develops the following symptoms:

- abdominal pain
- diarrhea (which may contain blood)
- vomiting (possibly containing blood)
- difficulty breathing
- sweating
- salivation
- tearing
- dizziness.

Symptoms arise within several minutes to 24 hours, depending on the type and amount of mushrooms eaten.

What to do for mushroom poisoning

If you suspect someone has eaten toxic wild mushrooms, call the doctor or poison control center at once. If medical treatment isn't available, induce vomiting. Keep the person's head down so he or she doesn't choke on the vomit.

An object that becomes lodged in a person's ear — typically a bean, an insect, or a small toy — can damage the ear's delicate structures.

It poses a serious problem if it can't be easily removed.

FOREIGN BODY IN EAR

An object that becomes lodged in a person's ear can damage the ear's delicate structures. That's why a foreign body in the ear — typically a bean, an insect, or a small toy — can pose a serious problem if it can't be easily removed. (See *A look inside the ear.*)

What are the symptoms?

A foreign body in the ear can cause:

- pain in the ear
- a buzzing sound
- puslike discharge
- bleeding from the ear
- decreased hearing.

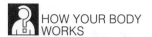

HOW YOUR BODY
WORKS

A look inside the ear

Divided into the external, middle, and inner ear, the human ear is a masterpiece of sound engineering. However, it's vulnerable to damage from infections, environmental stressors such as loud noises, and the intrusion of foreign objects.

External ear

The outside of the ear is made up of cartilage. You can feel the mastoid process, a bone located behind and below the ear, in back of your earlobe. However, this bone isn't part of the external ear.

External auditory canal

Thin, sensitive skin covers the cartilage that forms the outer third of the external auditory canal. Bone covered by a thin layer of skin forms the inner two-thirds. The adult's external canal leads inward, downward, and forward to the middle ear.

Eardrum

The eardrum, or tympanic membrane, separates the external ear from the middle ear. It appears pearly gray, shiny, and translucent. The auditory canal stretches most of the membrane tightly inward.

Middle ear

The external canal leads into the middle ear, a small, air-filled cavity in the temporal bone. Within this cavity, three small bones called *auditory ossicles* link together to transmit sound. As you may remember from health class, these bones are the malleus (hammer), incus (anvil), and stapes (stirrup).

Pressure equalizer

During an ear exam, the doctor uses an otoscope to see your eardrum. The eustachian tube equalizes pressure between the inner and outer surfaces of the eardrum. In children, the eustachian tube is shorter and wider than in adults — one reason why children are more susceptible to ear infections.

Inner ear

A bony labyrinth and a membranous labyrinth combine to form the inner ear. The *bony labyrinth* is made up of the vestibule, cochlea, and semicircular canals. These canals help maintain the body's balance.

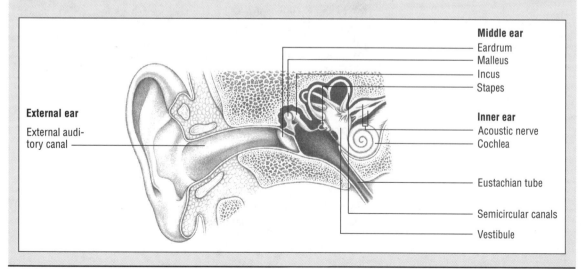

External ear

External auditory canal

Middle ear
Eardrum
Malleus
Incus
Stapes

Inner ear
Acoustic nerve
Cochlea

Eustachian tube

Semicircular canals

Vestibule

Instruct the person to shake the head with the affected ear facing downward. If the person is a young child, turn the child's head so the affected ear faces downward, and then have the child shake the head gently.

What should you do?

Instruct the person to shake the head with the affected ear facing downward. If the person is a young child, turn the child's head so the affected ear faces downward, and then have the child shake the head gently.

⊗ Never flush the ear with water when trying to remove a bean that's stuck in the ear canal. Adding water will cause the bean to swell.

If the foreign object is a live insect, place a few drops of mineral oil in the ear canal. The mineral oil should make breathing difficult for the insect, and it may then crawl out of the ear. If the insect doesn't crawl out, don't try to remove it. You could break off a piece of the insect, leaving the rest in the ear to cause an infection.

When to call the doctor

If your attempts to remove the foreign body from the ear fail, get immediate medical assistance. Also, call the doctor right away if a pointed object has been pushed into the ear or if the person shows signs of injury, such as bleeding, sudden difficulty hearing, or a swollen earlobe.

⊗ Avoid sticking your finger into the ear, and don't let a child stick a finger in the ear.

⊗ Don't try to pull the foreign object out with your fingers or tweezers.

⊗ Never touch a pointed foreign object that's lodged in the ear. Instead, get medical help immediately.

⊗ Don't insert a cotton swab into the ear.

How is a foreign body in the ear treated?

The person's ear canal is irrigated with water and hydrogen peroxide. Sometimes the object is removed beforehand, using forceps or a suction device.

What else should you know?

After a foreign object has been removed from the ear, the person's eardrum should be evaluated by a doctor.

FOREIGN BODY IN EYE

A foreign body lodged in the eye is the most common type of eye injury. It can be quite painful.

Typically, the foreign body is a tiny piece of dirt or metal, a cinder, or a bit of dust. Usually, the person unknowingly blinks the object into a position along the eyelid, where it can be removed with a clean gauze pad or tissue. Until it's removed, it can cause discomfort, inflammation, and even infection.

Damage to the cornea
If the particle scratches the surface lining of the cornea (the transparent front portion of the eye), a *corneal abrasion* occurs. Even if tears later wash out the particle, the cornea may still suffer injury.

What are the symptoms?
The person may have:
- pain, redness, and a burning sensation in the eye
- tearing of the eye (in an attempt to remove the foreign object)
- sensitivity to light
- a sensation of something being in the eye, which may persist even after the particle is removed (because the eye is still irritated).

With a *corneal abrasion,* the person may have impaired vision.

What should you do?
First, wash your hands with soap and water. This helps prevent any dangerous germs on your hands from infecting the person's eye. Your next step depends on where the foreign body is lodged.

Removing a particle that's floating on the eyeball or resting in the upper eyelid
- If you can see the foreign body floating on the person's eyeball or resting on the inside of the upper eyelid, gently pull the upper eyelid down over the lower eyelid.
- Wait a moment, then release the lid. This may help the flow of tears wash out the foreign body. Or it may cause the eyelashes to brush the object off the inside of the upper lid.
- Another way to remove a foreign body that's on the eyeball or resting inside the upper lid is to gently turn the eyelid inside out over a cotton-tipped swab. (See *Removing a particle from the eyelid,* page 249.)

Until the foreign body is removed from the eye, it can cause discomfort, inflammation, and even infection.

> *If the particle still seems to be in the eye but isn't visible, have the person hold his or her head under a gentle stream of clean, warm running water. Tell the person to move the eye in different directions as it's being flushed.*

Flushing the eye

- If the particle still seems to be in the eye but isn't visible, have the person hold his or her head under a gentle stream of clean, warm running water.
- Tell the person to move the eye in different directions as it's being flushed.

Removing a particle from the lower eyelid

- If the particle remains in the eye after flushing, gently pull the lower eyelid down and examine the inside of the lid.
- Then ask the person to look up. If you can see the foreign object on the inside of the lid, remove it with the corner of a moistened sterile gauze pad or a clean cloth or tissue.

If eye irritation continues or the particle is still in the eye

- Ask the person to close the eye.
- Cover the eye with several gauze pads.
- Tape the pads in place.
- Take the person to the doctor, clinic, or hospital emergency department.

⊗ Don't let the person rub the eye. Rubbing may force a sharp object deeper into the eye or scratch delicate eye tissues.

⊗ Never try to remove an object that's embedded or impaled in the eyeball. Doing so could force the object deeper into the eye, causing further damage. Instead, place a compress made of bandages over both eyes; make sure the compress doesn't exert pressure on the eyeball. Keep the person calm and get medical help immediately. (See "Eye injuries," page 223.)

⊗ Be sure not to use an instrument, such as tweezers, or dry cotton to remove the foreign body. Tweezers could cause injury if they graze the eyeball; dry cotton fibers may stay in the eye, causing irritation.

How is a foreign body in the eye treated?

If the particle is deeply embedded, the doctor anesthetizes the eye and tries to remove the particle with a spadelike device. After the particle has been removed, antibiotic eyedrops must be instilled in the eye every 3 to 4 hours. The doctor may also recommend using a pressure patch to prevent further irritation of the cornea when the person blinks. (See *Be kind to your injured eye,* page 250.)

Removing a particle from the eyelid

To remove a foreign body that's resting on the inside of the upper eyelid, follow these steps.

Examine the upper eyelid
Gently pull the upper eyelashes upward. Tell the person to look down, and examine the inside of the upper eyelid.

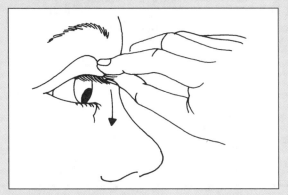

Turn the eyelid over
If you see the particle, ask the person to close the eye. Then place a cotton-tipped swab or similar object across the back of the upper eyelid. Turn the eyelid over the swab.

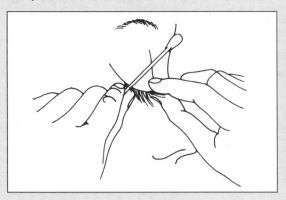

Remove the particle gently
Next, gently pull the lashes upward again. Tell the person to open the eye and look down. If you see the object on the inside of the upper lid, remove it with the corner of a moistened sterile gauze pad or a clean cloth or tissue.

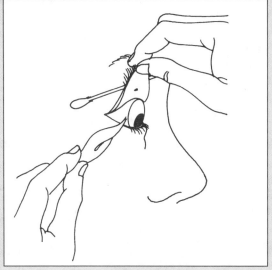

Be kind to your injured eye

After a foreign body has been removed from your eye, take the following precautions to help your eye heal without complications.

Use a patch if directed
If the doctor instructs you to wear an eye patch, be sure to leave the patch in place as long as directed — usually 12 to 24 hours. The patch will alter your depth perception, so use caution in everyday activities, such as stepping off a curb and climbing stairs.

Instill eye medicines properly
Use the proper technique when instilling antibiotic eyedrops or other prescribed eye medicine. Using the eyedrops exactly as the doctor directs will help prevent infection of the cornea — a condition that sometimes causes corneal ulcers and even vision loss.

Prevent eye infections
Be sure to wash your hands before and after using eyedrops or touching anything else that will come in contact with your eye.

What else should you know?

A tiny piece of metal that becomes lodged in the eye may quickly form a rust ring on the cornea, causing a corneal abrasion. Typical victims of this injury are metal workers who don't wear protective eyewear. To remove a rust ring, the doctor uses an abrasive device called an ophthalmic burr.

Permanent corneal scarring
Falling asleep while wearing hard contact lenses can cause a corneal abrasion too. So can a scratch from a piece of paper or a fingernail. If the eye doesn't heal properly, a persistent wound or ulcer may develop and the cornea may become permanently scarred.

FOREIGN BODY IN NOSE

Typically, a foreign body in the nose is a bead or a pea, placed there by an exploring young child. But even an adult may accidentally get a foreign body in the nose. The object can damage the lining of the nasal passages and interfere with breathing.

What are the symptoms?
If the foreign body causes a broken bone or displaces cartilage in the nose, the person's nose becomes swollen, tender, and discolored. Unless treated, these symptoms may make breathing impossible.

What should you do?
Try to keep the person calm. Have him or her breathe through the mouth to avoid inhaling the foreign body. Then try to have the person expel the object by blowing the nose, if possible. If the object remains lodged in the nose, call the doctor.

❌ Don't try to remove a foreign object that is lodged in the nostril unless it is sticking out.

How is a foreign body in the nose treated?

The doctor may administer a nasal decongestant to reduce swelling, apply a topical anesthetic to numb the tissues, and then try to remove the foreign object with forceps.

What else should you know?

A foreign body that stays in the nose for a prolonged time can lead to respiratory problems. How? By depriving the person of the benefits of nasal breathing. Nasal breathing is good for your lungs because it:

- moisturizes and warms inhaled air
- removes dust particles before the inhaled air reaches the lungs.

If you can't breathe through your nose, you must breathe through your mouth instead. But mouth breathing delivers dry, cold, unfiltered air to your lungs. This sets the stage for respiratory problems.

FRACTURES (BROKEN BONES)

A fracture — a break or crack in a bone — occurs when a bone is subjected to excessive force. A broken bone can damage nearby muscles, nerves, and other soft tissues. (See *How a bone breaks,* page 252.)

A broken arm or leg typically results from a major injury, such as a fall on an outstretched arm or a skiing accident. In people with certain diseases, a normal, everyday activity can cause a fracture. (See *Can a sneeze break a bone?* page 253.)

Types of fractures

A fracture can be closed (simple) or open (compound). In a *closed fracture,* the skin over the broken bone stays intact — the bone doesn't jut through.

In an *open fracture,* parts of the broken bone protrude through the skin and an open wound extends down to the bone. Usually, an open fracture is more serious than a closed fracture because it can cause severe bleeding and infection. (See *Is the fracture open or closed?* page 254.)

A fracture can be closed or open. In a closed fracture, the skin over the broken bone stays intact. In an open fracture, parts of the broken bone protrude through the skin.

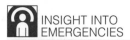
INSIGHT INTO
EMERGENCIES

How a bone breaks

Bones are elastic enough to absorb some pressure without breaking. But excessive force can cause a bone to break.

Types of bone-breaking forces

The force that breaks a bone may be direct or indirect — and it may be high or low energy. Read what follows to learn how different types of forces can break a bone.

Direct force

This violent, high-energy force can cause a serious fracture. Types of direct force include:
- *wedging force*, which breaks the bone and forces a bone fragment into another fragment or into a joint

- *compression force*, which propels bones together
- *crushing force*, which splinters bones into fragments.

Indirect force

This less violent, lower-energy force can break a bone at a distance from where the force is applied. Types of indirect force include:
- *torsion force*, a strong twisting force
- *shearing force*, a force exerted when part of the bone is fixed in place, breaking the part above or below
- *angulatory force*, a force exerted on an angle so that the bone breaks at that angle.

What are the symptoms?

It's not always easy to tell if a bone is broken. To be on the safe side, always *assume* a fracture has occurred whenever someone has been in a serious accident.

When to suspect a fracture

Looking for key fracture symptoms can help determine if the injury is a fracture. Here are some questions you should try to answer.

- Did the person hear or feel the bone snap, or feel a grating or crackling sensation? If the answer is yes, suspect a fracture.
- Does the injured area look swollen? Does the skin over it look blue? Swelling and discoloration are symptoms of a fracture.
- Does the injured bone look deformed? Does it differ in length or shape from the same bone on the other side of the body? A yes answer suggests the bone is broken.
- Does the person complain of pain and tenderness — especially when you gently feel along the bone? Can the person point to the painful area? If so, there's a good chance the bone is broken.
- Is the person unable to move the injured part? Or does the part move in an abnormal or unnatural way? Moving a broken bone causes pain, so reluctance to move it is a good indication that it's broken.

But this isn't always true. Sometimes a person can move a broken bone with little or no pain.

What should you do?

 WHEN SECONDS COUNT

If the person has been in a severe accident, check for a clear airway, feel for a pulse, and look, listen, and feel for breathing.

⊗ Don't open the airway by moving the head if there's any chance the person may have a neck or spinal cord injury.

If the person isn't breathing and has no pulse, start CPR at once, if you know how. Otherwise, call for emergency medical help immediately. (See *Performing CPR on an adult,* page 579, *Performing CPR on a child,* page 585, or *Performing CPR on an infant,* page 590.)

If you think the person might have a neck or spinal cord injury, stabilize the spine by placing rolled blankets or similar materials on either side of the neck and torso. Wait until professional help arrives. Tell the person not to move.

⊗ Don't let the person's body bend or twist if you suspect a neck or spinal cord injury.

What to do for a less serious injury

Most broken bones are minor and don't pose a serious threat to life or limb. If the person has symptoms of a fracture but is conscious with no trouble breathing, your key goals are to prevent further injury and keep the person calm and stable until medical help arrives.

To achieve these goals, follow the steps below.

■ Raise the person's legs 8 to 12 inches. This allows blood to drain from the legs to the heart, helping to prevent shock. Then, wrap the person with blankets or other material to halt loss of body heat.

⊗ Be sure not to raise the person's legs more than 12 inches. If the person is lying on a bed, don't lift the foot of the bed. Doing these things could impair breathing.

⊗ Don't raise the person's legs if he or she is unconscious or having trouble breathing or if you suspect a chest injury.

Can a sneeze break a bone?

A healthy bone can withstand some forceful pressure without breaking. But sometimes a fracture occurs when only slight force is applied.

Pathologic fractures

For example, if minimal force is exerted on a bone weakened by disease or a tumor, a *pathologic fracture* may occur. That's why a person with osteoporosis, a bone tumor, or a metabolic disease can break a bone merely by sneezing or coughing.

Stress fractures

A *stress fracture* may occur when fatigue and exercise have caused a small crack in a bone. Then, only slight force may extend the crack to a complete fracture. Prolonged standing, walking, or running can lead to stress fractures of the foot and ankle.

Stress fractures are most common in:
■ joggers
■ nurses
■ postal workers
■ soldiers.

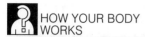

Is the fracture open or closed?

In a *closed (simple) fracture,* the skin at the fracture site isn't broken, and the broken bone doesn't protrude through the skin.

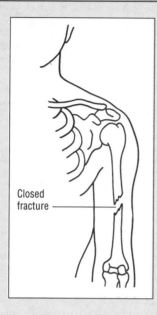

Closed fracture

In an *open (compound) fracture,* the overlying skin is broken. The broken bone may poke through the skin, or the skin may have been torn by a direct blow during the injury.

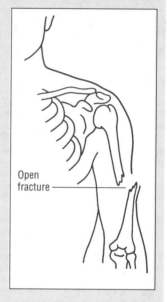

Open fracture

■ Next, check for severe bleeding. If you don't see any, check further by gently removing or cutting away any clothing covering the wound. If you see a bleeding wound, place gauze or the cleanest material available against it. Then apply direct pressure to the site with your fingers or palm.

■ If this doesn't stop the bleeding, elevate the injured part. If the bleeding persists, apply pressure to a pressure point while keeping direct pressure on the bleeding site. (See *Using pressure points to stop bleeding,* page 76.)

Important: Use protective equipment whenever you're likely to be exposed to another person's blood or other body fluids. This will help prevent exposure to blood-borne diseases, such as hepatitis and HIV (the virus that causes AIDS). Latex gloves offer the best protection. If they aren't available, use any waterproof material — plastic bags, plastic wrap, several layers of gauze pads, or even clothing.

■ Next, check movement by asking the person to wiggle the fingers or toes. If the person can't do this, bone fragments may have damaged a nearby nerve.

✖ Avoid moving the injured area unless it's absolutely necessary.

✖ Never try to push back any part of the bone that's sticking out. If you do, you might push foreign matter into the wound, causing further tissue damage.

Splint the injured bone

■ If you must move the person or wait a long time for medical help, splint the injured part. A splint supports and immobilizes the bone. It also protects muscles, nerves, and blood vessels from damage caused by broken bone ends.

■ Always splint a broken bone in the position in which you found it. (For information on what materials to use as splints, see *All about splints,* page 595. For details on splinting a specific type of fracture, see *How to splint a broken bone or dislocated joint,* page 596.)

✖ Don't move the person until the broken bone has been splinted, unless you fear imminent danger from an explosion, fire, or some other threat.

Dress the wound

■ If the injured area is still bleeding after you've splinted it, cover it with a pressure dressing or a clean pad or cloth. Then press firmly. Hold the pad firmly in place with such materials as cloth strips, neckties, or strong gauze. If these materials aren't available, close the wound with your gloved hands or fingers, and then apply pressure directly over the wound.

■ If a sterile dressing is available, place it over the first dressing. If the closest medical facility is more than 2 hours away, rinse the wound with clean water before applying the sterile dressing.

■ As soon as you've finished splinting the broken bone, get the person to a hospital emergency department or a doctor. If the person can't be moved, keep him or her warm while you wait for professional rescuers to arrive.

✖ Don't give the person anything to eat or drink; if the person needs surgery, the stomach should be empty.

How are fractures treated?

In the hospital, the doctor evaluates the injured bone to determine

If the injured area is still bleeding after you've splinted it, cover it with a pressure dressing or a clean pad or cloth. Then press firmly, holding the pad in place.

if it's broken. After asking about recent injuries, the doctor gently feels the injured area and has the person cautiously try to move the limb below the injury site. To confirm that the bone is broken, X-rays are taken of the injury and the joints above and below.

Treating an open fracture

To prevent infection, a person with an open fracture receives a tetanus shot and antibiotics, and the wound is thoroughly cleaned. Sometimes surgery is needed to repair damage to soft tissues or to wash out the wound to prevent infection.

Reducing the fracture

A displaced fracture is reduced — that is, the displaced bone segments are replaced to their normal position. Then the broken limb is immobilized with a splint or cast. Sometimes the person needs traction.

Reduction may be open or closed. In *closed reduction,* the doctor manipulates the bone fragments by hand after giving the person a local anesthetic, a pain reliever, and a sedative or muscle relaxant. The drug helps relax the muscle so the bone can be realigned.

If closed reduction isn't possible, *open reduction* is done in the operating room. The surgeon uses rods, plates, or screws to reposition bone segments and immobilize the fracture. Sometimes a plaster cast is applied afterward.

Applying traction

If a splint or cast alone won't reduce the fracture, traction is applied using weights and pulleys. In *skin traction,* traction devices are attached to the skin with elastic bandages and sheepskin covers. In *skeletal traction,* a pin or wire is inserted through the bone beyond the fracture and attached to a weight. This allows more prolonged traction.

What else should you know?

Most broken bones heal fully, without deformity — especially in children. But the bones of adults in poor health or with poor circulation may never heal properly.

A broken bone starts to heal as soon as the fracture occurs. Healing takes place in four main stages.

Stage one: A clot forms

First, blood collects around the broken bone ends, forming a sticky

If a splint or cast alone won't reduce the fracture, traction is applied. Traction involves the use of weights and pulleys.

mass called a clot. A meshwork forms from the clot. This becomes the framework for growing new bone tissue.

Stage two: Healing cells invade the clot

Soon, cells that heal the bone — osteoclasts and osteoblasts — invade the clot. *Osteoclasts* start smoothing the jagged bone edges, and *osteoblasts* begin bridging the gap between the bone ends. Within a few days, these cells form a granular bridge that links the bone ends.

Stage three: A callus forms

About 6 to 10 days after the fracture has occurred, the granular bridge of cells becomes a bony mass called a *callus.* The callus is fragile, and abrupt motion can split it. That's why a broken bone must be kept immobile during healing. Later, the callus hardens into solid bone.

Stage four: Bone ends fuse

Three to ten weeks after the injury, new blood vessels start bringing calcium to the area. The calcium hardens the new bone tissue. Called *ossification,* this process "knits" the bone ends together.

After ossification, the bone becomes solid and is considered healed. Although the cast may be removed, the healed bone may take up to 1 year before it's as strong as it was before the break.

FROSTBITE

Frostbite is the effect of extreme cold on the skin and the tissues near the skin surface. The nose, cheeks, ears, fingers, and toes are most often affected. Ice crystals form within and between the cells of the frostbitten area.

How cold injures body tissues

Here's how frostbite happens: Cold damages the blood vessels of exposed parts. This narrows the vessels, which in turn impairs blood flow to the limbs. With less blood, the limb or other area doesn't get enough oxygen. Lack of oxygen causes swelling and blisters, along with some tissue death.

Frostbite most often affects the nose, cheeks, ears, fingers, and toes. Ice crystals form within and between the cells of the frostbitten area.

Types of frostbite

If the damage is limited to the skin and the tissue just under it, the frostbite is called *superficial.* If deeper tissues are damaged, the frostbite is considered *deep.* Deep frostbite may lead to gangrene (tissue death) and loss of the frostbitten part.

What are the symptoms?

Symptoms depend on whether the frostbite is superficial or deep. Some people don't notice symptoms until they get indoors and start to warm up.

Symptoms of superficial frostbite

These may include:

- burning
- numbness
- tingling
- itching
- coldness.

Symptoms of deep frostbite

These may include:

- swelling
- blisters
- white or yellowish skin that looks waxy and turns purplish blue as it thaws
- hardening of the skin
- dead, blackened skin.

What should you do?

WHEN SECONDS COUNT

If the person has symptoms of deep frostbite — blackened skin and loss of feeling in the affected part — seek immediate medical help.

What to do for less severe symptoms

- Call for emergency medical help. Keep the frostbitten part elevated at all times.
- Move the person to a warm spot.
- Remove constrictive clothing and jewelry.
- Rewarm the affected part by immersing it in tepid water — about 100° to 104° F (37.8° to 40° C). Keep the part in the water until the skin regains its normal color and feels warm. This usually takes 20 to

If the person has symptoms of deep frostbite — blackened skin and loss of feeling in the affected part — seek immediate medical help.

Myths about treating frostbite

Some of the things you may have heard about how to treat frostbite could do the person more harm than good. For instance, someone may have told you that rubbing a frostbitten area with ice or snow is a good idea. Don't believe it; rubbing will only cause further tissue damage. Read what follows to learn more about what *not* to do for frostbite.

Rewarm wisely
- *Don't* rewarm the affected area too quickly because this could cause pain.
- *Don't* rewarm the affected area with dry heat, such as from a heat lamp, radiator, or hot stove. This could cause permanent tissue damage.
- *Don't* immerse the person's whole body in warm water. Heart problems could arise.

Promote good circulation
- *Don't* give the person a caffeinated beverage like coffee, tea, or hot chocolate. Caffeine impairs the circulation.

- *Don't* let the person drink alcohol. Like caffeine, it impedes the circulation — although the person may feel warmer after drinking it.
- *Don't* let the person smoke or use tobacco. It, too, cuts down the blood flow.

Other instructions
- *Don't* break any blisters; the open wound could become infected.
- *Don't* let a person with frostbitten feet walk. Again, this could worsen tissue damage. If necessary, the person should be placed on a stretcher for transport.

30 minutes. If warm water isn't available, wrap the frostbitten part in wool.
- Give the person warm, noncaffeinated fluids to drink. (See *Myths about treating frostbite.*)
- Next, loosely bandage the area with a dry sterile dressing.
- Give the person a mild pain reliever, such as aspirin. This will reduce swelling and relieve the pain that the person will feel when the frostbitten part is rewarmed and sensation returns.
- Finally, get the person to a medical facility promptly. It's hard for a nonprofessional to gauge how severe frostbite is.

> Be sure not to rewarm the frostbitten part if there is a chance it will freeze again. This could increase tissue damage.
>
> Don't rewarm the part too quickly because this may cause pain.
>
> Be sure not to rub the frostbitten area; this can worsen tissue damage.
>
> Avoid breaking any blisters. Place dry sterile cotton or gauze between the person's fingers or toes if they're frostbitten.

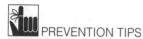

Fighting off frostbite

Dressing for the weather is the best prevention against frostbite. Specialty clothing catalogs are filled with ads for high-tech fabrics that will keep you warm and dry during your favorite winter activity. But some old-fashioned advice on winter dressing and winter activities is still indispensable.

Keep your trunk, hands, and feet warm
- Dress in layers. If you plan to be outdoors for a long time, wear windproof, water-resistant clothing as your outermost layer.
- Wear mittens, not gloves, to keep your hands warm.
- Wear two pairs of socks — a cotton pair next to your skin to wick the water away, and a wool pair over the cotton.
- Wear waterproof shoes or boots.

Keep your head covered
- Always wear a scarf and a hat that covers your ears; most of your body heat is lost through your head.

- If it's extremely cold, wear something over your face, nose, and ears too.

Use common sense outdoors
- Pace yourself during outdoor activities. Don't let yourself get sweaty or wet because this cause chilling.
- Don't touch bare flesh to cold metal.
- If you're caught in a severe snowstorm, find shelter early or increase your physical activity to help you stay warm and alert.
- Don't go winter hiking or ice-fishing alone. Take along someone who knows how to manage the cold weather, or read up on the topic.

Other instructions
- Don't drink alcohol or smoke when outdoors. Smoking cuts down blood flow to the limbs; alcohol leads to heat loss.
- Get adequate food and rest before prolonged exposure to the cold. You'll need to be energetic and rested if you get stranded outdoors.

How is frostbite treated?

Rewarming the frostbitten area is always the priority. The person may also receive antibiotics and a tetanus shot to prevent infection and a narcotic to relieve pain.

After rewarming, the affected part is kept elevated and uncovered at room temperature. It may be covered with a bulky dressing, with cotton or gauze placed between frostbitten fingers or toes.

The doctor may recommend whirlpool treatments for the next 3 weeks. These treatments clean the skin and remove dead tissue.

What else should you know?

To prevent frostbite, always dress for the weather. (See *Fighting off frostbite*.)

G

GENITAL SORES

Sores in the genital area can come from many causes. Among the most common are sexually transmitted diseases — particularly herpes and syphilis.

Genital herpes
Caused by herpesvirus, genital herpes spreads during oral, vaginal, or anal intercourse. You can get it from direct skin-to-skin contact with an infected person who has a visible sore, or you can catch it a day or two before the person's sore appears.

Syphilis
Although now less common and less serious than in past decades, syphilis infects about 100,000 Americans every year. If left untreated, the disease can be devastating. Caused by a tiny bacteria-like organism called a spirochete, syphilis spreads during sexual contact.

What are the symptoms?
The appearance of genital sores and the person's other symptoms vary with the underlying cause.

Symptoms of herpes
A herpes sore is fluid-filled and may look like a blister. It may start out painless and then rupture and become an extensive, shallow, painful ulcer with a yellow, oozing center. The sores may tingle or itch. In some people, herpes sores form in clusters. (See *What does herpes look like?* page 262.) Most herpes sores crust over and clear up on their own in 7 to 10 days.

In women, the sores may appear in the following regions:
- vaginal lips
- clitoris
- area between the vagina and the anus
- cervix

A herpes sore is fluid-filled and may look like a blister. It may start out painless and then rupture and become a shallow, painful ulcer with a yellow, oozing center.

What does herpes look like?

Often, genital herpes starts out as a swollen, slightly itchy, raised, firm, reddened lesion and then becomes a group of small blisters, as you see here.

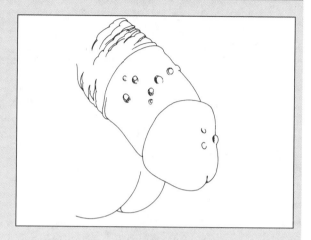

- buttocks
- thighs
- inside of the vagina.

In men, the sores typically appear in these areas:

- shaft or head of the penis
- foreskin
- testicles
- thighs
- anus
- buttocks
- area between the penis and the anus.

The sores may make urination painful.

A herpes sore can occur on the mouth too. Oral herpes can be passed during kissing or oral-genital contact, causing mouth sores.

During a herpes outbreak — especially the initial one — the person may have a fever, swollen glands, and an overall ill feeling. Once the sores crust over and disappear, they may arise in the same area months or years later. Later outbreaks typically are less severe than the initial one.

Symptoms of syphilis

A genital sore that remains painless is probably syphilis. In this disease, one or more syphilis sores, called *chancres,* erupt on the genitals. Other sores may appear on the:

- anus

- fingers
- lips
- tongue
- nipples
- tonsils
- eyelids.

In women, syphilis sores may be overlooked because they often develop only on internal structures, such as the cervix and the inside of the vagina.

Symptoms during the stages of syphilis
The syphilis sore starts as a pimple. Small and fluid-filled, it has raised edges. Eventually it erodes, forming a painless, firm, shallow ulcer. It disappears on its own without treatment. During this *primary stage* of syphilis, the person usually has swollen lymph nodes on one or both sides of the body.

Unfortunately, the disease itself doesn't go away. It just enters the next stage within a few days or weeks. During this *secondary stage*, the person may develop an all-over body rash. Small, flat discolorations may erupt between rolls of fat on the trunk, arms, palms, soles, face, and scalp. In warm, moist body areas, these lesions grow bigger and erode, becoming highly contagious.

Other symptoms of secondary-stage syphilis include:
- headache
- overall ill feeling
- poor appetite
- weight loss
- nausea
- vomiting
- sore throat
- mild fever
- pitted, brittle nails
- hair loss (which is usually temporary).

The third stage, *latent syphilis,* doesn't cause noticeable symptoms. *Late syphilis* is the final stage (although the disease is noncontagious at this point). The disease now attacks body organs and bones, eventually causing death.

The syphilis sore starts as a small, fluid-filled pimple. Eventually it erodes, forming a painless, firm, shallow ulcer.

What should you do?
If you have a genital sore, see your doctor promptly — unless you have a history of genital herpes and you're certain the current sore is

from herpes. (If the sore doesn't clear up within 2 weeks, call your doctor — what you have may not be herpes but some other condition.)

Seeing a doctor is especially important if you're pregnant: You could transmit syphilis to your fetus in the womb; you could transmit herpes to your baby during delivery.

Avoid sexual contact

Avoid sexual contact until your condition has been diagnosed and successfully treated. And be sure to tell your sexual partners so they can get treated. Otherwise, you could pass the disease back and forth.

How are genital sores treated?

To diagnose herpes, the doctor may want to obtain a culture from a sore during the first few days after the sores appear. Often, though, the disease is diagnosed from its characteristic symptoms.

Treating an initial herpes outbreak

The doctor may prescribe aspirin or Tylenol (or another acetaminophen product) to reduce fever and relieve pain as well as a drying agent like calamine lotion to ease pain from genital sores.

For a severe case, the doctor may prescribe Zovirax. An antiviral drug, Zovirax may shorten the first outbreak by a few days. Zovirax cream is also available to apply directly on the sores. Some doctors prescribe Zovirax capsules to be taken daily for people with frequent or severe herpes recurrences.

For an initial herpes outbreak, the doctor may prescribe aspirin or Tylenol to reduce fever and relieve pain as well as a drying agent to ease pain from genital sores.

Diagnosing and treating syphilis

Syphilis can be diagnosed by a blood test called VDRL. But because the disease has a long incubation period, the person may need to repeat this test over several months.

To treat syphilis, the person gets an injection of penicillin. Someone who is allergic to penicillin will probably receive tetracycline or Vibramycin by mouth instead; these drugs are taken for 15 days for early syphilis or 30 days for advanced infections. (Pregnant women shouldn't take tetracycline.)

What else should you know?

Other causes of genital sores include:
- chancroid, a sexually transmitted disease
- granuloma inguinale, a rare chronic venereal infection
- lymphogranuloma venereum, a sexually transmitted disorder

■ cancer of the penis, which causes a painless ulcer or an enlarging "wart"

■ scabies, in which mites burrow under the skin and may cause crusted lesions

■ drugs, including tetracycline and some other antibiotics, as well as barbiturates. Usually, a genital sore that comes from a drug reaction is bright red to purple.

GUNSHOT WOUNDS

A gunshot wound to the abdomen or chest can pose an immediate threat to the person's life by damaging major blood vessels and internal organs. Sometimes a bullet travels from the chest to the abdomen or from the abdomen to the chest.

How a bullet causes internal injuries
Depending on the size of the wound, the person may suffer varying degrees of damage to bones, soft tissue, nerves, and blood vessels.

The high energy from the bullet creates pressure waves within the person's body. These waves may create a cavity many times the size of the bullet. Also, combustion burns from gunpowder may cause serious internal tissue and bone damage. (See *The gun and the damage done,* page 266.)

What are the symptoms?
These differ with the wound location.

Symptoms of an abdominal wound
A gunshot wound to the abdomen causes obvious abdominal discomfort or pain, which may spread to the shoulders (called referred pain). The person's skin may appear pale or bluish. You may see blood coming from the abdomen as well as bruises, scrapes, and abdominal swelling. Other symptoms may include:
■ abdominal rigidity
■ holding the body as if to "guard" the wound
■ shortness of breath or trouble breathing

A gunshot wound to the abdomen or chest can pose an immediate threat to the person's life. Depending on the size of the wound, the person may suffer varying degrees of damage to bones, soft tissue, nerves, and blood vessels.

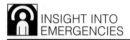 INSIGHT INTO
EMERGENCIES

The gun and the damage done

Before lodging in the back, a bullet ricocheting through the abdomen may injure the liver, intestines, and kidneys, as shown in the illustration below.

BULLET PATH

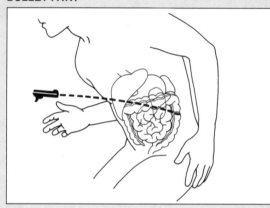

What are the victim's chances?

The amount of damage caused by a gunshot wound depends on:
- the type of firearm used
- the bullet's physical features
- bullet velocity (speed)
- the tissue the bullet strikes
- the range at which the gun was fired.

Close-range catastrophe
A bullet fired at close range causes more damage than one fired from further away. For example, a shotgun fired at less than 3 yards causes massive tissue injury that proves fatal for about 85% to 90% of victims.

Caliber size counts
Also, a large-caliber gun like a .45 causes more damage than a .22 or another small-caliber gun.

- dizziness and weakness (from low blood pressure)
- bloody urine.

Symptoms of a chest wound
A gunshot wound to the chest can cause severe pain. The person may guard the chest with the arms if breathing is painful. You may see an obvious wound that makes a sucking sound as air passes through it into the chest cavity. Other symptoms may include:
- pale or bluish skin
- decreased level of consciousness
- dizziness and weakness (from low blood pressure)
- fast or weak pulse (from anxiety and blood loss)
- rapid breathing.

If the wound has led to lung collapse, the person may have difficulty breathing, rapid breathing, anxiety, bluish skin, and shortness of breath.

What should you do?

WHEN SECONDS COUNT

■ Call for emergency medical assistance at once, or have someone else do this. Try to keep the person calm and quiet. Check the person's airway, breathing, and pulse to make sure they're adequate. If you don't detect a pulse or breathing, start CPR at once, if you know how. (See *Performing CPR on an adult,* page 579, *Performing CPR on a child,* page 585, or *Performing CPR on an infant,* page 590.)

■ If you see air being sucked into the lungs through a chest wound, cover the wound at once, using, for example, plastic wrap, wax paper, or your hand.

Important: Use protective equipment whenever you're likely to be exposed to another person's blood or other body fluids. This will help prevent exposure to blood-borne diseases, such as hepatitis and HIV. Latex gloves offer the best protection. If they aren't available, use any waterproof material — plastic bags, plastic wrap, several layers of gauze pads, or even clothing.

■ If the person's breathing becomes more labored after you've covered the wound, briefly remove the covering to allow accumulated air to escape.

Dress the wound

■ Dress the wound with a clean cloth, a gauze pad, or your bare hand if no dressing is available.

■ If you can see the person's intestines protruding through a large abdominal wound, place him or her on the back with something under the knees to help relax the abdominal muscles. Then cover the exposed intestine with aluminum foil, plastic wrap, or a moist saline dressing. On top of this, place a light outer dressing to preserve heat.

■ Cover any other open wounds with a dry, sterile dressing.

■ Try to keep the person from moving until medical help arrives.

■ Avoid putting pressure on the protruding intestinal part or trying to push it back into the abdominal cavity.

■ Don't give the person anything to eat or drink. He or she will probably need surgery, so the stomach should remain empty.

Dress the wound with a clean cloth, a gauze pad, or your bare hand if no dressing is available. Try to keep the person from moving until medical help arrives.

How are gunshot wounds treated?

With a gunshot wound to either the abdomen or the chest, the person receives intravenous fluids and blood components immediately to control massive blood loss and help prevent shock. The medical team may also need to insert a breathing tube, administer oxygen, or put the person on a mechanical ventilator.

Treating an abdominal wound

The person is usually admitted to the hospital. Most people need surgery to repair the injury. The medical team gives pain relievers, antibiotics, and a tetanus shot.

Treating a chest wound

Emergency medical treatment focuses on keeping the person's airway open and supporting breathing. The doctor may insert a tube into the person's chest to reinflate the lung and allow blood to drain from the chest. Other treatments include pain relievers to reduce pain and antibiotics and a tetanus shot to prevent infection. Usually, the person needs surgery to repair the wound.

What else should you know?

After the gunshot wound has been treated, the doctor typically prescribes respiratory therapy. The person needs to learn breathing exercises to help the lungs work effectively as well as special methods called splinting techniques to avoid injury when turning, deep breathing, and walking. During recovery, the person should avoid smoking and participating in contact sports.

What symptoms to report

Get medical help if the person experiences any of the following symptoms during recovery from a gunshot wound:

- worsening pain
- fever
- productive cough
- shortness of breath.

These symptoms may indicate infection or a collapsed lung.

Get medical help if a person experiences worsening pain, fever, a productive cough, or shortness of breath during recovery from a gunshot wound.

H

HAND INJURIES

Every day, as the human hand manipulates objects and explores the environment, it risks injury from a host of potentially harmful experiences. Sports pose special dangers to the hand — among them such injuries as skier's thumb and baseball finger.

Skier's thumb
This injury tears the ligament that joins the thumb to one of the bones of the palm. In severe cases, the ligament is severed.

Skier's thumb typically occurs when a skier falls and the ski pole forces the thumb away from the fingers, or when someone catches a baseball, football, or basketball traveling at high speed. (See *What happens in skier's thumb,* page 270.)

Baseball finger
This injury tears a tendon at the joint located at the end of the finger. If the injury is severe, the person can't straighten the finger. The usual cause of baseball finger is sudden force exerted on the end of the finger — for example, from a hit or pitched baseball.

What are the symptoms?
Skier's thumb causes immediate pain and swelling at the base of the thumb. A few hours later, the pain may get worse and bruising may occur.

Baseball finger also causes immediate pain in the finger, along with swelling and bruising.

What should you do?
For either injury, put ice on the finger right away. This will reduce pain and swelling. Then call the doctor.

How are hand injuries treated?
The doctor evaluates the finger to find out the extent of the injury.

Both skier's thumb and baseball finger cause immediate pain and swelling. For either injury, put ice on the finger right away.

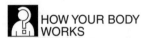

HOW YOUR BODY WORKS

What happens in skier's thumb

The *phalanges*, shown in this illustration, are the tapering bones of the fingers and thumb. The five bones that make up the framework of the palm are called *metacarpal bones*. The *collateral ligaments* attach the thumb to a metacarpal bone.

A tearing force
As a skier falls, the ski pole may force the thumb away from the fingers. This tears the ulnar collateral ligament, which attaches the thumb to one of the palm bones.

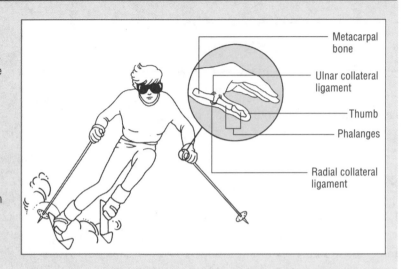

- Metacarpal bone
- Ulnar collateral ligament
- Thumb
- Phalanges
- Radial collateral ligament

To immobilize it and promote healing, the finger may be splinted. The doctor may recommend that the person take aspirin, ibuprofen (such as Motrin or Advil), or another mild pain reliever to reduce pain and swelling.

Don't give aspirin to a child under age 16 who also has a cold, flu symptoms, or chickenpox. Doing so could cause Reye's syndrome — a life-threatening condition that affects the brain.

Self-treatment
To ease discomfort and promote a fast recovery, take these steps:
- Apply an ice pack to reduce swelling.
- Avoid the activity that caused the injury, until the injured part heals.
- Do exercises that strengthen tendons in the finger or hand.

What else should you know?
For a severe injury, the person may need surgery to repair the torn ligament (in skier's thumb) or to reattach the tendon to the bone (in baseball finger).

HEADACHE

A headache usually isn't an emergency. The vast majority of headaches come from either scalp muscle tension or changes in the size of blood vessels in the head — migraine headache, for instance. Both headache types involve the layer of tissues on the outside of the skull. (See *How headaches happen*, page 272.)

Something more serious?
So when *is* a headache something to worry about? When it involves a structure on the inside of the skull. Although rare, this may be a warning sign of one of the following emergencies:
- severe inflammation or swelling of the brain, known as *encephalitis*
- inflammation of the brain or the membranes covering it, called *meningitis*
- stroke
- ballooning of a blood vessel segment in the brain, which doctors call *cerebral aneurysm*
- brain abscess, a brain cavity filled with pus and surrounded by inflamed tissue
- bleeding inside the skull.

How can you tell the difference between a harmless headache and one that could be a medical emergency? From the headache features and any accompanying symptoms.

A headache may be something to worry about when it involves a structure inside the skull. Although rare, this may be a warning sign of a brain inflammation or another emergency.

What are the symptoms?
Even a harmless headache can throb, create the feeling of a vise around the head, or send the person to a dark, quiet room to rest. But if the person has any of the warning signs below, suspect an emergency.

Serious warning signs
Call the doctor right away if the headache:
- follows a head injury
- is sudden, severe, and unlike any the person has had before
- affects a specific part of the head
- recurs in the same general area
- causes constant or persistent pain or pressure lasting a day or longer

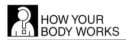

HOW YOUR BODY WORKS

How headaches happen

The inside of your skull barely feels pain. In contrast, just about everything on the outside of your skull *can* feel pain. Outer skull structures include the:

- skin
- muscles just beneath the skin
- arteries
- the skull's thin covering
- eyes
- ears
- sinuses
- nasal cavities.

Where the pain comes from

When a headache involves an outer skull structure, as most harmless headaches do, the pain usually stems from:

- muscle tension or inflammation
- an inflamed scalp artery
- allergy
- minor illness
- eye or ear disorders
- sinus infection
- heat exhaustion
- high blood sugar or certain other metabolic problems
- conditions that trigger migraines.

Inner structures that feel pain

Inside your skull, pain-sensitive structures include arteries, some blood-collecting spaces called venous sinuses, parts of the outer membrane at the brain's base, and the cranial and cervical nerves.

A more ominous headache

In the rare cases when headache involves an inner skull structure, the underlying cause may be a brain inflammation or infection, stroke, or some other serious condition. For instance, a brain tumor causes pain by displacing pain-sensitive structures like blood vessels.

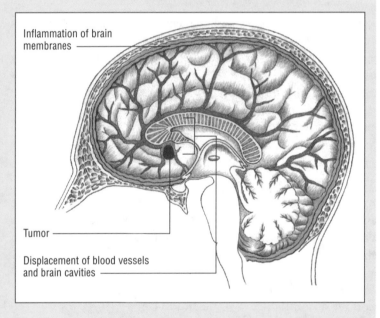

Inflammation of brain membranes

Tumor

Displacement of blood vessels and brain cavities

- causes unusually severe head pain, possibly with a painful or stiff neck
- tends to occur in the morning; this may indicate dangerously high blood pressure

Headache and pregnancy: A warning combination

Severe or persistent headache late in pregnancy could warn of danger to both mother and baby. That's because headache is a common symptom of *toxemia of pregnancy*.

A mysterious malady
In this relatively rare condition (also called *preeclampsia*), the mother's body reacts badly to having the baby inside her. No one knows exactly what causes the condition.

Who's at risk?
Toxemia of pregnancy most commonly affects women who are having their first baby. Although the disorder is known worldwide, it's most prevalent in the southeastern United States. The risk seems to be lower among women who get adequate protein, calories, and essential nutrients plus rest and exercise.

Stay alert for symptoms
Symptoms of toxemia of pregnancy include:
- swelling of the face and fingers
- high blood pressure
- kidney problems
- blurred vision
- rapid weight gain.

A dangerous progression
If toxemia of pregnancy progresses to its more severe phase, called *eclampsia*, the mother experiences seizures and may lapse into a coma. Other symptoms of eclampsia include:
- anxiety
- stomach pain
- severe headache
- blurred vision.

How common is it?
Eclampsia develops in about 2 pregnancies in every 1,000. About 10% of those mothers die, along with 25% of the babies.

Understanding the treatment
Treatment of toxemia of pregnancy involves bed rest and drugs to help the mother relax and reduce her blood pressure. If the condition threatens to get worse, the doctor may need to induce labor or do a cesarean section. As soon as the baby is delivered, symptoms begin to subside.

- is severe and coupled with tingling sensations, nausea, weakness, a diminished mental state (such as drowsiness or confusion), vision changes, or speech changes. This combination may indicate bleeding and increasing pressure inside the skull.

Another potentially dangerous situation is when a pregnant woman has a headache. (See *Headache and pregnancy: A warning combination.*)

Read what follows to learn about symptoms of specific headache emergencies.

Symptoms of meningitis
The person with this bacterial or viral brain infection has a severe,

constant headache that affects the entire head. The pain starts suddenly and worsens with movement. Other symptoms may include:

- fever
- chills
- stiff neck
- decreased level of consciousness
- seizures
- facial and eye weakness.

The person with encephalitis has a severe headache throughout the entire head. Over the course of about 48 hours, the person may show a lack of energy and then lapse into a coma.

Symptoms of encephalitis

With this viral brain inflammation, the person has a severe headache that's felt throughout the entire head. Over the course of about 48 hours, the person may show a lack of energy and then lapse into a coma. Other symptoms include:

- fever
- stiffness
- irritability
- seizures
- nausea
- vomiting
- unusual light sensitivity
- weakness or paralysis on one side of the body
- swollen or protruding eyes.

Symptoms of a brain tumor

Usually, the person first has a headache in an area near the tumor. Then, as the tumor grows, the headache pain spreads. The pain is usually intermittent, deep-seated, and dull. At its worst in the morning, the headache is aggravated by coughing and stooping. The person may also show:

- personality changes
- altered consciousness
- problems with movement and senses.

Symptoms of a brain aneurysm

In this life-threatening emergency, part of an artery in the brain swells up due to a weakness in the artery's wall. The person suffers sudden, excruciating pain, possibly just on one side of head. Within minutes, the headache peaks and the person may become unconscious. Other symptoms may include:

- nausea
- vomiting

- difficulty walking
- one eye that drifts downward
- blurred vision.

Symptoms of a brain abscess
The headache typically intensifies over a few days, affects a particular spot, and worsens when the person strains. It may be accompanied by nausea, vomiting, seizures, drowsiness, or coma. Depending on the location of the abscess, the person also may have:

- loss of memory or balance
- vision changes
- tremors
- personality changes.

Symptoms of bleeding in the brain
Typically, the person develops a sudden or increasingly severe headache. After a brief "blackout," he or she may become unconscious. Other symptoms may include:

- fever
- drowsiness
- confusion
- agitation
- nausea
- vomiting
- seizures
- stiff neck
- weakness or paralysis on one side of the body
- decreased sensations
- dizziness.

What should you do?
The harmless headache usually succumbs to Tylenol or a similar pain reliever. Some people get relief by applying ice or cold packs to the back of the neck or massaging the neck and scalp.

What to do if symptoms are more severe
If the person's symptoms suggest the need for prompt medical attention, be prepared to provide the doctor with important information, such as:

- a detailed description of the headache
- when the headache started

If the person's symptoms suggest the need for medical attention, be prepared to provide the doctor with a detailed description of the headache, including when it began and what makes it better or worse.

- the type of pain — steady, throbbing, dull, aching, boring, shooting, or stabbing, for instance
- whether anything makes it better or worse
- whether other symptoms are present, such as fever, nausea, vomiting, stiff neck, weakness, tingling or decreased sensation in limbs, drowsiness, confusion, vision disturbances, eye pain, light sensitivity, or dizziness.

WHEN SECONDS COUNT

Get immediate medical help for a person who has a severe or steadily worsening headache or a headache along with any of the warning symptoms listed under "What are the symptoms?"

How is a headache treated?

The doctor may order computed tomography (commonly called a CAT scan) or magnetic resonance imaging (called an MRI) to detect abnormalities inside the person's skull. A person who has suffered a recent injury may have neck and spine X-rays taken.

Sometimes the person undergoes a spinal tap so the doctor can obtain a sample of the fluid surrounding the spine. This helps to determine whether the person has a brain inflammation, infection, or bleeding. In some instances, the doctor orders neurologic tests to find the cause of the headache.

What else should you know?

The doctor may prescribe a muscle relaxant or a narcotic like codeine for someone who gets muscle tension headaches. However, many muscle relaxants and narcotics are habit-forming and shouldn't be used to treat chronic headache. Better choices may be nonnarcotic pain relievers, like ibuprofen (Motrin or Advil).

Medicine for migraine

To prevent migraine in a chronic migraine sufferer, the doctor may prescribe a beta blocker, such as Inderal. Ergotamines, a new class of drugs, can stop migraines once they've begun. Unfortunately, they may raise the blood pressure and cause headaches to recur when the person stops taking them.

> *The medical team may obtain a CAT scan or MRI to detect abnormalities inside the person's skull. Sometimes the doctor orders neurologic tests to find the cause of the headache.*

HEARING LOSS

Sudden hearing loss — the abrupt loss of hearing in someone with no previous hearing difficulty — may be caused by disease, injury, a drug reaction, or exposure to loud noise. This condition is considered a medical emergency because prompt treatment may restore full hearing.

Noise-induced hearing loss

This form of hearing loss, which can be temporary or permanent, may occur in someone who is exposed to loud noise (85 to 90 decibels) for a long time or to extremely loud noise (greater than 90 decibels) for a short time.

Noise-induced hearing loss is common in workers subjected to constant industrial noise as well as in military personnel, hunters, and rock musicians. For instance, rock musician Pete Townshend of The Who suffered hearing loss from overly amplified sound and now advocates turning down the volume. (See *How to preserve your hearing,* page 278.)

Noise-induced hearing loss may occur in someone who is exposed to loud noise for a long time or to extremely loud noise for a short time.

Understanding the causes

Conditions linked to sudden hearing loss include:
- acute infections, especially bacterial infections and viral infections like measles, mumps, German measles, the flu, shingles, and infectious mononucleosis
- buildup of earwax
- diabetes
- an underactive thyroid gland
- high blood fat and cholesterol levels
- high blood pressure
- atherosclerosis (hardening of the arteries)
- head injury
- brain tumor
- nervous system disorders, such as multiple sclerosis (MS) and neurosyphilis
- blood diseases, such as leukemia
- certain drugs, such as streptomycin.

What are the symptoms?

Symptoms vary with the type of hearing loss — conductive, sensorineural, or mixed.

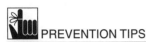

How to preserve your hearing

Overexposure to loud noise is one of the main causes of hearing loss. We're constantly bombarded by environmental noise. If you don't take steps to prevent hearing loss, you're risking your hearing.

Harmless din or dangerous noise?
Sound is measured by frequency (pitch) and intensity (loudness). *Frequency* is measured in sound vibrations per second, or hertz (Hz). For example, a boat whistle has a frequency of about 250 Hz, and a bird singing has a frequency of about 4,000 Hz.

Intensity is measured in decibels (dB). A conversational voice measures about 65 dB. A shout measures 90 dB or more. A jackhammer registers 100 to 120 dB. Loud rock music is 120 to 130 dB, and an explosion registers 140 dB or more.

The lower, the better
Low-intensity sounds are harmless and often quite pleasant. Sounds at or above the 85- to 90-dB range — called the caution or action zone — are dangerous.

How to estimate loudness
To estimate how loud a sound is, use this benchmark: If the noise occurs 3 feet (1 meter) away and you need to raise your voice to be heard, the level is probably about 85 dB. Constant exposure to noise at this level can cause permanent hearing loss. So can short exposure to extremely loud noise (greater than 140 dB) — a condition called *acoustic trauma.*

Lower your noise dosage
Another way to lose your hearing is by being exposed to a large *dosage* of noise. Dosage equals intensity (amount of noise exposure) times duration (over a period of time). The louder the noise and the longer it lasts, the greater the damage to the hair cells in the ear's organ of Corti — and the greater the hearing loss.

How to protect your ears
On the job, at home, or at play, you can protect yourself from hearing loss by wearing earplugs or earmuffs to muffle environmental noise.

Create a buffer
Always wear hearing protectors when you'll be exposed to sounds above the caution zone — for example, when using loud appliances, power tools, lawnmowers, tractors, or jackhammers. And don't forget your earplugs when shooting a gun or when you're around or on motorcycles, snowmobiles, speedboats, or other noisy vehicles. Although hearing protectors may seem inconvenient or uncomfortable at first, wearing them now will preserve your hearing.

Disposable plugs
Placed inside the ear canal to block out noise, disposable plugs also keep dirt out of the ear. Almost invisible, the plugs are available in several styles. Try different plugs and pick the ones you find most comfortable. Look for pliability and a snug fit. Never break off the tips.

Reusable plugs
Like disposable plugs, reusable plugs are placed inside the ear canal to block out noise and help keep dirt from entering the ear. They should fit snugly in the ear canal and feel comfortable. Also available in several styles, these plugs may be joined by a string to prevent loss.

Keep them clean
Before inserting disposable plugs, wash your hands and inspect the plugs for dirt. Wash them, if

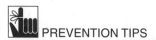

PREVENTION TIPS

How to preserve your hearing *(continued)*

necessary. If you use earplugs all day at work, wash them every day. Then rinse, dry, and store them in a plastic case or clean pill bottle. Replace them when they harden or discolor.

Headband plugs

These plugs are placed in your ears with the headband under your chin. The plugs should fit comfortably.

Wash the entire headband often. Don't twist or bend it because this will interfere with the fit of the earplugs. Store the headband safely.

Earmuffs

Earmuffs are worn over the ears with the band over your head. Cushioned muffs form a seal around the ear that completely blocks out noise. The cushions are foam- or liquid-filled. Loosening the earmuffs reduces their effectiveness. If you wear glasses, they may not fit correctly.

Replace hardened cushions

Remove the cushions and wash them often. Peri-odically inspect the cushions to see if they need replacing because they harden with use. Store the earmuffs in a safe place.

Other tips

Here are some hints that will help you protect your hearing.

Block out loud noises

■ Cover your ears when you're near noise, such as that from sirens or subways. If you commute daily, obtain and wear earplugs for your comfort and safety.

■ Avoid loud music, and don't listen to music with earphones. Turn down the volume on your television, stereo, and car radio.

■ Give your ears a vacation. Turn off the television and read a book.

Reduce appliance din

■ When shopping for appliances, ask about the decibel levels of competing products.

■ Run appliances one at a time. The combined sound of more than one loud appliance can put you well into the danger zone.

Symptoms of conductive hearing loss

In conductive hearing loss, the function of the external and middle ear structures is impaired. The person has decreased sensitivity to sound but no change in sound clarity.

Hearing is normal if the volume is increased to compensate for the loss. Typically, the person speaks quietly and can discriminate sounds but may have trouble hearing when chewing.

Symptoms of sensorineural hearing loss

In this condition, the person has suffered damage to inner ear structures or the pathway leading from the inner ear. (Noise-induced hearing loss produces symptoms of sensorineural hearing loss.) Symptoms include:

- poor sound discrimination
- poor hearing in noisy areas
- difficulty hearing high-frequency sounds
- the perception that others are mumbling or shouting
- tinkling or ringing in the ears (tinnitus). (See *When ringing isn't music to the ears.*)

Symptoms of mixed hearing loss

The person with mixed hearing loss has symptoms of both conductive and sensorineural loss. At first, the person can't hear certain frequencies (around 4,000 hertz). With continued exposure, he or she eventually loses hearing of all frequencies.

What should you do?

Prompt treatment is important. Let the doctor know if the person has had recent head or neck trauma, surgery, or exposure to loud environmental noise. Also tell the doctor if the person is taking antibiotics; some of these drugs can cause hearing loss.

What to do if hearing loss follows an infection

If the hearing loss follows a cold or an ear infection, a perforated eardrum may be the cause. Call the doctor, who will examine the person's ear with an otoscope to check the eardrum. The doctor may prescribe antibiotics to treat the underlying infection. Make sure the person finishes the full course of antibiotics and returns to the doctor for follow-up visits.

> Don't underestimate the long-term damage caused by environmental noise.
>
> Never turn the volume on headphones all the way up. Years of ear abuse can cause permanent hearing loss.
>
> Be sure not to leave your earplugs at home if you're exposed to high-decibel machinery on the job. Always wear them when exposed to loud noises.

How is hearing loss treated?

The sooner the doctor can identify and treat the underlying cause of sudden hearing loss, the better the outcome. For example, when high blood pressure is the underlying cause, controlling blood pressure can restore full hearing.

Prompt treatment is important if a person experiences sudden hearing loss. Let the doctor know if the person has had recent head or neck trauma, surgery, or exposure to loud noise.

When ringing isn't music to the ears

Chances are, you've heard someone complain of tinnitus — or maybe you've had it yourself.

Although tinnitus means *ringing in the ears,* many other abnormal sounds fall under this term. For example, some people describe tinnitus as the sound of escaping air, running water, or the inside of a seashell. Others say it's a sizzling, buzzing, or humming noise or a roaring or musical sound.

A threat to sanity?

Tinnitus may affect one or both ears, and it may be constant or intermittent. Although the brain can adjust to or suppress constant tinnitus, some people with intermittent tinnitus find it so disturbing that they contemplate suicide as their only source of relief.

Common causes

Usually, tinnitus results from a disorder that affects the external, middle, or inner ear.

External ear disorders

External ear disorders that can cause tinnitus include:
■ blockage of the ear canal by wax or a foreign object
■ inflammation or infection of the external ear canal
■ perforation of the eardrum.

Middle ear disorders

Middle ear disorders that can produce tinnitus include:
■ dislocation of an ossicle, a tiny bone inside the ear
■ inflammation or infection of the middle ear
■ otosclerosis, an inherited condition marked by irregular bone development within the ear.

Inner ear disorders

Inner ear disorders linked to tinnitus include:
■ a tumor of the eighth cranial nerve, called acoustic neuroma
■ atherosclerosis, or hardening, of the carotid artery in the neck
■ labyrinthitis, or inflammation of the labyrinthine canals of the inner ear
■ Ménière's disease, a chronic disease of the inner ear.

Other causes

Tinnitus can also come from severe high blood pressure, chronic exposure to noise (especially high-pitched sounds), drugs, and alcohol. For example, the pain reliever Indocin, alcohol, and an overdose of salicylates, such as aspirin, can cause reversible tinnitus. Irreversible tinnitus is a possible side effect such antibiotics as streptomycin, gentamicin, and vancomycin.

Treating the problem

Although tinnitus tends to resist treatment, some people get relief from tranquilizers, vasodilators, and antiseizure drugs. These drugs may help the person tolerate the condition. Other people try biofeedback.

Masking the problem

Some people with tinnitus use a tinnitus masker. The masker produces a band of noise measuring about 1,800 Hz, which helps block out tinnitus without interfering with hearing.

Other treatments

The doctor also may recommend:
■ a hearing aid, which obscures tinnitus by amplifying environmental sounds
■ a device that combines the features of a masker and a hearing aid to block out tinnitus.

Helping a family member cope with hearing loss

Coping with hearing loss is frustrating enough. But having to deal with the reactions and attitudes of others at the same time puts an extra burden on the person with impaired hearing.

If someone in your family has suffered hearing loss, you can take steps to smooth communication and avoid hurting his or her feelings. Read over these suggestions.

Speak distinctly

- If the person is older, speak slowly and distinctly in a low tone. Avoid shouting.
- If the person can read lips, stand directly in front of him or her when speaking and speak slowly and distinctly.

Approach the person carefully

- Approach within the person's range of vision.

- Try raising your arm or waving to get the person's attention. Touching may startle the person.
- Provide emotional support and encouragement to the family member who is learning how to use a hearing aid.

What to do if your child can't hear

You'll need to decide how to proceed with your child's treatment. Expect to face challenging choices, depending on the level of the child's hearing loss and the options available.

Learn how to sign

If your hearing-impaired child uses sign language, consider learning how to sign. This can prevent your child from feeling isolated or rejected and will help ensure communication among family members.

Treating noise-induced hearing loss

The doctor advises the person to rest overnight. A good night's sleep usually restores normal hearing in people who've been exposed to noise levels above 90 decibels for several hours, but not in those who've been repeatedly exposed to such noise. The best prevention is to reduce further exposure, if possible.

As hearing worsens, the person must undergo speech and hearing rehabilitation. Hearing aids seldom help a person with noise-induced hearing loss.

What else should you know?

To reduce the risk of hearing loss, read over these suggestions.

- Decrease your exposure to excessive noise.
- Use protective hearing devices in noisy environments.
- Immunize your children against measles, mumps, and rubella. (See *How vaccinations can prevent deafness.*)

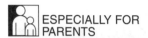

ESPECIALLY FOR
PARENTS

How vaccinations can prevent deafness

Throughout history, mumps has been the leading cause of sensorineural hearing loss in children. Measles and German measles (rubella) can lead to hearing loss too.

Reduce the threat with vaccines
The development of the measles, mumps, and German measles vaccine has greatly diminished these threats to children's hearing. But no matter what the socioeconomic background, some parents neglect to have their children immunized.

Follow the immunization schedule
Don't make the mistake of neglecting your child's immunizations. Preventing deafness is just one of many reasons why you should make sure your

child gets all immunizations at the appropriate times.

Check with the pediatrician
Measles shots are scheduled at age 15 months and again at ages 11 to 12. (A child who gets a measles vaccination at age 5 for school admission usually doesn't have to repeat it at ages 11 to 12.) These recommendations may vary, though, so check with the pediatrician for the recommended immunization schedule in your community.

Keep track of your child's shots
Remember to keep track of your child's immunizations. You'll need proof of immunization for entrance to kindergarten.

How to help a family member
If a family member suffers hearing loss, you can help the person to cope by being sensitive to the loss. (See *Helping a family member cope with hearing loss.*)

Heart attack

You've probably watched the scene countless times on TV or in the movies: A person grimaces, clutches the chest, and keels over.

A massive heart attack *can* cause this intense reaction. But a heart attack isn't always severe. Some heart attacks are mild; others don't cause any symptoms. Many people aren't even aware of the drama taking place within their chests. And some people who *do* have symptoms dismiss or deny them.

> *The developments leading to a heart attack represent coronary artery disease — a major cause of death in the United States. Sometimes, the heart attack is the person's first sign that something is wrong.*

How the crisis builds

Usually, a heart attack climaxes a chain of developments that began many years earlier. These developments represent coronary artery disease — a major cause of death in the United States. Despite the long-standing disease, a heart attack commonly is the person's first sign that something is wrong with the heart.

Here's what happens: Over the years, the coronary arteries that supply the heart with blood and oxygen become increasingly clogged with atherosclerotic plaques — pearly, white areas containing fats and other substances.

Then a piece of plaque breaks off, or a blood clot that has formed along the artery's wall breaks loose. The heart attack occurs as the plaque or the loosened blood clot blocks the artery, preventing adequate blood from reaching the heart. If the blood shortage is prolonged, part of the heart muscle dies. (See *What happens in a heart attack?*)

Predicting the damage

How much damage a heart attack does depends on two things:
- the size of the coronary artery involved
- the location of the damaged area of the heart.

If a clot blocks a large artery, it can cause extensive damage by cutting off blood flow to a large portion of the heart's muscle tissue. But even a small blockage can be threatening if it injures muscle tissues that control the heart valves or the heartbeat. (See *The starving heart,* page 287.)

What are the symptoms?

Typically, a heart attack causes crushing, constant, aching, constricting, or burning pain in the chest, under the breastbone. The pain may spread to the shoulders, left arm, neck, or jaw. Some people describe the sensation as pressure or indigestion rather than pain.

Other symptoms to watch for

Many people also have other symptoms, such as:
- a cold sweat
- nausea
- weakness
- dizziness
- shortness of breath
- fear or anxiety
- feelings of dread or impending doom
- pale skin

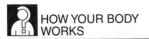

HOW YOUR BODY WORKS

What happens in a heart attack?

Once a heart attack begins, no one can predict how long it will last or how much damage it will do. Here are the steps that lead up to a heart attack and the events that typically occur during the attack.

1. Arteries become narrow

Over time, the heart's arteries become narrow as injury to their walls causes buildup of fats, blood cells, and fibrin (a substance that aids blood clotting).

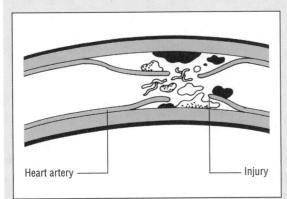

Heart artery ——⌐   ⌐—— Injury

2. New vessels grow

As the artery narrows, the body tries to bypass the narrowed area by developing new vessels to carry blood to the heart. This new vessel system is called collateral circulation.

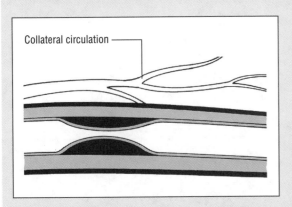

Collateral circulation ——⌐

3. Too little oxygen reaches the heart

If the new vessels can't deliver the oxygen-rich blood the heart needs, lactic acid is produced. Lactic acid stimulates nerve endings in the heart muscle, causing pain.

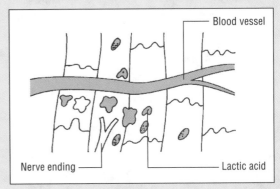

                                    ⌐—— Blood vessel

Nerve ending ——⌐   ⌐—— Lactic acid

4. Blood pressure drops

Without oxygen, heart muscle cells die and the heart can't pump enough blood at sufficient pressure. This makes the person's blood pressure drop.

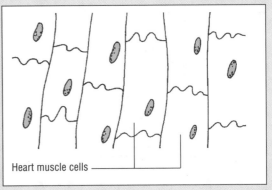

Heart muscle cells ——⌐

(continued)

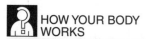

HOW YOUR BODY WORKS

What happens in a heart attack? *(continued)*

5. The heart beats faster

Decreased blood pressure triggers a chain of events that cause the adrenal gland to produce epinephrine. This chemical makes the heart beat faster and raises the blood pressure. Irregular heartbeats may result.

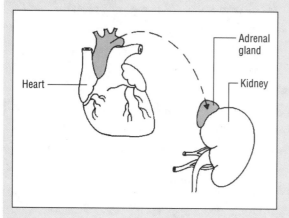

6. Enzymes flood the bloodstream

Dead heart muscle cells release their contents into the bloodstream. These show up in blood tests as increased levels of certain enzymes or potassium.

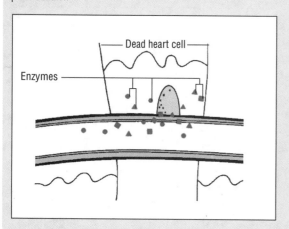

7. Electrical system goes awry

Damage to heart tissue can interfere with the heart's electrical system, triggering an abnormal heart rhythm.

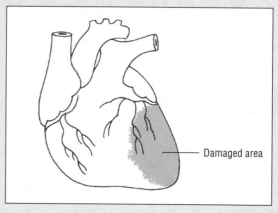

8. Blood backs up

If the heart muscle suffers extensive damage, some of the heart's chambers lose their pumping power. Blood then backs up in the other chambers and into vessels leading to the lungs or other areas of the body. These complications may cause swelling (edema) and difficulty breathing.

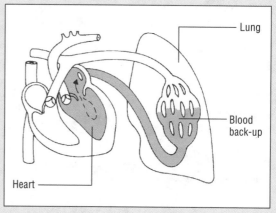

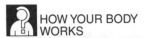

HOW YOUR BODY WORKS

The starving heart

During a heart attack, blockage or narrowing of one of the coronary arteries cuts off the supply of blood and oxygen to a portion of the heart muscle.

Heart tissue dies

All heart muscle fed by the blocked or narrowed artery dies. In this picture, the blocked artery and the affected heart tissue are shaded.

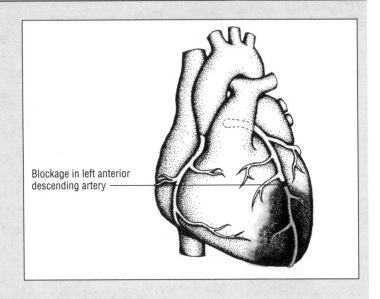

Blockage in left anterior descending artery

■ blue fingernails and lips. (See *Crisis on a downtown train,* page 289.)

What should you do?

 WHEN SECONDS COUNT

If you're alone and you think you're having a heart attack, try to stay calm. Call for medical help immediately. (See *Alone with chest pain: What should you do?* page 132.)

If someone you're with starts to have heart attack symptoms, call for medical help immediately. If this isn't possible, take the person to the nearest hospital emergency department.

Don't wait too long to get medical help. More than half the deaths caused by heart attacks occur before the person reaches the hospital — frequently in the first hour.

What to do if the person is unconscious

If the person becomes unconscious or unresponsive, check for an open airway, feel for a pulse, and look, listen, and feel for breathing. If a pulse and breathing are absent, start CPR if you know how. (See *Performing CPR on an adult,* page 579, *Performing CPR on a child,* page 585, or *Performing CPR on an infant,* page 590.)

What to do if the person is conscious

Help the person to rest comfortably in a sitting or semi-sitting position, and try to calm the person. Loosen any tight clothing, especially around the neck. Cover the person with a blanket or coat.

> ⊗ Be sure not to let the person lie down because this could make breathing more difficult.

When in doubt, get help

Even if you're not sure how serious the problem is, get medical help. Remember — any chest pain warrants immediate medical attention. Don't try to diagnose the condition yourself. Doing so can have deadly consequences: During the early stages of a heart attack, the heart starts beating in rapid, uncoordinated contractions. Without treatment, the person may die within minutes.

How is a heart attack treated?

The medical team tries to:
- stabilize the person's heartbeat
- restore blood flow to the coronary arteries
- preserve heart muscle tissue and ease the heart's workload
- relieve chest pain.

Stabilizing the heartbeat

A person having irregular heartbeats — the main problem during the first 48 hours after a heart attack — may need drugs and possibly an artificial pacemaker. Drugs used to steady the heartbeat include lidocaine, Pronestyl, Cardioquin, Bretylol, and Norpace. Some people require an emergency procedure called cardioversion, in which an electrical current is delivered to the heart through two paddles placed on the chest.

To speed up an abnormally slow heart rate, the person may receive the drug atropine or a temporary pacemaker.

Restoring blood flow to coronary arteries

If the person gets to the hospital within 6 hours after heart attack symptoms begin, the doctor may administer a "clot buster" — a

Even if you're not sure how serious the problem is, get medical help. Remember — any chest pain warrants immediate medical attention.

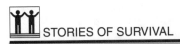

STORIES OF SURVIVAL

Crisis on a downtown train

Three friends were riding the commuter train into New York City when a 58-year-old man in their car suffered a heart attack. This is their story.

Laurie: We were out for a day of fun and shopping, that's all. What a wild trip it turned out to be.

Terri: I remember seeing this guy fidgeting, like his clothes were uncomfortable. Then he grabbed at his chest. He was sitting across the aisle, facing the opposite direction, so we had a pretty clear view of what happened, right Maureen?

Maureen: Yes, right.

Terri: He turned blue — well, grayish, really — and he was sweating through his suit. And he had this really pained look on his face.

Laurie: Terri asked him if he was all right but he didn't say anything. He just sat there and clutched his chest. Then, all of a sudden, he slumped in his seat.

Terri: His head hit the window, that's how fast he went over. We didn't know what to do. Next thing I know, Maureen is beside me, telling me to help get him on the floor. You tell it, Maureen.

Maureen: No, that's all right, you're doing fine.

Terri: Come on, Maureen, don't be modest. Well, OK then. I'll tell them: First, she listened for breathing and felt his neck for a pulse. Then she started CPR, which I've seen on TV but never learned. But Maureen had just learned it in a class, right? She was wonderful, really.

Laurie: Absolutely. She was absolutely wonderful. She just went ahead and did it. I took off and found the conductor in the next car and told him to call an ambulance and have it meet us at the next stop.

Terri: Right. Meanwhile, Maureen showed me how to do the chest thing, so while she breathed for the man, I pushed on his chest. We kept that up for what seemed like forever but what Maureen says was just a few minutes. Then the guy woke up.

Laurie: Yes, he just woke up. It was startling, really. By that time, we had arrived at the station and the paramedics took over. I understand the man recently had a bypass operation and is doing fine, thanks to Maureen.

Terri: She's a hero. I mean, she saved his life.

Laurie: Oh, she did, she absolutely did. She truly is a hero.

AfterWords

Maureen and her friends did everything right. Maureen knew CPR and didn't hesitate to use it. Laurie ran immediately for help, and Terri kept enough composure to follow Maureen's instructions. The heart attack victim survived, and in a situation like that, no better outcome is possible.

---

drug that breaks up clots in the arteries. These drugs include Kabikinase, alteplase (tPA), and urokinase.

Percutaneous transluminal coronary angioplasty (PTCA) may be an option for some people. In this procedure, the doctor threads a catheter with a balloon at its tip into the narrowed coronary artery. After injecting contrast dye through the catheter to pinpoint the narrowed site, the doctor inflates the balloon to expand the artery. If PTCA is done soon after heart attack symptoms arise, a "clot buster" may then be injected directly into the artery.

Resuming activity after a heart attack

If you're recuperating after a heart attack, the doctor will probably recommend exercise programs and suggest lifestyle changes. Here are the answers to questions you may have about resuming activity after a heart attack.

How soon can you have sex again?
Usually, the doctor will allow you to resume sex several weeks after your heart attack. Sex uses up about as much energy as climbing two flights of stairs.

When can you start driving again?
Wait 3 to 4 weeks before driving, and then start out with short trips. Driving increases stress and makes you tense your arm muscles — neither of which is good for your healing heart.

How will you know if you're overdoing your exercise program?
You're overdoing it if you feel chest pain, dizziness, or extreme shortness of breath during exercise, or if you're tired for more than 45 minutes after exercising.

Take your pulse
To monitor your heart during exercise, take your pulse. If your pulse exceeds 110 beats per minute or if you notice a new heartbeat irregularity, you're probably overdoing it. (If you're taking a drug called a beta blocker, though, your pulse rate may not rise to 110 beats per minute during exercise.)

Go easy on your heart
If your pulse rate changes or if you develop the symptoms mentioned above, just go back to a more comfortable exercise level.

Giving other drugs
Some people also receive oxygen and such drugs as nitroglycerin or a calcium channel blocker to relieve pain, send blood to blood-starved areas of the heart, help the heart pump more blood, and lighten the heart's workload.

Heparin or aspirin may be given to prevent blood clots. Morphine may be used for pain relief and sedation.

Monitoring the person's response
To monitor the response to treatment or to detect heart failure, some people undergo pulmonary artery catheterization. In this procedure, the doctor threads a thin, hollow tube through the heart and into the pulmonary artery. This allows measurement of various pressures within the circulatory system.

Performing surgery
Many people eventually have coronary artery bypass graft surgery. In this operation, the doctor removes a portion of a healthy blood vessel from another part of the body and attaches it above and below the blocked coronary artery. This surgery eliminates angina pain,

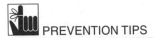

PREVENTION TIPS

Lowering your heart attack risk

Certain conditions may make you more vulnerable to heart attack. Of course, you can't alter risk factors like advanced age or a family history of coronary artery disease. But you *can* reduce others by changing your habits. Here are some examples.

Make lifestyle changes
If you smoke, stop. If you're overweight, talk to your doctor about starting a weight-loss program.

If you lead a sedentary lifestyle, look for ways to become more active. Ask your doctor about starting a walking program or some other form of exercise that interests you.

Eat right
Eat a heart-healthy diet. Ask your doctor or a dietitian to recommend a meal plan that's low in saturated fats, carbohydrates, and salt.

Other instructions
■ If you have high blood pressure, follow the treatment plan your doctor prescribes to control the condition.
■ Try to reduce stress in your life. If you have a Type A personality (aggressive, competitive, addicted to work, chronically impatient), ask your doctor or a therapist for help in learning to modify or moderate your behavior.

---

improves heart function, and may increase life expectancy by restoring normal blood flow to the heart.

Other treatments
Along with these treatments, the doctor usually prescribes an exercise program, and certain lifestyle changes. (See *Resuming activity after a heart attack*.)

What else should you know?
Typically, the underlying cause of heart attack is arteriosclerosis (hardening of the coronary arteries).

Risk factors
The following conditions increase a person's risk for developing arteriosclerosis:
■ family history of heart disease
■ high blood pressure (See *Lowering your heart attack risk*.)
■ smoking
■ high blood cholesterol and fat levels
■ diabetes
■ obesity
■ diet high in saturated fats, carbohydrates, or salt

- sedentary lifestyle
- aging
- use of drugs, especially cocaine
- stress or Type A personality.

A growing threat to women

Although men seem to be more susceptible to heart attacks than women, the heart attack rate is rising in women — especially for those who smoke or take oral contraceptives.

HEARTBURN

Heartburn has nothing to do with the heart. It occurs when stomach acids and partially digested food move upward from the stomach into the lower end of the food tube, or esophagus.

If you've ever had heartburn, you know it has nothing to do with the heart. An ailment of the digestive tract, heartburn occurs when stomach acids and partially digested food move upward from the stomach into the lower end of the food tube, or esophagus. This causes a burning sensation, which feels like it's near the heart. Doctors call this condition *gastroesophageal reflux.*

An untimely opening

Normally, everything we eat and drink moves *down* the esophagus with the help of wavelike, involuntary muscle contractions called peristalsis. These contractions cause the lower esophageal sphincter — a ring of muscle at the lower end of the esophagus just above the stomach — to relax and open. This action lets food into the stomach.

At all other times, the sphincter normally stays closed so the stomach contents don't come back up into the esophagus. If the sphincter opens, the person experiences heartburn.

Understanding the causes

Often heartburn comes from:

- emotional stress or nervous tension
- increased pressure in the abdomen, such as from tight clothes, pregnancy, straining, or swallowing air
- eating foods or taking drugs (such as aspirin and the diabetes drugs Orinase and Dimelor) that decrease pressure in the lower esophageal sphincter

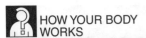 HOW YOUR BODY WORKS

What is a hiatal hernia?

Heartburn sometimes comes from a condition called hiatal hernia. This condition occurs when the muscular tissue around the hiatus (an opening in the diaphragm) weakens.

Chest intrusion
Weakening of the tissue allows the abdominal portion of the esophagus and part of the upper stomach to move through the hiatus into the chest.

Often a "silent" condition
Hiatal hernia affects about 40% of the population. However, most people have few if any symptoms.

SLIDING HIATAL HERNIA

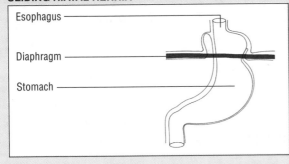

NORMAL STOMACH AND ESOPHAGUS

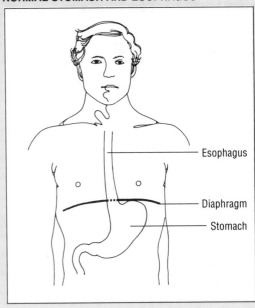

- surgery on the valve at the bottom of the stomach, called the *pylorus*
- being hospitalized with tubes going through the nose and into the stomach for 4 or 5 days
- certain illnesses, such as hiatal hernia. (See *What is a hiatal hernia?*)

What are the symptoms?
The major symptom of heartburn is a burning sensation at the base of the throat or in the chest or upper abdomen. The person may also experience increased burping.

How to relieve heartburn

Most people can eliminate simple heartburn by following these suggestions.

Keep abdominal pressure low
- Avoid activities that increase abdominal pressure. For instance, try to avoid coughing, straining, and vigorous exercise if possible.
- Don't wear tight clothes.

Stay upright
- During the day, sit upright when resting and napping, if possible.
- At night, use extra pillows or raise the head of your bed.
- Wait at least 2 hours after you eat before lying down.

Take medicines and eat meals on time
- If the doctor prescribes an antacid, take it at the correct times. Many doctors recommend taking an antacid 1 hour and 3 hours after meals and at bedtime.
- Eat regularly. Try eating four to six small meals a day instead of three large meals.
- Don't eat within 3 hours of bedtime.

Eat right
- Avoid highly seasoned foods, acidic juices, caffeinated coffee or tea, alcohol, carbonated beverages, and foods high in fat or carbohydrates.
- Be sure to eat slowly.
- Go on a weight-loss diet if you need to.

What should you do?

For occasional mild heartburn, the person should take an antacid and make dietary changes. (See *How to relieve heartburn.*) Severe or long-term heartburn warrants a call to the doctor.

When to suspect a heart attack

Occasionally, a person may dismiss the chest pain of a heart attack as heartburn. But keep in mind that a heart attack usually causes other symptoms besides chest pain — shortness of breath, a pounding or rapid heartbeat, palpitations, or nausea and vomiting. Anyone who has these symptoms *plus* heartburn that doesn't respond to antacids should seek medical attention right away.

How is heartburn treated?

Heartburn treatment can involve a wide range of medical and behavioral approaches. Mild heartburn may call for nothing more than occasional antacid use and simple dietary changes.

Using antacids and other drugs

If these treatments aren't effective, the doctor may prescribe regular antacid use or a drug that strengthens the lower esophageal sphincter, neutralizes stomach acid, and reduces abdominal pressure.

Checking for other conditions
To make sure the person doesn't have an ulcer or other disorder affecting the lining of the esophagus or stomach, the doctor may also order a series of X-rays using barium. The barium lines the esophagus and stomach, helping these organs to show up better on the X-ray.

What else should you know?
Cigarette smoking makes the stomach produce more acid and may cause or aggravate heartburn. So if you're a smoker and you suffer frequent heartburn, try to quit or at least cut down. Alcohol and spicy or fatty foods can be troublesome, too, so reduce your consumption of these.

Heat exhaustion

After prolonged exposure to high temperatures and high humidity, a person may lose fluids and body salts through sweating or from not drinking enough. When that happens, heat exhaustion occurs. Overexertion on a hot, humid day exaggerates the process, especially if the person is obese, overdressed, or not used to the heat.

Don't confuse heat exhaustion with heatstroke — a much more serious condition. If you aren't sure whether a person has heat exhaustion or heatstroke, respond as though the person has heatstroke. (See "Heatstroke," page 297.)

What are the symptoms?
A person with heat exhaustion is alert and rational, usually with a body temperature between 98.6° and 104° F (37° and 40° C). Other symptoms of heat exhaustion typically include:
- pale, clammy skin
- excessive sweating
- rapid pulse

Don't confuse heat exhaustion with heatstroke — a much more serious condition. If you aren't sure whether a person has heat exhaustion or heatstroke, assume the person has heatstroke.

Helping a person who has heat cramps

For reasons we don't completely understand, some people get heat cramps instead of heat exhaustion. These painful muscle spasms occur suddenly, usually in the legs but sometimes in the stomach.

How heat cramps develop

Typically, heat cramps arise after several hours of strenuous activity and profuse sweating in the heat. The person may have been drinking fluids that didn't contain salt.

How to relieve the cramps

Move the person to a cool place. Have the person sit or lie down and gently stretch out the cramped leg.

Give fluids

Give the person one of the following:
- weak salt water ($\frac{1}{4}$ teaspoon to 1 teaspoon of salt in a quart of water)
- a sports drink
- cold water.

Don't give the person salt tablets because they can irritate the stomach and cause nausea or vomiting.

Massage the muscle

Gently massage or rub the cramped muscle to relieve the cramp and reduce the pain.

- weakness
- headache
- nausea
- dizziness or fainting
- cramps in the legs or stomach (see *Helping a person who has heat cramps*).

When to suspect heatstroke

As heat exhaustion progresses toward heatstroke, the person may experience:
- muscle twitches or spasms
- enlarged pupils
- emotional instability
- seizures
- delirium
- fainting or collapse.

If the person is confused, delirious, or unconscious, assume you're dealing with heatstroke.

What should you do?

Move the person to a cooler place, preferably into air conditioning. Have the person lie flat and elevate the legs 8 to 12 inches. Loosen or remove any tight or excess clothing.

Cool the person's body

Put cool, moist cloths on the person's forehead and upper body, then fan the wet skin. If the person is conscious and has no trouble breathing, give sips of weak salt water (1 teaspoon salt to 1 quart water) or a commercial sports drink containing salt and electrolytes. Try to get the person to drink about half a glass of water every 15 minutes for 1 hour.

Don't give any more to drink if the person vomits, because the liquid could enter the lungs.

Be sure not to give the person alcohol or caffeinated beverages.

Avoid giving the person salt tablets.

WHEN SECONDS COUNT

If the person's symptoms progress to heatstroke or last more than 1 hour, get emergency medical help.

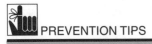

Heading off a heat disorder

The advice below can help you avoid heat exhaustion.

Increase your fluid intake
- Drink plenty of liquids.
- If you expect to be sweating a lot, drink a commercial sports drink that contains electrolytes and salt.

Wear protective clothing
- Wear loose, lightweight, cotton clothes during the summer.
- Wear a hat or other covering to protect your head from direct sun.

Use common sense
- Exercise sensibly in hot or humid weather.
- Spend time in air-conditioned places.

How is heat exhaustion treated?

Depending on the severity of the person's symptoms, the medical team may administer oxygen and may give oral fluids, intravenous fluids, or both. They continuously check the person's heartbeat, temperature, and breathing. They also may apply ice packs or special cooling blankets that contain coils through which chilled fluid can flow.

What else should you know?

Older people who don't have home air conditioning are at high risk for heat exhaustion on hot summer days. To help prevent heat exhaustion in older relatives and acquaintances, regularly check on them and encourage them to seek air-conditioned places, such as libraries, movie theaters, and shopping malls. (See *Heading off a heat disorder.*)

HEATSTROKE

Heatstroke is a life-threatening emergency that occurs when the body's temperature-regulating system goes haywire. This can happen after prolonged exposure to the sun or to high temperatures.

The higher the temperature and humidity, the higher the risk of heat stroke. (See *Heat plus humidity: Recipe for heatstroke*.)

The two types of heatstroke

Heatstroke occurs in two types. *Classic heatstroke* affects the elderly, obese people, children, and those with long-term illness, alcoholism, or circulation problems. About half of the people who get this type of heatstroke die, even with medical treatment.

Exertional heatstroke occurs in healthy adults who overdo it in the heat. Although still life-threatening, exertional heatstroke is easier to treat than classic heatstroke. That's because symptoms usually arise before the body becomes severely — and perhaps irreversibly — dehydrated.

What are the symptoms?

Suspect heatstroke if a person gets confused or delirious or stops sweating after a long time in excessive heat. Other symptoms of heatstroke include:

- body temperature above 104° F (40° C)
- flushed, hot, dry skin (although a person with exertional heatstroke may be sweating)
- strong, fast pulse
- rapid breathing
- anxiety
- hallucinations
- combativeness
- delirium
- poor coordination
- seizures
- enlarged pupils
- loss of consciousness.

Suspect heatstroke if a person gets confused or delirious or stops sweating after a long time in excessive heat. Other symptoms of heatstroke include a body temperature above 104° F (40° C) and flushed, hot, dry skin.

What should you do?

WHEN SECONDS COUNT

Call for emergency medical help. Check the person for an open airway, feel for a pulse, and look, listen, and feel for breathing. If pulse and breathing are absent, start CPR if you know how. (See *Performing CPR on an adult,* page 579, *Performing CPR on a child,* page 585, or *Performing CPR on an infant,* page 590.) If you think there's a chance of vomiting, lay the person on his or her side.

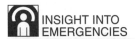

INSIGHT INTO EMERGENCIES

Heat plus humidity: Recipe for heatstroke

Depending on the humidity, your body may feel a temperature that's higher or lower than what registers on a typical outdoor thermometer. That's because humidity levels affect your body's ability to cool itself by evaporating sweat.

The table below shows the temperatures your body feels when you take humidity into account.

Danger zone
When the apparent temperature is 130° F (54.4° C) or higher, the risk of heatstroke is high no matter what your activity level. Here are some other guidelines to follow.

Between 105° and 130° F (40.5° and 54.4° C), you're at high risk for heat cramps and heat exhaustion. Long exposure or strenuous activity in this temperature range puts you at risk for heatstroke.

Between 90° and 105° F (32.2° and 54.4° C), long exposure or strenuous activity raises the risk of heat cramps or heat exhaustion.

HEAT INDEX

Relative humidity	Air temperature*										
	70	75	80	85	90	95	100	105	110	115	120
	Apparent temperature*										
0%	64	69	73	78	83	87	91	95	99	103	107
10%	65	70	75	80	85	90	95	100	105	111	116
20%	66	72	77	82	87	93	99	105	112	120	130
30%	67	73	78	84	90	96	104	113	123	135	148
40%	68	74	79	86	93	101	110	123	137	151	
50%	69	75	81	88	96	107	120	135	150		
60%	70	76	82	90	100	114	132	149			
70%	70	77	85	93	106	124	144				
80%	71	78	86	97	113	136					
90%	71	79	88	102	122						
100%	72	80	91	108							

*Degrees Fahrenheit

Source: National Weather Service

Put the person in a tub of cold water (not ice). If that's not possible, spray or soak the person with water and then fan the wet skin.

Cool the person's body

Get the person out of the heat. Put him or her in a tub of cold water (not ice). If that's not possible, spray or soak the person with water and then fan the wet skin. Or cover the person with a sheet, continuously spray the sheet with water, and vigorously fan the sheet. If the humidity exceeds 75%, place ice packs on the person's neck and groin and in the armpits.

Track the person's temperature

If possible, keep track of the person's body temperature. Once it falls to about 102° F (38.9° C) and the person becomes conscious and alert, stop vigorous cooling efforts. Otherwise, you could cool the person *too* much. Also reduce your cooling efforts if the person starts to shiver.

Don't use a glass thermometer to monitor temperature if the person is delirious, having seizures, or otherwise apt to break the thermometer and be injured.

Be sure not to give Tylenol or other drugs that contain acetaminophen or aspirin to try to lower the person's temperature.

Avoid giving the person anything to drink because he or she could breathe the fluid into the lungs.

How is heatstroke treated?

The medical team administers oxygen and gives oral or intravenous fluids to restore lost body fluids. They also monitor the person's heartbeat, body temperature, and breathing continuously. To lower the temperature, they apply ice packs or special cooling blankets that contain coils through which chilled fluid can flow.

Other treatments

The doctor may prescribe drugs to control shivering, such as intravenous Ativan or Valium. A breathing tube may be inserted to keep the windpipe open if the doctor is concerned about the person's continued ability to breathe or the risk of seizures.

What else should you know?

Unlike heat exhaustion, which typically clears up in about 12 hours, heatstroke may have long-lasting effects. The medical team watches for acute complications while the person is in the hospital. Afterwards, the person must be cautious about further heat exposure.

Many people remain sensitive to the effects of heat for weeks after suffering heatstroke.

Drugs to watch out for
Certain drugs may make a person more sensitive to the heat. They include:
- antihistamines, used for colds and allergies
- thyroid medicines
- amphetamines
- Haldol
- beta blockers, used to control blood pressure or to steady an irregular heartbeat
- anticholinergics, such as belladonna and Pro-Banthine
- phenothiazines, such as thorazine and Stelazine.

HEMORRHOIDS

A hemorrhoid is a painful, enlarged, bleeding vein in the lower rectum or anus. It can be inside the rectum or protrude from it. (See *Comparing internal and external hemorrhoids,* page 302.) Hemorrhoids are most common in adults between ages 20 and 50.

Types of hemorrhoids
Doctors sometimes classify hemorrhoids as:
- first degree, the least serious
- second degree
- third degree, the most serious.

Understanding the causes
Hemorrhoids probably result from increased pressure in the veins around the anus. Conditions that contribute to the development of hemorrhoids include:
- straining to defecate
- constipation
- prolonged sitting
- pregnancy.

Hemorrhoids probably result from increased pressure in the veins around the anus. Such conditions as constipation and straining to defecate can contribute to the development of hemorrhoids.

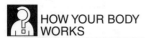

HOW YOUR BODY WORKS

Comparing internal and external hemorrhoids

A hemorrhoid may be internal or external. The illustrations below show each type.

Internal hemorrhoid
Covered by a thin sheet of tissue called mucous membrane, an internal hemorrhoid bulges into the rectal opening and may sink a bit during bowel movements.

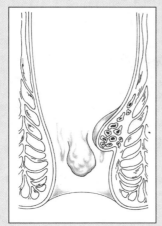

External hemorrhoid
Covered by skin, an external hemorrhoid protrudes from the rectum.

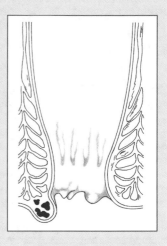

What are the symptoms?

Hemorrhoids usually cause painless, intermittent bleeding that can be seen in bowel movements. Bright red blood appears on the stool or on toilet paper when the hemorrhoid's fragile covering is broken.

First-degree hemorrhoids may cause itching. *Second-degree* hemorrhoids bulge out of the rectum during bowel movements and then return; they are usually painless. *Third-degree* hemorrhoids cause constant discomfort. They bulge even more with any abdominal pressure and must be pushed back into the rectum by hand.

What should you do?

Simple, at-home measures can help relieve the discomfort of hemorrhoids. To reduce swelling and pain, try local anesthetics, available in lotions, creams, and suppositories. Astringents and a cold compress followed by a warm sitz bath or a thermal pack are soothing, too. (See *Getting the most from a sitz bath*.) If hemorrhoids cause constant pain, call the doctor.

Getting the most from a sitz bath

A warm-water sitz bath can decrease pain and swelling in the rectal area. It can also ease discomfort and promote healing after hemorrhoid surgery.

How often to take sitz baths
Take three or four sitz baths a day, especially after bowel movements and before bedtime. Continue the baths until your symptoms disappear.

Step-by-step instructions
If you've just had surgery, the hospital may give you a sitz bath kit, or you can buy one at a drugstore. The kit contains a plastic pan and a plastic bag with attached tubing. To take a sitz bath, follow these steps.

Prepare the plastic pan and bag
■ Raise the toilet seat and fit the plastic pan over the toilet bowl. Be sure the drainage holes are in back and the single slot is in front.
■ Close the clamp on the plastic bag's tubing and fill the bag with warm water. If the doctor ordered medication for the bath water, add it to the bag now.
■ Insert the free end of the tubing into the slot at the front of the pan. Then hang the bag on a doorknob or towel bar, keeping the bag higher than the toilet.

Fill the pan and soak
■ Sit over the pan and open the clamp on the tubing. The warm water will flow from the bag and fill the pan. The excess water will flow out the drainage holes.
■ Continue to sit in the pan until the water begins to cool.

Aftercare
After you've finished the sitz bath, dry yourself completely. Apply an ointment or dressing if the doctor orders it.

How are hemorrhoids treated?
Treatment depends on the person's general health and the severity of the hemorrhoids. Generally, treatment focuses on easing pain, relieving anal swelling and congestion, and regulating bowel habits. Sometimes the doctor reduces or removes the hemorrhoid.

Reducing a hemorrhoid
Sometimes, the doctor reduces a hemorrhoid by hand or with a laser, or injects a solution to produce scar tissue, which keeps hemorrhoids from bulging.

Removing the hemorrhoid
Someone with a serious hemorrhoid — for example, one that causes bleeding, intolerable pain, or infection — may need a surgical procedure called *hemorrhoidectomy* to remove the hemorrhoid.

After surgery, the person should keep the wound clean to prevent infection and irritation. Here are some other tips.

- Use care when washing the wound.
- Avoid harsh soaps.
- Use white toilet paper (chemicals in colored paper can irritate the skin).
- Don't use stool softeners after surgery. A firm stool is a natural dilator and will help prevent scar tissue from tightening the anal canal.

What else should you know?

To help prevent hemorrhoids, take these steps:
- Avoid constipation.
- Eat more raw vegetables, fruits, and whole grain cereal.
- If the doctor approves, use a stool softener.
- Spend less time sitting on the toilet. This will reduce pressure in the veins around the anus.
- If the doctor prescribes a fiber medication, such as Metamucil, take it about 1 hour after your evening meal to ensure a daily bowel movement.

HIGH BLOOD PRESSURE

The effects of high blood pressure depend on which blood vessels have been damaged. For instance, damage to blood vessels in the brain can cause a stroke; damage to the eyes' vessels can cause blindness.

In high blood pressure, or hypertension, blood exerts too much pressure against the walls of arteries as it travels throughout the body. This increased pressure taxes vital organs, especially the heart, kidneys, brain, and eyes.

The effects of high blood pressure depend on which blood vessels have been damaged. For instance, damage to blood vessels in the brain can cause a stroke; damage to the eyes' vessels can cause blindness. Heart attack and kidney failure result from damage to the heart and kidney vessels, respectively. (For information on heart attack, stroke, and blindness, see "Heart attack," page 283, "Stroke," page 494, and "Vision loss," page 547.)

A silent affliction

In North America, roughly 15% to 20% of adults have high blood pressure, but many are unaware of the condition until they have symptoms of organ damage, such as vision problems and chest pain.

Hypertensive crisis occurs in about 1% of people with high blood pressure. In this emergency, the blood pressure may soar dangerously high. Brain damage and death may occur unless the person receives prompt treatment. (See *What brings on hypertensive crisis?*)

What are the symptoms?

Many people with high blood pressure have no symptoms. Some learn they have high blood pressure only when blurred vision, headaches, or seizures prompt them to seek medical treatment, or when an eye exam reveals the changes typically caused by high blood pressure.

Other symptoms to watch for

The most devastating complication of high blood pressure, hypertensive crisis, is signaled by:
- severe headache, nausea, and vomiting in the early stages
- seizures and changes in mental status, such as sluggishness, confusion, stupor, and coma
- nervous system problems, such as sudden blindness, speech difficulties, and muscle twitching.

What should you do?

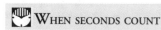 WHEN SECONDS COUNT

If someone has the symptoms of hypertensive crisis listed above, get medical help immediately. Ask the person if he or she takes blood pressure medicine and, if so, when the last dose was taken. (Hypertensive crisis may occur when a person abruptly stops taking prescribed blood pressure medicine.) If possible, send all drugs to the hospital with the person to help speed the diagnosis.

> Don't let the person take extra doses of medicine in an attempt to decrease the blood pressure. This practice can cause dangerous reactions.

> Be sure that the person doesn't take medicine prescribed for someone else.

How is high blood pressure treated?

The emergency rescue team provides supportive treatment to a person with symptoms of hypertensive crisis on the way to the hospital. For instance, they may insert an artificial airway, give oxygen, and start an intravenous line to administer fluids. They may also

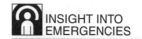 INSIGHT INTO EMERGENCIES

What brings on hypertensive crisis?

Many conditions can bring on the high blood pressure emergency known as hypertensive crisis. Here are some of them.

Medical conditions
Medical causes of hypertensive crisis include:
- abnormal kidney function
- bleeding within the brain
- heart failure
- lack of blood to the heart (such as from a heart attack)
- seizures or coma occurring in a pregnant woman or one who has just given birth
- a tumor of the adrenal gland, called *pheochromocytoma*.

Drugs
Hypertensive crisis can occur if a person takes a type of antidepressant called a monoamine oxidase (MAO) inhibitor along with certain other medicines.

Healthy habits: The key to controlling your pressure

If you have high blood pressure, you can take many positive steps to keep your blood pressure under control and avoid complications. Here are some dietary and stress-reducing suggestions.

Cut down on salt

Because salt causes your body to retain water, you need to cut down on it. If you're sensitive to salt, even a moderate amount can make your blood pressure rise. And the more salt you eat, the more medicine you'll need to take to control your blood pressure.

Here are some facts about salt, plus some suggestions on how to reduce your salt intake.

Facts about salt consumption

- Table salt is about 40% sodium.
- Americans consume about 20 times more salt than their bodies need.
- About three-fourths of the salt you consume is already in the foods and beverages you eat and drink.
- One teaspoon of salt contains 2 grams (2,000 milligrams) of sodium — the recommended daily amount for people with high blood pressure.

Tips for reducing salt intake

Even a moderate reduction in salt intake can significantly lower your blood pressure. It's easy to reduce your intake to a healthful level. Simply stop salting your food during cooking or before eating. Here are some other guidelines that will help you cut your salt intake to 1 teaspoon or less each day.

- Read labels on medicines and food containers.
- Put your salt shaker away (if you must use salt, use "light salt").
- Eat fresh meats, fruits, and vegetables instead of canned, processed, and convenience foods.
- Substitute spices and lemon juice for salt.
- Watch out for sources of hidden sodium — for example, carbonated beverages and iced teas, nondairy creamers, cookies, and cakes.
- Avoid salty foods, such as bacon, sausage, pretzels, potato chips, mustard, pickles, and some cheeses.

Read consumer labels

You're probably aware that fast foods are loaded with sodium, but did you know that ketchup is high in salt? Even some foods that don't taste salty contain a large amount of sodium. You can get nearly half your total recommended daily intake of sodium from a dill pickle. A hot dog or a cheeseburger would bring you to one-third of your total daily intake. And a can of tomato soup provides nearly 45% of your sodium intake for the day.

Other salt sources

Other high-sodium sources include baking powder, baking soda, barbecue sauce, bouillon cubes, celery salt, chili sauce, cooking wine, garlic salt, onion salt, softened water, and soy sauce.

Many medicines and other nonfood items contain sodium, among them indigestion remedies, laxatives, aspirin, cough medicine, mouthwash, and toothpaste.

Cut down on fats

Because fats cause narrowing of the blood vessels, you need to cut down on your fat intake too. Be especially miserly with saturated fats, found in eggs, dairy products, and fatty meats. In the grocery store, read food labels before choosing an item. Try to pick items with less than 30% of calories from fat.

Tips for reducing fat intake

- Eliminate egg noodles, pies, cakes, doughnuts, and high-fat crackers and cookies from your diet. Replace these items with pasta, rice, angel food cake, and low-fat cookies and crackers.
- Avoid whole milk, cream, whole-milk yogurt

Healthy habits: The key to controlling your pressure *(continued)*

and cottage cheese, cream cheese, sour cream, and ice cream. Instead, choose skim milk, nonfat or low-fat yogurt, 1% or 2% cottage cheese, and sherbet.

■ Stay away from fatty cuts of beef, lamb, or pork as well as organ meats, hot dogs, ribs, cold cuts, bacon, and sardines. Instead, eat lean cuts of beef, lamb, pork, poultry, and fish (such as sole and salmon.)

Take your medicine, eat right, and exercise

■ Take your blood pressure medicine as prescribed, even when you feel fine. Establish a daily routine for taking it so you won't forget. Always notify the doctor if you experience side effects. Don't stop taking the medicine without consulting your doctor.

■ If directed, begin a weight-loss diet.

■ Get regular exercise to help reduce stress and lower your blood pressure.

■ Have the doctor check your blood pressure at frequent, regular visits.

■ Learn to relax and meditate or have a quiet time daily. Find new ways of coping with stress — for example, learn how to manage your time better or handle your anger assertively.

apply electrodes and take an electrocardiogram.

In rural areas, or if the trip to the hospital will take more than 30 minutes, the team may have to start drug therapy too. Usually, they're in radio contact with a doctor who advises them on which drugs to give.

What else should you know?

For most people, the cause of their high blood pressure remains unknown; this type of high blood pressure is called *primary hypertension.* Risk factors for primary hypertension include:

■ a family history of high blood pressure
■ race (most common in African-Americans)
■ stress
■ obesity
■ diet high in saturated fats or salt
■ tobacco use
■ sedentary lifestyle
■ aging. (See *Healthy habits: The key to controlling your pressure.*)

In some people, high blood pressure comes from another condition, such as pregnancy, a nervous system or endocrine disorder, or kidney disease. This type of high blood pressure is called *secondary hypertension.* Use of drugs like birth control pills, cocaine, Epogen, and Sandimmune can also raise a person's blood pressure to a dangerous level.

*H*IP *POINTER*

A hip pointer is a bruise or tear in a muscle or in a tendon that attaches a muscle to the top of the ilium — the largest of the three hip bones. A common injury from contact sports, a hip pointer results from a blow to or a fall on the hip. (See *How a hip pointer occurs.*)

What are the symptoms?
A hip pointer causes pain, bruising, and possibly swelling at the hip. The pain may get worse several hours after the injury. With a severe injury, the person may have trouble walking or bearing weight on the affected side.

What should you do?
If the person complains of severe pain or can't walk easily, get medical help right away.

Apply ice
With a less severe injury, place an ice pack on the hip bone as soon as possible. This will decrease swelling by reducing internal bleeding and fluid buildup at the injury site.

Give pain relievers
To relieve pain and inflammation, give the person aspirin, ibuprofen (such as Advil or Motrin), or acetaminophen (Tylenol).

> Don't give aspirin to a child under 16 who also has a cold, flu symptoms, or chickenpox. Doing so may cause Reye's syndrome — a life-threatening condition that affects the brain.

How is it treated?
Treatment for a hip pointer aims to reduce pain, inflammation, and swelling and to allow the injured area to heal.

Using cold and heat treatments
Usually, the doctor advises the person to use cold treatments, then heat treatments, as described below.
■ First, apply an ice pack to the injured hip at least once a day for 2 to 4 days after the injury to reduce swelling.

A hip pointer causes pain, bruising, and possibly swelling at the hip. The pain may get worse several hours after the injury.

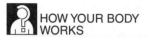

HOW YOUR BODY WORKS

How a hip pointer occurs

A person can get a hip pointer by falling on the hip or when an object makes hard contact with the hip, as you see in the large picture here. In this injury, the muscle at the top of the ilium (the largest hip bone) becomes bruised or torn, as shown in the closeup.

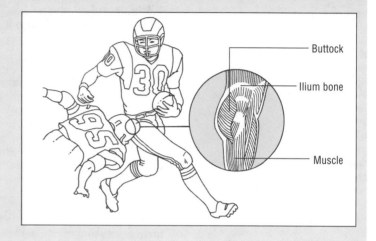

Buttock

Ilium bone

Muscle

■ Once the swelling goes down, apply a heating pad to the hip at least once a day until the injury heals. The heat widens small blood vessels, improving blood circulation and speeding recovery.

If you don't have a heating pad, you can use a chemical hot pack, available at most drug stores. Usually, you have to slap or knead the hot pack to release the chemical that causes the heat reaction. Before placing the hot pack on the person's skin, be sure to wrap it in a towel.

What else should you know?

The person should avoid athletic activities until the injury heals and the pain disappears. Depending on the severity of the injury, a hip pointer may take 3 to 6 weeks or longer to heal.

Follow a rehabilitation program

After the injury heals, the doctor may recommend an exercise program in which the person gradually and carefully stretches the muscles in the upper legs and waist. If necessary, the person should continue to use an ice pack to reduce swelling and should keep taking a mild pain reliever to reduce pain and inflammation. If the pain persists or the injury recurs, the person should call the doctor.

HIVES

Hives are smooth, raised bumps that erupt rapidly on the skin, usually as part of an allergic reaction. During such a reaction, the body releases a compound called histamine and similar substances. These substances enlarge tiny blood vessels in the skin, causing fluid to leak into the tissues. Hives caused by a minor allergic reaction involve just the top layer of skin.

Hives and Lyme disease
Sometimes hives result from Lyme disease, an infection spread by tick bites. The hives may erupt along with the rash that often heralds Lyme disease.

Brief or long-term condition?
Typically, hives last about 12 to 24 hours. However, new ones may form as existing ones clear up. Hives that keep surfacing for 6 weeks or more are considered chronic.

A more serious form of hives
An inherited condition called *angioedema* also causes hives — but these are larger, deeper, and involve additional skin layers. Hives associated with angioedema tend to erupt on the eyelids, hands, feet, lips, and genitals.

Angioedema also causes swelling of loose tissue under the skin, and may affect the person's digestive system and ability to breathe. Hives and angioedema affect about 20% of the population at one time or another. The two conditions can occur separately or together, but angioedema typically lasts longer.

A life-threatening allergic reaction
Hives can also accompany a life-threatening allergic reaction called *anaphylaxis*. Unless treated immediately, this condition can be fatal within 5 to 30 minutes, typically by causing throat swelling that prevents the person from breathing. For more information on this emergency, see "Allergic reaction to a drug," page 27.

What are the symptoms?
Hives can range in size from pinpoint to palm size or larger. Several small hives may join together to form one large, raised patch. Each

> *Typically, hives last about 12 to 24 hours. However, new ones may form as existing ones clear up. Hives that keep surfacing for 6 weeks or more are considered chronic.*

hive has a well-defined red border and a pale center.

Hives tend to sting and itch, except in angioedema, where they may burn and tingle. Because hives itch, people tend to scratch at them. Eventually, the hives may become scabs or infected areas.

Symptoms of angioedema

The person with angioedema may have hives plus swelling of the face, limbs, and genitals. Other symptoms may include:
- stomach discomfort
- nausea
- vomiting
- gasping for breath (if the throat or airway swells up).

Symptoms of Lyme disease

Besides hives, the person may have:
- an overall ill feeling
- fatigue
- an intermittent headache
- fever
- chills
- aches
- swollen lymph nodes
- joint pain
- heart and nervous system problems.

What should you do?

A person with hives needs prompt medical attention if he or she has never had the condition before or if hives are accompanied by trouble breathing, a change in the tone of voice, or a lump in the throat.

Self-treatment

For less serious symptoms, the person usually can relieve hives by:
- taking a lukewarm bath
- putting cool compresses or ice on affected areas
- removing known allergy-causing substances from the immediate environment.

WHEN SECONDS COUNT

Call for emergency medical assistance if the person has hives along with symptoms of a life-threatening allergic reaction, such as:
- anxiety
- weakness

A person with hives needs prompt medical attention if he or she has never had the condition before or if hives are accompanied by trouble breathing, a change in the tone of voice, or a lump in the throat.

- sweating
- sneezing
- shortness of breath
- runny or stuffy nose
- increasing trouble swallowing and breathing.

Then find out if the person has an anaphylaxis kit nearby. (Many people know they're at risk for severe allergy and carry the kit with them at all times.) The kit includes an injector that contains Adrenalin. Use the injector according to the package instructions. Then massage the injection site to speed the spread of the drug into the person's body.

If the person loses consciousness, check for an open airway, feel for a pulse, and look, listen, and feel for breathing. If pulse and breathing are absent, start CPR at once if you know how. (See *Performing CPR on an adult,* page 579, *Performing CPR on a child,* page 585, or *Performing CPR on an infant,* page 590.)

How are hives treated?

If the person is experiencing a life-threatening allergic reaction, the medical team takes steps to keep the airway open, maintain blood pressure, and keep the heart beating. They may need to perform CPR if the heart stops beating. A tube may be inserted into the person's windpipe to keep it open. The person typically receives oxygen and intravenous medications and fluids.

Treating less serious hives

To treat hives stemming from a minor allergic reaction, the doctor usually prescribes a soothing skin ointment, such as one that contains a cooling ingredient like menthol. Other helpful drugs may include an antihistamine to reduce itching and a steroid to reduce inflammation. If hives seem to be stress-related, the doctor may prescribe a tranquilizer, too.

What else should you know?

To help prevent future episodes of hives, the person should try to find out what substances trigger them. To do this, he or she may need to undergo extensive skin testing and eliminate foods systematically from the diet while keeping a diet diary.

Reduce contact with offending substances

Once the offending substances are identified, the person must reduce contact with these as much as possible. Usually, the hives then

To help prevent future episodes, the person should try to find out what substances trigger hives. The doctor may recommend extensive skin testing and systematic elimination of foods from the diet.

disappear within a few days. If the person is allergic to a certain drug, the hives will persist as long as the drug stays in the person's body. Many people need repeated skin injections to develop tolerance for substances to which they're allergic.

HOARSENESS

Hoarseness — a rough or harsh-sounding voice — usually comes from simple inflammation of the vocal cords. This inflammation is called laryngitis. (See *How laryngitis causes hoarseness*.) Other common causes of hoarseness are:

- a cold
- overusing the voice
- excessive alcohol use
- smoking
- infection
- allergic reaction
- anxiety.

When hoarseness stems from one of these causes, it's typically short-lived, disappearing within a week or so.

Long-lasting hoarseness
Hoarseness that lasts more than 2 weeks may indicate a serious problem, such as a growth on the larynx (laryngeal cancer) or on the vocal cords (vocal cord polyps).

What are the symptoms?
The person's voice typically sounds rough or harsh. Depending on the cause of the hoarseness, other symptoms may include:

- shortness of breath
- sore throat
- dry mouth
- cough
- difficulty swallowing dry food.

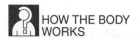

HOW THE BODY WORKS

How laryngitis causes hoarseness

The vocal cords are folds of tissue that line the inner walls of your voice box (larynx). The cords stretch in various ways to make the different sounds of speech.

Voice distortion
In laryngitis, irritation or infection of the larynx causes the vocal cords to become swollen and inflamed. When a person speaks, air passes over the swollen cords, distorting the voice and making it sound hoarse.

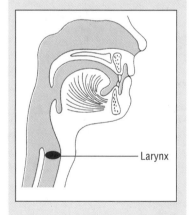

Larynx

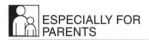

Helping your child cope with hoarseness

Some childhood diseases can make a child hoarse. For instance, *croup* causes severe inflammation and blockage of the upper airways. In *epiglottitis,* the flap that covers the larynx when a person swallows food or fluids becomes severely inflamed and swollen.

Encourage your child to rest the voice
If your child is hoarse, help him or her to rest the voice. For instance, try to anticipate the child's needs so he or she won't have to use the voice to ask for things. To help your child communicate without talking, suggest writing, drawing pictures, pointing to items, or gesturing.

How to help an infant
If your infant is hoarse, follow these suggestions:
- Try to minimize crying.
- Play quiet games with the child.
- Use a room humidifier.

What should you do?

Call for emergency medical help right away if the person develops a harsh, vibrating sound, called *stridor,* heard during breathing. (Stridor often occurs in children with croup.) Keep the person calm and place a humidifier in the room. If you don't have a humidifier, run a hot shower and have the person inhale the steam.

What to do if symptoms are less serious

Mild to moderate hoarseness doesn't require immediate medical care. Encourage the person to rest the voice. Talking — even whispering — further strains the vocal cords and can prolong hoarseness. Suggest using other ways to communicate, such as writing or gesturing. To relieve laryngitis, use a room humidifier. (See *Helping your child cope with hoarseness.*)

Don't let the person drink alcohol, smoke, or enter a smoke-filled room. These factors can make hoarseness worse. (See *Kicking a nasty habit.*)

Kicking a nasty habit

Even if you've smoked heavily for years, stopping now can help relieve hoarseness and reduce many serious health risks. Your doctor can suggest ways to stop smoking, such as hypnosis, relaxation therapy, the nicotine patch, and self-help groups. But if you really want to stop smoking, you can do it yourself by following these steps.

Track your smoking pattern
Prepare yourself to quit: Chart every cigarette you smoke for 2 weeks. Then look over your chart. Pay special attention to those times when you "light up" automatically, like after a meal or when you start work. Train yourself to notice every puff you take.

Psych yourself up
Convince yourself that quitting is worth the effort. Make a list of its benefits, such as being able to taste your food better, not coughing in the morning, and most of all, staying alive.

Choose a good time
Pick a date to quit smoking and circle it on your calendar. To make it easier, try quitting with several other smokers or quitting on a date when your routine will change, like when you go on vacation.

Find a substitute
As a cigarette substitute, try chewing gum or over-the-counter anti-smoking tablets, such as Bantron. If your appetite increases, consume plenty of low-calorie foods and drinks. Hold a pencil or pen in your fingers instead of a cigarette.

Reward yourself
Spend your "cigarette money" on a gift for yourself.

Keep saying no
Remember that you should lose your craving for cigarettes in about 8 weeks. After that, don't be tempted to have "just one" cigarette because you think you've kicked the habit. Keep saying "no." It gets easier each time you say it.

When to consult the doctor
Call the doctor if hoarseness lasts more than 2 weeks or if the person has several attacks of hoarseness over a 6-month period.

How is hoarseness treated?
If hoarseness lasts longer than 2 weeks, the doctor may examine the inside of the person's throat using a special mirror to observe the larynx at rest and during speaking. This helps to find the cause of hoarseness. Depending on the underlying disorder, treatment for hoarseness varies greatly.

What else should you know?

Sometimes a medical treatment leads to hoarseness. For example, surgery that cuts a nerve that controls the larynx can cause hoarseness by permanently paralyzing the vocal cords on one side. A person who has a breathing tube inserted to aid breathing may also suffer temporary hoarseness.

I

INCONTINENCE

Urinary incontinence is the involuntary passage of urine. It occurs in people of all ages but is most common in elderly adults. Altogether, nearly 10 million Americans (more women than men) have the disorder.

Urinary incontinence can be temporary or permanent. It may involve large volumes of urine or just scant dribbling.

An embarrassing condition
Although incontinence doesn't necessarily signal a serious disease, it is an embarrassment. It may lead to depression and to reclusive behavior if the incontinent person hesitates to leave home for fear of having an "accident."

Urinary incontinence may be short-term or long-lasting. Typically associated with a severe illness, *short-term incontinence* usually subsides with successful treatment of the illness. *Long-term incontinence* can take the form of stress, urge, overflow, or functional incontinence.

Stress incontinence
In this disorder, the person has intermittent urine leakage resulting from a sudden physical strain, such as coughing, sneezing, laughing, or a quick movement.

Stress incontinence results from weak pelvic muscles or from weakness or damage to the *urinary sphincter,* a circular band of muscles that constricts the urinary passage. Typically, stress incontinence affects:
- mature women who've borne several children
- young or middle-aged women who've just experienced a difficult childbirth
- women who've had recurrent pelvic or bladder surgery.

Men who suffer damage to the structure that drains urine from the bladder, called the *urethra,* during prostate surgery may also have stress incontinence. (See *Looking at the urinary tract,* page 318.)

Although incontinence doesn't necessarily signal a serious disease, it is an embarrassment. It may lead to depression and to reclusive behavior.

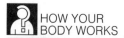

HOW YOUR BODY WORKS

Looking at the urinary tract

The urinary tract, shown here, includes all the organs that help to produce urine and eliminate it from the body.

The path of urine

After urine forms in the kidneys, it flows through the ureters into the bladder, where it's stored. Urine leaves the body through the urethra, the tube that extends from the bladder to the outside of the body.

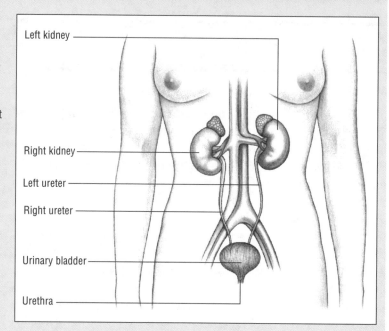

Left kidney

Right kidney

Left ureter

Right ureter

Urinary bladder

Urethra

Urge incontinence

With this form of incontinence, the person can't suppress a sudden urge to urinate. Urge incontinence results from uncontrolled or excessive contractions of the bladder muscle.

Overflow incontinence

This condition causes a dribble of urine. It results from urine retention, or buildup of urine in the bladder. The full bladder is unable to contract with enough force to expel a stream of urine.

Overflow incontinence may come from a structural abnormality or a blockage that impairs normal bladder contraction and prevents normal urine passage. Sometimes, it comes from faulty nerve stimulation of the bladder.

Functional incontinence

This form of incontinence comes with age, as the function of the lower urinary tract deteriorates. It affects mostly elderly people.

What are the symptoms?

Depending on the type of incontinence the person has, either small or large amounts of urine pass uncontrollably from the bladder. Incontinence may be intermittent or continuous throughout the day and night.

Other symptoms to watch for

Urinary incontinence may be accompanied by:
- a need to urinate more often (urinary frequency)
- a feeling of having to urinate immediately (urinary urgency)
- a feeling of having to urinate but being unable to start the urine stream (urinary hesitancy).

What should you do?

If this is the first episode of urinary incontinence, urge the person to see the doctor to determine what is causing it. Many people wrongly assume that urinary incontinence is an inevitable result of aging that must be endured. However, the condition can be treated and possibly reversed.

How is incontinence treated?

To find out the cause of the condition, the doctor performs a physical exam, checking for inflammation or defects of the opening of the urethra. Then the doctor evaluates the person's nervous system and tests the pelvic muscles for strength and tone.

Performing bladder tests

Usually the doctor orders a test to determine whether the person's bladder retains urine, called a *post-void residual urine volume test*. The person may also undergo other tests, such as instillation of sterile water into the bladder through a catheter. Called *cystometry*, this test assesses bladder sensation and capacity and helps evaluate muscle contractions.

Treating an infection or other cause

The doctor may prescribe drugs to treat the condition that's causing urinary incontinence. For instance, if incontinence comes from a bacterial infection, the doctor may prescribe an antibiotic, such as Bactrim or Septra.

Increasing muscle tone and relieving muscle spasms

Various medicines may help treat incontinence that results from an

If this is the first episode of urinary incontinence, the person should see the doctor to determine what is causing it. The condition can be treated and possibly reversed.

unstable bladder muscle — Pro-Banthine, for instance. If excessive bladder muscle contractions are the cause of incontinence, antispasmodic drugs may help. Examples include Ditropan and Urispas.

Treating shrinkage of vaginal tissue

If shrinkage of vaginal tissue is causing urinary incontinence, the doctor may prescribe estrogen.

Treating bladder problems

To treat stress incontinence or incontinence caused by an unstable bladder, the doctor may recommend an antidepressant whose side effects include increased bladder capacity and improved sphincter tone. Tofranil is one such drug.

Easing nighttime incontinence

Recently approved to treat bedwetting, the drug DDAVP may be prescribed as a nasal spray. It treats some forms of incontinence by drastically reducing the amount of urine produced overnight.

Special procedures

The doctor may order various procedures and devices to improve or manage urinary incontinence. At first, the person may undergo habit training and bladder retraining. These programs teach the person how to regain urinary control by establishing a regular voiding pattern. A person with stress incontinence may be taught how to do exercises that strengthen the pelvic floor muscles. (See *How to strengthen your pelvic muscles.*)

Next, the doctor may suggest use of a pessary or a condom (external) catheter. Then, depending on the cause of incontinence, the doctor may recommend an artificial sphincter implant.

If a nervous system disorder is the cause of the incontinence, the person may need to use a urinary catheter from time to time to prevent urine retention.

Surgery

In women, treatment of stress incontinence may include surgery to repair the front wall of the vagina or to restore the bladder and urethra to their proper positions within the abdomen. In some women, the operation may be effective for only a short time.

Men with urge incontinence resulting from an enlarged prostate may undergo prostate surgery.

To help manage incontinence, the doctor may recommend habit training and bladder retraining. These programs teach the person how to regain urinary control by establishing a regular voiding pattern.

How to strengthen your pelvic muscles

Exercising your pelvic muscles every day can make them stronger and help prevent urinary incontinence. The following exercises, called *Kegel exercises*, are easy to learn and simple to do.

When should you exercise?
If you have stress incontinence, try to perform these exercises just before a sneeze or a cough. Also try to do a few exercises before you lift something heavy or cumbersome.

By exercising faithfully and correctly, you'll notice an improvement in about 4 weeks. In 3 months, you'll see an even greater improvement. To do the exercises, follow these instructions.

Find the right muscle
The muscle you want to strengthen is the one that controls the flow of urine. You can find this muscle in two ways:
- by voluntarily stopping the stream of urine
- by pulling in on your rectal muscles as you would to retain gas.

Once you've mastered these motions, you've mastered the exercises.

Practice the exercises
Strengthen and tone your pelvic muscles by performing one of the two motions described above. Hold the muscle tight for up to 10 seconds. Then relax the muscle for 10 seconds.

Do them morning, noon, and night
Do 15 exercises in the morning, 15 in the afternoon, and 20 at night. Or exercise for about 10 minutes three times a day.

Exercise almost anywhere
You can do Kegel exercises almost anywhere and at any time. Most people sit in a chair or lie on a bed to do them. You can also do them standing up.

What else should you know?
Self-care for urinary incontinence includes wearing protective devices and taking steps to prevent skin irritation.

Use protective devices
Protective pads and garments are absorbent devices that augment habit training and bladder retraining. Besides making the person feel more comfortable and secure, they provide greater mobility during treatment of urinary incontinence. These devices include:
- thin panty liners
- sanitary pads
- disposable adult-size diapers
- washable incontinence briefs.

Prevent skin irritation and breakdown
After each episode of incontinence, the person should wash the skin exposed to urine, using mild soap and water. Then he or she should pat the area dry and apply a protective barrier cream, such as Sween.

INFECTION

Infection is the process by which one organism invades and grows in another. An infection is harmful because the infecting organism can kill body tissues or compete with the host organism in its drive to reproduce.

Infection also may produce substances that are toxic to the body. And it may prompt the person's immune system to respond by attacking the invader and trying to kill it. Unfortunately, the body sometimes harms itself in the process.

Limited reaction or whole-body ailment?
People are vulnerable to infection by many different organisms — nearly all of them too small to detect without a microscope or a chemist's lab. But whether or not we can see these invaders, we feel their effects.

Infection can be limited to a specific area, as in a cut finger that becomes infected. Or it can affect the entire body, as in the flu.

Still a serious cause of illness
Despite improved methods for treating and preventing infection — potent antibiotics, immunization programs, and modern sanitation — infection still causes much serious illness. This is true even in highly industrialized countries. In developing countries, infection is one of the most serious health problems. (See *How infections spread.*)

When is an infection an emergency?
An infection becomes an emergency when it grows severe enough to threaten the life of one person, an entire population, or any number of people in between. This can happen if:
■ the infectious agent gets into the bloodstream, causing a condition called septic shock (see "Shock," page 452)
■ the infectious agent resists our medicines, as is the case with a new tuberculosis strain
■ the infection progresses so quickly that it does great damage before doctors can treat it, as with gangrene and certain strains of *Streptococcus* bacteria
■ the infection seems to go away or goes unnoticed until it becomes a serious problem, as in syphilis and Lyme disease.

Despite improved methods for treating and preventing infection, infection still causes much serious illness. This is true even in highly industrialized countries.

What are the symptoms?

Symptoms depend on whether the infection is localized or affects the entire body, as well as on which infectious organism is involved.

Symptoms of a localized infection

A person with a localized infection, such as an infected cut on a finger, may have these symptoms at the wound site:

- pain
- redness
- swelling
- tenderness
- pus.

Symptoms of a body-wide infection

The person typically has fever, chills, and joint pain. Swollen lymph nodes are common, too; for instance, the person may have a lump in the groin.

What should you do?

Prevention is the best treatment for infection. Always wash cuts and other wounds thoroughly with soap and water. Then apply an antibiotic ointment and cover with a sterile dressing.

Watch wounds closely

Be sure to keep a close eye on a wound. If it becomes swollen, red, painful, or pus-filled, call your doctor. Chances are the wound is infected and you'll need to take an antibiotic. Also seek prompt medical attention if you notice red streaks in the area of the wound or feel lumps in your groin or armpit.

Use self-treatment

If you have a generalized infection like the flu, self-treatment includes:

- resting
- drinking clear liquids
- taking aspirin or ibuprofen (such as Advil or Motrin) to ease joint pain.

Be sure not to delay getting medical attention if you're diabetic or elderly and have symptoms of an infection.

Don't hesitate to call the doctor if your infant or young child shows infection symptoms.

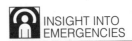

INSIGHT INTO EMERGENCIES

How infections spread

Most infections spread in one of four ways.

Contact transmission

This type of transmission occurs when you come into contact with the infectious agent. The contact can be *direct,* as in a sexually transmitted disease, or *indirect,* as when you use an infected person's towel or shake an infected person's hand and then rub your eyes.

Airborne transmission

With this type of transmission, you inhale the infectious agent from airborne droplets.

Enteric transmission

With enteric transmission, the infection spreads to a person who ingests food or water contaminated with feces that harbors an infectious agent.

Vector transmission

In this process, a third organism such as a mosquito or flea physically transports and transfers the infectious agent.

How is an infection treated?

Treatment depends on the type of infection and the organism causing it.

Treating a local infection

A local skin infection, such as a cut, may require only a topical antibiotic ointment. For a bacterial infection, the doctor may prescribe one or more antibiotics, based on which ones are known to be most effective against the suspected organism.

Treating a generalized infection

For a viral infection, such as the flu, no drugs are available, so the doctor prescribes simple measures like bed rest and aspirin.

For a bacterial infection, the doctor usually prescribes an antibiotic. Be sure to take every dose and complete the entire course of medicine. If you decide to stop taking the antibiotic early — say, because you feel better — you're giving the infection a second chance to sicken you. That's because you may still have a few "bugs" in your system. These bugs can reinfect you — only this time, they'll be more resistant to the antibiotic and you'll have a harder time getting rid of them.

What else should you know?

You can get an infection anywhere just by being exposed to an infectious agent. Specific ways to get an infection include:
- traveling to an area known for a certain infection
- being exposed to an animal or insect that carries an organism that's infectious to humans
- getting a contaminated blood transfusion
- undergoing surgery or another invasive procedure
- being injured or burned.

> *If the doctor prescribes an antibiotic, be sure to take every dose and complete the entire course of medicine. Otherwise, you could get reinfected and have a harder time fighting the infection the second time around.*

INSULIN SHOCK

Insulin shock (also called low blood sugar crisis) occurs when the body has too little sugar and too much insulin. A hormone made by the pancreas, insulin helps the body use the energy in food.

Normally, the body continuously balances its insulin and sugar (glucose) levels. Diabetes mellitus, a disease affecting the body's use of nutrients, throws off this balance. If the disease isn't controlled, insulin shock and other complications may occur.

Understanding the causes

Insulin shock can occur when a person with diabetes:
- doesn't eat and thus doesn't take in enough sugar
- exercises too much, which makes the body burn sugar too fast
- takes too much insulin
- doesn't prepare the insulin properly
- injects insulin into a site with irregular insulin absorption (see *Rotating insulin injection sites,* page 326).

What are the symptoms?

Insulin shock comes on suddenly. Symptoms include:
- personality changes, such as confusion and combativeness
- dizziness
- hunger but no thirst
- trembling
- headache
- profuse sweating
- rapid, weak pulse
- moist mouth and tongue
- cold, sweaty skin
- shallow breathing (although in some people, breathing remains normal)
- seizures
- eventual loss of consciousness.

Insulin shock comes on suddenly. Symptoms include personality changes, dizziness, hunger, trembling, headache, and profuse sweating.

What should you do?

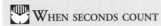 **W**HEN SECONDS COUNT

If the person is unconscious, call for emergency medical help at once. Check for a pulse and look, listen, and feel for breathing. If a pulse and breathing are absent, start CPR. if you know how. (See *Performing CPR on an adult,* page 579, *Performing CPR on a child,* page 585, or *Performing CPR on an infant,* page 590.) Call for medical help immediately.

Give glucagon

If glucagon, a hormone used to raise blood sugar level, is available

Rotating insulin injection sites

If you're taking insulin to control your diabetes, you can help avoid a low blood sugar crisis by making sure your body absorbs the insulin properly after you inject it. One way to do this is by rotating injection sites.

What are the benefits?
Rotating injection sites helps to:
- reduce injury to the skin and underlying fatty tissue
- prevent swelling, lumps, and buildup of scar tissue
- minimize a slow insulin absorption rate. Why? Repeated injections in the same site can lead to fibrous tissue growth, which reduces blood supply to that area.

Better insulin absorption after exercise
Rotating injection sites can also offset changes in insulin absorption caused by exercise. Exercise boosts blood flow to the body part being exercised, which increases the insulin absorption rate. (That's why you shouldn't inject yourself in an area you're about to exercise. For instance, don't inject yourself in the thigh before you go walking or bike riding.)

Where can you inject insulin?
You can inject insulin into these areas:
- outer part of the upper arm
- right and left areas of the stomach, just above and below the waist (except for a 2-inch [5-centimeter] circle around the navel)
- right and left areas of the back below the waist, just behind the hip bone
- front and outsides of both thighs, from 4 inches (10 centimeters) below the top of your thigh to 4 inches above the knee.

Keep insulin absorption steady
Try to rotate injections between sites with similar absorption rates, because different parts of the body absorb insulin at different rates. For instance, the stomach absorbs insulin best, then the upper arm, and last, the thighs.

Points to remember
To correctly rotate injection sites, follow these guidelines.

Use one area at a time
- Inject into the same body area for 1 to 2 weeks, depending on the number of injections you need daily. For instance, if you need four injections a day, use one area for only about 5 days.
- Cover the entire area within an injection site, but don't inject into the same spot.

Other instructions
- Don't inject into spots where you can't easily grasp fatty tissue.
- Have a family member give you injections in hard-to-reach areas.
- Check with your doctor if a site becomes especially painful or if swelling or lumps appear.

INJECTION SITES

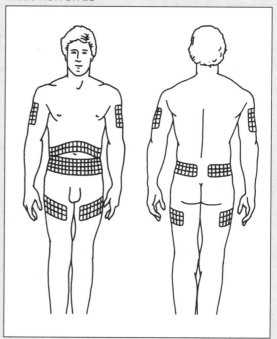

and you've been trained to give it, inject the drug directly under the person's skin. This will raise the blood sugar level rapidly. Then get immediate medical attention for the person.

❎ Never try to give an unconscious person anything to eat or drink.

What to do if the person is conscious

If a glucose product, such as Glutose, Glutol, or Instant Glucose, is available, squeeze it into the person's mouth. (But be careful not to block the person's airway.) If you can't obtain one of these products, place some honey on the person's tongue or squeeze prepared cake-decorating icing between the person's gum and cheek.

Other foods you may give include:
- a glass of fruit juice (such as apple or orange juice)
- nondiet soft drink (such as cola or ginger ale)
- water with 3 tablespoons of table sugar added to it
- corn syrup
- grape jelly
- six jelly beans
- 10 gumdrops.

After giving the sugary food, call for medical help at once.

When in doubt, give sugar

If you know the person is a diabetic but don't know if the crisis stems from high or low blood sugar, give sugar anyway to a conscious person. You could save the person's life if he or she is in insulin shock. And even if the crisis stems from the opposite problem — high blood sugar — you won't be doing any harm by giving sugar.

❎ Be sure not to give diet soda or other diet drinks. They don't contain the sugar the person needs.

❎ Don't worry about giving too much sugar; the medical team will correct any blood sugar excess when the person gets to the hospital.

How is insulin shock treated?

In the hospital, the person who is still unresponsive receives drugs — intravenous dextrose or glucagon — to make the blood sugar level rise quickly.

After regaining consciousness, the person is monitored closely, especially for changes in the blood sugar level. After symptoms sub-

If the person is conscious, give a glucose product, a glass of fruit juice, a nondiet soft drink, water with 3 tablespoons of table sugar added to it, or another sugary food.

STORIES OF SURVIVAL

The runner stumbles

Chuck was a runner. He ran everyday, rain or shine. Our company newsletter printed an article about him a few months ago, describing how he was trying to break a record for the number of consecutive days he ran. He just passed the 1,000-day mark.

Valentine's day crisis

Yes, Chuck was a runner. He was also a diabetic. I knew that; we all did. But none of us were prepared for what happened one Valentine's Day.

Chuck had just returned from his ritual lunchtime run. I passed him in the hall as he was heading into the men's room. He looked sweaty, but I figured he had just finished a run, right?

I picked up my mail and decided to stop by the men's room on the way back to my office. When I walked in, I saw the stall door open. Chuck was sitting fully clothed on the toilet, his head slumped and his hands dangling at his knees.

"Are you all right?"

"Chuck, are you all right?" I asked.

"Get... gotta, um... stuff... kit," came the mumbled reply.

He was shaking and sweat was dripping off his forehead. "What do you need?" I asked. How could I help him if I didn't know what was going on?

"Sugar," he said. "Sugar low."

"Bring something sweet — fast"

So *this* is what low blood sugar looks like, I thought. I ran into the hall, flagged down Jill, one of the analysts, and told her to bring something sweet — fast.

She returned with a half-eaten candy bar she

had been saving and a can of cola. But she hesitated to come inside the men's room. "It's all right, Jill!" I yelled. "We're all dressed in here!"

Walking into walls

While Jill had been hunting for sweets, Chuck had seemed to gain energy. His eyes were wild, and he was mumbling incoherently. I was trying to get him to sit still, but he kept trying to get away from me and walking into walls.

"Should we call the ambulance?" Jill asked when she saw the scene.

"Yeah," I said. "I think maybe we'd better."

Beginning to talk sense

I managed to pour some cola into Chuck's mouth and to get him to swallow small pieces of candy, but it wasn't easy. Then I just waited; I didn't know what else to do.

By the time the ambulance arrived, Chuck had come around a bit. His skin wasn't as clammy, and he was beginning to talk sense. The EMTs took him to the hospital anyway, just to be sure.

I'm prepared now, just in case

Chuck hasn't had any low blood sugar reactions since. For its part, the company purchased a blood-sugar testing kit and some tubes of rapid-acting sugar.

And I now keep a couple of those juice boxes for kids in my desk drawer. Just in case.

AfterWords

As a diabetic and a regular runner, Chuck probably knows that exercise makes his body burn sugar faster. And he probably also knows that to

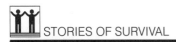

The runner stumbles *(continued)*

make up for this, he must adjust his insulin dosage.

Perhaps he neglected to adjust the dosage that day, or maybe he hadn't eaten enough. Whatever the cause of Chuck's low blood sugar crisis, it's a good thing that his colleagues were aware he was a diabetic and one of them happened to see him slumped over in the men's room. Although this man eventually figured out what Chuck's problem was, he might not have recognized the low blood sugar crisis if Chuck hadn't managed to blurt out a few pertinent words before he became incoherent.

Learn to recognize the symptoms

Chuck probably feels safer and his colleagues feel better prepared now that they're keeping a blood-sugar testing kit and rapid-acting sugar on hand. But to ensure quick detection of a blood sugar crisis, Chuck should make sure they all know how to recognize the symptoms of low and high blood sugar.

---

side, the person receives a snack of complex carbohydrates, such as peanut butter and crackers, cottage cheese and fruit, a small sandwich, or milk and graham crackers.

What else should you know?

Anyone who has diabetes should be prepared for insulin shock and other emergencies. Here are some suggestions.

Wear medical identification

Wear medical identification jewelry, such as a Medic Alert bracelet, that indicates your illness. This way, health care workers and others will know you're a diabetic if you're unable to communicate. This information will help them to decide what actions to take in an emergency.

Be prepared

■ Teach family members and friends about the symptoms of high or low blood sugar. (See *The runner stumbles*.)
■ Keep a supply of glucagon at home. Make sure someone in your family knows how to prepare and administer a glucagon injection.
■ Always carry a fast-acting carbohydrate with you to take in case of

a low blood sugar crisis. Examples include:

- sugar packets
- cookies
- chocolate bars
- jelly beans
- hard candy
- gumdrops.

Jaundice

Jaundice is a yellow tinge of the skin or mucous membranes (the tissue that lines the mouth and other body cavities). You're most likely to notice jaundice when looking at someone in natural sunlight. In artificial or poor light, the discoloration may be hard to detect.

Jaundice occurs when a person's blood contains too much bilirubin. A yellow pigment, bilirubin is found in a fluid secreted by the liver, called *bile*. When the liver is damaged, bilirubin builds up in the body and skin, turning the skin yellow and itchy.

Understanding the causes

Jaundice usually comes from a liver disorder, such as cirrhosis or hepatitis, or a disease of the gallbladder or pancreas. But it can be a symptom of other disorders, including severe heart failure and some types of anemia. Some people get jaundice after upper abdominal surgery or after prolonged surgery in which they experienced shock or blood loss or received a blood transfusion.

Sometimes jaundice results from taking a drug that damages the liver. (See *Drugs that can cause jaundice,* page 332.)

What are the symptoms?

Jaundice is fairly obvious from the person's yellow-tinged skin and mucous membranes. In fair-skinned people, you can see the yellow tinge best on the face and trunk and in the whites of the eyes. In dark-skinned people, you can notice it mostly in the whites of the eyes and on the roof of the mouth.

Other symptoms to watch for

Some people with jaundice also have:
- itching
- dark urine

You're most likely to notice jaundice when looking at someone in natural sunlight. In artificial or poor light, the discoloration may be hard to detect.

Drugs that can cause jaundice

You may experience the yellow skin discoloration of jaundice if you're taking any of the drugs below:
- antibiotics used to treat urinary tract infections, such as Bactrim, Gantrisin, and Microsulfon
- Laniazid, a tuberculosis medicine
- oral contraceptives (birth control pills)
- niacin
- phenothiazines (used for anxiety, nausea and vomiting, or mental illness), such as Prolixin and Stelazine
- Purinethol, a drug used to fight leukemia
- steroids such as Android and Anavar.

- light-colored stools
- fatigue
- fever
- chills
- appetite loss
- abdominal pain
- nausea
- vomiting
- shortness of breath
- palpitations.

What should you do?

Call the doctor if you notice symptoms of jaundice.

How is jaundice treated?

To find the cause of jaundice, the doctor usually orders blood tests and studies of the liver, gallbladder, and bile ducts. Some people need to undergo special tests, such as:
- ultrasound
- X-rays of the bile ducts
- removal of liver tissue for analysis (liver biopsy)
- laparotomy (incision into the abdominal cavity).

Treating bile duct stones

If jaundice is caused by stones blocking the bile duct — a condition called *obstructive jaundice* or *cholestasis* — the doctor may recommend surgery to remove the stones or a procedure called *lithotripsy* to crush them.

Treating a liver disorder

If jaundice stems from a liver disorder, the person may benefit from consuming fewer meats and other proteins and eating more carbohydrates such as bread.

Treating other conditions

Other underlying causes of jaundice call for different treatments. For instance, someone with a tumor of the pancreas may undergo surgery to remove the tumor.

Self-care

Self-care for the person with jaundice includes:
- eating small, frequent, nutritious, low-fat meals

- bathing frequently
- applying an anti-itch lotion, such as calamine, to ease itching.

What else should you know?

Don't get alarmed if your baby develops jaundice a few days after birth. About half of all full-term newborns and 90% of premature newborns have some degree of jaundice.

Usually, the jaundice is harmless and disappears by the seventh day. However, babies who have *pathologic jaundice* may experience serious problems.

JAW PAIN

Jaw pain may come from the upper jaw bone, called the *maxilla,* or the lower jaw bone, called the *mandible.* For some people, jaw pain originates where the two bones are hinged, a location called the *temporomandibular joint (TMJ).*

What jaw pain may mean

Jaw pain is seldom the main symptom of any one disorder. It usually results from disorders of or medical treatment on the teeth, soft tissue, or glands of the mouth or throat. These problems are seldom emergencies.

But sometimes jaw pain stems from an injury or infection that, if serious enough, could be an emergency. Finally, jaw pain may come from a disease or problem completely unrelated to the jaw itself. (See *What does a child's jaw pain mean?* page 334.)

Understanding the causes

A few of the disorders known to cause jaw pain include:
- angina pectoris (chest pain)
- heart attack
- TMJ syndrome — a malfunction of the joint that opens and closes the mouth
- tetanus (lockjaw) — a rare, life-threatening nervous system disease caused by a bacterial toxin
- tetany — a potentially fatal disorder of calcium metabolism that

Sometimes jaw pain stems from an injury or infection that could be an emergency.

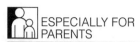

What does a child's jaw pain mean?

Jaw pain in children some-times stems from disorders that are uncommon in adults.

Causes of jaw pain in children

Mumps can cause swelling at the jaw level on one or both sides of the head. *Cystic fibrosis* can cause the parotid glands — large salivary glands just in front of the base of the ears — to become swollen and painful.

Detecting clues

Be alert for nonverbal signs of jaw pain in your child. These could include rubbing the painful area or wincing while talking or swallowing.

Symptoms of tetany in an infant

In an infant, early symptoms of tetany (an abnormality in calcium metabolism) may include fussiness and episodes of breathing stoppage. Later symptoms include:
- facial grimaces
- rigid muscles
- seizures.

causes cramps, seizures, and muscle twitching
- trigeminal neuralgia — a condition that causes excruciating episodes of pain in the face.

Certain drugs can cause jaw pain, too, especially those used to treat mental illness, such as Stelazine and Thorazine.

What are the symptoms?

The person's symptoms depend on the underlying cause of the jaw pain.

Symptoms of angina pectoris

The person with this condition may have chest pain that spreads to the jaw or left arm. The pain typically follows exertion, emotional stress, or a large meal and usually subsides with rest and nitroglycerin. Accompanying symptoms may include:
- shortness of breath
- nausea and vomiting
- rapid pulse
- dizziness
- sweating
- belching
- palpitations.

Symptoms of a heart attack

This emergency usually causes crushing chest pain, unrelieved by rest or nitroglycerin. The pain may spread to the lower jaw, left arm, neck, back, or shoulder blades. Occasionally, a heart attack involves *only* jaw pain and no chest pain. Other symptoms of a heart attack are:
- pale, clammy skin
- shortness of breath
- excessive sweating
- nausea
- vomiting
- anxiety
- restlessness
- a feeling of impending doom.

Symptoms of TMJ syndrome

This condition causes jaw pain, spasms and pain of the chewing muscle, clicking or popping of the TMJ, and restricted jaw movement. The pain may spread to other head and neck areas. Some people also experience:

- ear pain
- headache
- deviation of the jaw to the affected side when opening the mouth
- jaw dislocation (especially after yawning).

Symptoms of tetanus

This serious disease causes jaw pain and stiffness along with difficulty opening the mouth. The person may not notice early symptoms — headache, irritability, restlessness, slight fever, and chills — or may mistake them for the flu. If the disease progresses, the person experiences painful, involuntary muscle spasms that spread to the abdomen, back, or face.

Symptoms of tetany

This condition leads to painful jaw and mouth contractions, numbness or tingling sensations and cramps in the hands, thumbs, or toes. The person may also complain of:

- weakness
- fatigue
- palpitations
- odd twitches or muscle movements.

Symptoms of injury to the face, head, or neck

Such an injury — especially a broken jaw — can produce pronounced jaw swelling and pain and difficulty moving the jaw.

Symptoms of trigeminal neuralgia

In this condition, the person has attacks of intense jaw pain on one side of the head or rapid-fire shooting sensations. The pain occurs mainly over the lips and chin and in the teeth, and can last from 1 to 15 minutes. Exposure to heat or cold and consuming hot or cold beverages can trigger an attack.

What should you do?

Get medical attention at once for a person with severe jaw pain or symptoms of trigeminal neuralgia. If the jaw is swollen, apply ice packs and discourage the person from talking or moving the jaw.

For a *non-emergency* medical problem that could be causing jaw pain, make sure the person sees the doctor as soon as possible.

> ❌ Don't give the person anything to eat or drink until he or she sees a doctor.

Get medical attention at once for a person with severe jaw pain or symptoms of trigeminal neuralgia. If the jaw is swollen, apply ice packs and discourage the person from talking or moving the jaw.

If the person has suffered a head injury or has symptoms suggesting a heart attack, tetanus, tetany, or a broken jaw, call for emergency medical help or get the person to the nearest emergency facility at once.

If the person has a head injury

If the jaw pain comes from a head injury, avoid moving the person's head or neck. This will help prevent further damage in case the neck or spine has been injured. Be sure to keep the person's airway open. Also take steps to control bleeding. (See "Bleeding," page 73.)

WHEN SECONDS COUNT

If the person has suffered a head injury or has symptoms suggesting a heart attack, tetanus, tetany, or a broken jaw, seek emergency medical help at once.

How is jaw pain treated?

If the doctor suspects jaw pain is a symptom of a heart attack, tetany, or tetanus, the person is treated for that disorder. (See "Heart attack," page 283.)

Treating a jaw problem

To treat a problem that affects only the jaw, the medical team typically gives the person pain relievers and orders jaw X-rays to determine the extent of the problem.

What else should you know?

TMJ syndrome is controversial. In fact, some authorities doubt the condition exists. Possible causes of TMJ include whiplash from a car accident, a blow to the chin or jaw, dental overbite, and grinding or clenching the teeth.

The person with symptoms of TMJ should see a dentist to find out the underlying cause. The dentist may recommend such treatment as adjusting the dental bite or wearing a tooth guard to prevent teeth grinding during sleep.

How to cope with TMJ

If you've been diagnosed with TMJ, following these suggestions may ease your discomfort.

■ Take aspirin, acetaminophen (Tylenol), or ibuprofen (such as Advil or Motrin) for chronic pain.
■ Apply heat or ice to relieve pain and soreness.
■ Reduce your caffeine intake (caffeine can cause you to clench your jaw).
■ Avoid chewing gum.
■ Relax your jaw whenever you think of it.
■ Massage your jaw, neck, and shoulders.

Knee injuries

When a knee is injured, it usually means the cartilage or the ligaments of the knee joint have been damaged, twisted, or torn. This often happens during sports in which the knee performs a repetitive motion, undergoes sudden stress, or is subjected to extreme pressure.

Types of knee injuries

Common sports-related knee injuries include runner's knee (chondromalacia), torn cartilage, and torn ligament. (See *Comparing knee injuries,* page 338.)
- With runner's knee, the cartilage covering the surface underneath the kneecap becomes rough or suffers damage.
- With torn cartilage, the curved band of elastic material (meniscus) that sits atop the tibia (shin bone) is injured.
- With a torn ligament, one of the two ligaments that cross behind the knee and give it added stability is damaged.

What are the symptoms?

The chief symptom of a sports-related knee injury is pain in and around the knee. Often, the pain is accompanied by swelling.

Symptoms of runner's knee

Pain caused by this injury may be:
- dull or sharp
- mild or severe
- intermittent or persistent.

The person may feel the pain in or behind the knee or on the outside of one or both knees. The pain may occur when the person sits with knees bent, squats, kneels, or walks upstairs or downstairs. Other symptoms of runner's knee include:
- weakness of the muscle in the front upper leg (quadriceps)
- grinding or popping of the knee.

The chief symptom of a sports-related knee injury is pain in and around the knee. Often, the pain is accompanied by swelling.

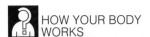

HOW YOUR BODY
WORKS

Comparing knee injuries

You don't have to be a football player to injure your knee. A hinge joint, the knee is vulnerable to a host of injuries. Read what follows to learn about three common knee injuries.

Runner's knee

This injury affects runners and other athletes of all abilities. Repetitive motion or sudden stress on the knee damages the cartilage that covers the kneecap's undersurface.

Rough spots and rubbing

Rough spots on the damaged cartilage then rub against the thighbone, causing pain on or behind the kneecap. The person may also feel pain on the outside of one or both knees.

Torn cartilage

A tear in the meniscus cartilage — the circular band of elastic material atop the shin bone — usually comes from a severe twist or blow to the knee when the person straightens the leg. This injury is common in football and soccer players.

TORN CARTILAGE

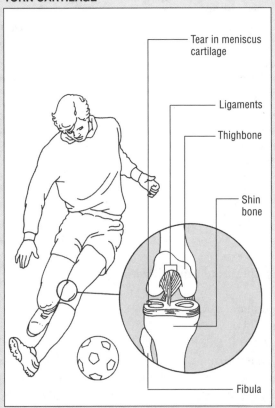

Tear in meniscus cartilage

Ligaments

Thighbone

Shin bone

Fibula

RUNNER'S KNEE

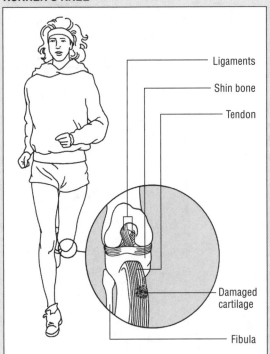

Ligaments

Shin bone

Tendon

Damaged cartilage

Fibula

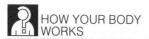
HOW YOUR BODY
WORKS

Comparing knee injuries *(continued)*

Torn ligament
Damage to the anterior cruciate ligament (some-times called an ACL injury) may range from a tiny tear to full separation of the ligament from the bone.

A sudden blow
Typically, this injury results from a sudden blow to the knee when the leg is straightened. Or it can happen from the force placed on the knee when a person plants the leg and then straightens it, as in basketball and skiing.

Symptoms of torn cartilage
The person may feel pain where the leg bones join to form the knee. At the time of injury, the knee may lock or buckle and make a popping sound.

Symptoms of a torn ligament
The person feels pain and swelling as fluid and blood build up inside the knee. The knee may become displaced or stiff and may have a limited range of motion. Depending on the severity of the tear, symptoms may not show up for 6 to 12 hours after the injury.

What should you do?
Have the person stop the activity that is causing the pain and apply an ice pack to the knee as soon as possible. Applying cold relieves the pain and reduces swelling by helping to stop internal bleeding and fluid accumulation. Also, tell the person to keep the injured leg still.

Get medical help to evaluate the extent of the injury — especially if the person complains of persistent or severe pain. Be sure to let the doctor know if walking upstairs or downstairs is difficult.

Use self-treatment
A person with runner's knee should apply ice for 2 to 4 days to reduce pain and swelling, and then rest the leg for 3 to 6 weeks. The leg should be kept slightly elevated. To increase the knee's stability, occasionally apply an elastic bandage to the knee.

Don't use an elastic bandage if you have diabetes or a blood vessel disease unless the doctor approves.

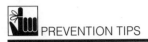

Safeguarding your knees

If you're recovering from a knee injury, you should expect some stiffness, swelling, or pain even after the injury heals. To minimize these symptoms and avoid a recurrence of the injury, take these precautions.

Resume activity gradually
- Wait until your knee has completely healed before resuming the activity that caused your injury.
- To avoid runner's knee, don't suddenly increase your running mileage or intensity.

Treat your feet well
- Wear shoes that fit properly.
- Check with your doctor about wearing shoe inserts to support your foot and to help you strike the ground properly while running.

Be kind to your knees
- Use caution when running on a different surface or terrain.
- When bicycling, don't strain your knees by "pushing the high gears."

Strengthen your legs
- If your doctor approves, work with a trainer or physical therapist to strengthen your leg muscles.
- Pay special attention to strengthening the hamstring muscles on the back of your upper leg and the quadriceps muscles on the front of your upper leg.

How are knee injuries treated?
To relieve pain and swelling, the doctor may prescribe a pain reliever like aspirin, ibuprofen (such as Advil or Motrin), or acetaminophen (Tylenol). Some people may need surgery to smooth out the roughness on the back of the kneecap, to repair a torn ligament, or to repair or remove damaged cartilage.

Resuming activity
Once the pain subsides, the person may resume the activity that caused the injury, if the doctor approves. However, the person should take steps to prevent the injury from recurring. (See *Safeguarding your knees.*)

What else should you know?
When applying ice, be sure to place a towel between the ice and the person's skin. Or use a chemical ice pack, available at most drug stores in different sizes and shapes. Because the ice pack doesn't freeze solid, it conforms to the injured area. It may be stored in the freezer.

Lead poisoning

Potentially fatal, lead poisoning occurs when a person's body contains dangerously high levels of lead. How does the lead get there? People, especially children, eat it, usually in the form of lead-based paint chips. (See *What you should know about lead,* page 342.)

Tracing the lead trail
Although usually associated with paint, lead is found in many other substances. Among other potential sources of lead poisoning are:
- water coming through lead pipes
- juice kept in an improperly fired ceramic pitcher coated with a lead-based glaze
- painted furniture
- color-tinted newspapers
- some painted toys.

What are the symptoms?
Symptoms of lead poisoning are subtle and may be confused with other conditions. Early symptoms include:
- listlessness
- irritability
- loss of appetite and weight
- constipation
- a bluish line in the gums.
    Later, you may notice clumsiness, vomiting, and stomach cramps.

What should you do?
If you suspect a person is suffering from lead poisoning, take him or her to a doctor immediately. A simple blood test will determine if your suspicions are correct.

How is lead poisoning treated?
A child who has absorbed enough lead to show symptoms will prob-

Although usually associated with paint, lead is found in many other substances, including water coming through lead pipes, painted furniture, and color-tinted newspapers.

INSIGHT INTO
EMERGENCIES

What you should know about lead

Until about 40 years ago, all house paint was manufactured with lead. Although laws now regulate the use of lead in new paint, layers of old, lead-based paint still cover the walls of millions of homes throughout the United States. This lead-based paint is responsible for most cases of lead poisoning. Why? Children eat it.

Here are some other facts you should know about lead.

Old paint: Loaded with lead

Lead was added to paint to make it dry faster and to give it a shinier, harder finish. The more lead, the better and more expensive the paint. Some paint contained as much as 50% lead.

A chip of lead-based paint about the size of a fingernail contains almost 100 times the amount of lead a person can safely consume in 1 day. A child who eats an average of three fingernail-sized chips a day for several months will become sick. The more lead the child eats, the more serious the effects.

Paint chips and pica

A child with pica (an unusual nonfood craving) will eat such potentially lead-containing items as paint chips and plaster, as well as crayons, chalk, wallpaper, newspaper, dirt, and cigarettes. Pica isn't restricted to children; pregnant women frequently develop pica.

How to find lead in your home

The first step in treating lead poisoning is to get the child away from the source of contamination. Locating the source of lead isn't always easy. It may be in the child's home or in a home or building the child visits frequently.

Have your home tested for lead

The paint in your home can be tested for lead. In the usual method, a meter is placed against the wall to measure the amount of lead in the paint. This test can be performed by local health authorities. Contact the nearest office of the U.S. Department of Health, Education, and Welfare.

Get the lead off your walls

If the paint in your home contains lead, repaint the walls. If you can, first scrape down the walls to get off all the old paint.

If you can't afford to repaint, keep your floors swept and look around to find paint that might be pulled off. Brush off the loose paint with a broom or stiff brush.

---

ably require hospitalization. Treatment usually consists of giving drugs to help the body eliminate the lead.

Getting rid of the lead

To cause increased urination and help excrete lead in the urine, the child may receive intravenous fluids. The doctor also may prescribe a medicine that binds with the lead, called a chelating agent, to make it easier for the body to eliminate lead.

What else should you know?

Lead poisoning is a long-term poisoning. If the child keeps ingest-

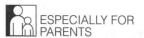

ESPECIALLY FOR
PARENTS

Keeping your kids safe from lead

The best way to prevent lead poisoning is to keep lead-based paint away from your children. Here are some tips.

Prevent lead ingestion
■ Teach your children not to eat anything they find, indoors or outdoors. Be clear that you mean *anything* — even things as small as paint chips.
■ If your child craves nonfood substances, he or she may have pica. Persistent pica can cause lead or other poisoning. Know that the chance of pica seems to increase when a child is teething. Discuss the problem with the doctor.

Keep a close watch on kids
■ Keep an eye on children outdoors. Many exte-

rior house paints, especially around windows, flake off easily.
■ Be alert for signs that your child is picking at painted surfaces.
■ Keep cribs away from windows that may be painted with lead-based paint.

Make your home lead free
■ Use only lead-free paint when you paint your home or anything in it.
■ Watch out for peeling paint. If your home is old enough, it may have layers of old, lead-based paint beneath the more recent layers of paint. If you suspect there's any lead-based paint on your walls, scrape off all the layers of old or peeling paint before repainting with lead-free paint. Don't just add another coat of paint.

ing lead, large amounts will accumulate and eventually reach a toxic level.

A child may ingest lead for 3 to 6 months before showing symptoms of poisoning. If the condition goes undetected, the child may suffer serious complications, such as mental retardation. (See *Keeping your kids safe from lead*.)

LEG INJURIES

Many sports place unusual stress on the legs, making them targets for potential injury. Three common sports-related leg injuries are Achilles tendinitis, hamstring muscle pull, and shin splints.

Achilles tendinitis

Tendons are strong, glistening white fibrous tissue bands that attach muscle to bone. The Achilles tendon attaches the calf muscles to the heel bone. It allows you to climb, run, and stand on your tiptoes.

Injury to the Achilles tendon can range from a strain or a tiny tear to a complete separation of the tendon from the heel bone (rare). Such an injury can come from:

- repetitive motion over time, as in running
- sudden stress placed on the tendon, as in sprinting
- tendon fatigue, as when a person places pressure on the tendon before it warms up sufficiently
- running or training on a hard surface
- wearing improper shoes during sports
- wearing athletic shoes with a stiff heel.

Many activities can lead to Achilles tendinitis — basketball, baseball, football, aerobics, hiking, tennis, soccer, rugby, track and field, and even running for the bus.

Hamstring muscle pull

The hamstring is the large muscle in the back of the thigh. Extending from the top of your knee to the bottom of your pelvis, the hamstring bends the leg. Most hamstring injuries occur in the muscle, although the tendons that attach the muscle to bone may also be torn.

A hamstring muscle pull may range from a tiny tear to a more serious tear. This injury happens to athletes of all abilities. The usual cause is making a quick start when the leg is straightened, as in sprinting. People who play baseball, football, basketball, rugby, soccer, or tennis are also vulnerable. So is anyone who engages in sports without warming up sufficiently beforehand. (See *Leg injuries: The inside story.*)

A hamstring muscle pull may range from a tiny tear to a more serious tear. It usually occurs when a person makes a quick start on a straightened leg, as in sprinting.

Shin splint

The shin is the front part of the leg below the knee. It consists of the tibia and fibula (the two large bones of the lower leg) and the muscles and ligaments attached to them.

A shin splint refers to one of several injuries:

- a tiny tear in a lower leg muscle
- a stress fracture in the tibia or fibula
- a tear or inflammation in the membrane covering the bone surface

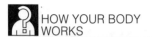

HOW YOUR BODY
WORKS

Leg injuries: The inside story

Most sports-related leg injuries involve a tear in a muscle or tendon. Typical causes include repetitive motion (as in running), sudden stress placed on the tendon or muscle (as in sprinting), and overuse (as in aerobics). Here's how three common sports injuries look from the inside.

Achilles tendinitis
In this injury, the tendon that attaches the calf muscles (gastrocnemius and soleus muscles) to the heel bone is torn or separates from the heel bone.

Hamstring muscle pull
The hamstring muscle can be injured during a quick start on a straightened leg. (Think of a sprinter leaving the starting block.) The injury may range from a tiny tear to a more severe one.

Shin splint
This injury, which affects the front of the leg below the knee, can take the form of:
- a muscle tear
- a stress fracture
- a tear or inflammation in the membrane that covers a bone
- anterior compartment syndrome (poor blood flow to and from the leg muscles).

HAMSTRING MUSCLE PULL

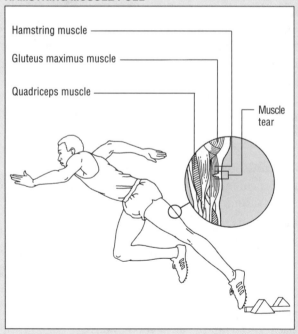

Hamstring muscle

Gluteus maximus muscle

Quadriceps muscle

Muscle tear

SHIN SPLINT

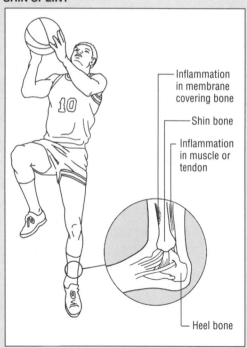

Inflammation in membrane covering bone

Shin bone

Inflammation in muscle or tendon

Heel bone

■ anterior compartment syndrome — a condition in which the muscles during exercise grow too large for the space they occupy. This syndrome may curb blood flow to and from the muscles.

Conditions that can lead to a shin splint include:
■ overuse, such as running without rest
■ running on a different surface than usual
■ changing the running routine
■ engaging in sports after a period of inactivity
■ weight gain.

Like Achilles tendinitis and hamstring pulls, shin splints occur in athletes of all abilities and in a wide range of activities — running, aerobics, baseball, tennis, basketball, soccer, rugby, and even walking.

What are the symptoms?
The chief symptom of a leg injury is pain. Depending on the extent of the injury, the pain may range from mild to severe. It may worsen several hours after the injury and may be coupled with swelling. Other symptoms vary with the specific injury.

Symptoms of Achilles tendinitis
This injury may cause pain that is centered above the back of the ankle, at the lowest part of the leg. With a mild tendon strain or tear, the pain may occur on awakening, disappear later in the day, and return the next morning.

A more serious tear or separation of the tendon from the bone may cause sharp, sudden pain that prevents the person from bending the foot or ankle downward.

Symptoms of a hamstring muscle pull
This injury causes pain in the back of the leg. The person may have difficulty walking, sitting, or bending.

Symptoms of a shin splint
This injury causes pain in the lower front part of the leg.

What should you do?
The person should stop the activity that is causing the pain and apply an ice pack to the injury site as soon as possible. Cold treatment helps to reduce pain and swelling.

If the pain is severe or prevents the person from walking or climbing stairs, call the doctor. As the doctor directs, the person should

The person should stop the activity that is causing the leg pain and apply an ice pack to the injury site as soon as possible. Cold treatment helps to reduce pain and swelling.

take aspirin, ibuprofen (Advil or Motrin), or acetaminophen (Tylenol) to relieve pain and inflammation.

> Don't apply a heating pad to the injured area until swelling subsides. Heat could increase the swelling.

How are leg injuries treated?

The doctor prescribes treatments to reduce pain, inflammation, and swelling — for instance, a mild pain reliever and ice application to the injury at least once a day for 2 to 4 days until swelling subsides.

Then, for a person with a hamstring pull or shin splint, the doctor may order heat treatments. Heat enhances blood circulation by enlarging the small blood vessels in and near the injury site.

Performing surgery

Rarely, a leg injury calls for surgery. For instance, a person with Achilles tendinitis may need surgery to remove scar tissue and part of the tendon. A person with severe anterior compartment syndrome may undergo surgery to cut the fibrous tissue covering the muscle.

What else should you know?

With proper treatment, rest, and rehabilitation, most leg injuries don't cause long-term effects. And by taking some simple precautions, the person can avoid recurrence of the injury. (See *How to avoid flare-ups.*)

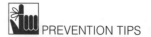
PREVENTION TIPS

How to avoid flare-ups

After a leg injury, be kind to your legs. Avoiding a flare-up of the injury can be as simple as taking the common-sense precautions described below.

Give your leg time to heal

■ Resume activities *gradually* — especially those that involve running.
■ Work with a trainer or physical therapist to strengthen the affected muscles.

Exercise with caution

■ Perform stretching and warm-up exercises before strenuous activity.
■ Run or train on a dirt track, not concrete.

Treat your feet well

■ Wear proper shoes when running.
■ Ask your doctor about wearing shoe inserts to take stress

LIGHTNING STRIKE

Lightning is a massive bolt of electricity that moves from one object — a thunderhead cloud — to another object of opposite charge — the earth. Lightning travels the path of least resistance. When it hits, it is more likely to strike an object sticking up from the earth's surface. This could be a tree, a telephone pole, or a person.

Direct and indirect targets

A person standing in a field may be the tallest thing around. A golfer

Most people aren't struck by lightning directly but are injured when lightning hits a nearby object, such as the tree they're standing under. On average, lightning strikes injure 300 Americans and kill 93 each year.

standing on a fairway not only may be the tallest thing around but may be holding a lightning rod — a golf club. (See *How to avoid a lightning strike.*)

However, most lightning strikes aren't direct. Typically, people are injured when lightning hits a nearby object, such as the tree they're standing under.

Your chance of being struck by lightning is roughly 1 in 600,000. On average, lightning strikes injure 300 Americans and kill 93 each year.

Lightning's path through the body

Lightning instantly travels a path through the body. Lightning that enters a person's body at the torso, leaving an entry burn, may exit one or both feet, leaving exit burns.

Along the path between entry and exit, lightning does considerable damage. Here are some examples:

■ Internal organs may be injured, especially those that contain air (the air heats up and conducts electricity poorly).
■ Muscles may be damaged.
■ Chemicals released by the injured muscles may harm the kidneys.
■ Bones may break, and violent muscle contractions may injure the spine.
■ The tympanic membranes — structures that transmit sound vibrations to the internal ear — may rupture.

What's more, lightning shocks the heart like a giant version of the paddles doctors use to shock a patient's heart in the hospital. And just like the patient's heart, the heart of someone who's been struck by lightning often starts beating again spontaneously.

What are the symptoms?

Lightning disrupts the brain's control over breathing. That's why a person who has been struck by lightning may not be breathing. Also, most people hit by lightning lose consciousness for some time. Almost all are confused and don't remember the event. Many suffer temporary paralysis of the legs; a few suffer permanent paralysis.

A lightning strike may also cause:

■ disorientation
■ dizziness
■ inability to speak
■ shock (which can cause such symptoms as anxiety, restlessness, a fast pulse, rapid breathing, and confusion).

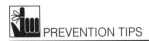 PREVENTION TIPS

How to avoid a lightning strike

Would you know what to do if you were caught outdoors during an electrical storm? Here's some advice worth remembering.

Find shelter

■ If you can hear thunder, you're close enough to the storm to be struck by lightning. Immediately take shelter in a sturdy building or a car with the windows rolled up.

■ If you're riding in a car, keep the windows closed.

■ If you're not near a sturdy building or a car, take shelter in a low spot away from trees, poles, and fences. If you're in the woods, find a short tree. Make sure the place you pick isn't likely to flood.

■ Don't run across an open area to seek shelter. Lightning can outrun you.

Avoid dangerous areas

■ Don't take shelter in a small shed, under an isolated tree, or in a convertible car.

■ Stay away from open water. If you're in a boat when an electrical storm comes up, immediately go to shore and get out.

Shrink the target

■ If you can feel your skin tingle or your hair stand on end, that means lightning's dangerously close. Make yourself the smallest target possible by squatting low to the ground on the balls of your feet, as you see in this picture. This will minimize your contact with the ground. Put your hands on your knees and lower your head.

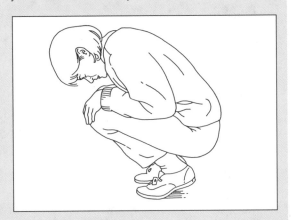

Other precautions

■ Don't touch metal objects, such as a golf club, a fishing rod, or an antenna, during an electrical storm. The object could become a lightning rod.

■ Don't use the telephone or an electrical appliance. You could be struck by lighting while talking on the phone.

■ Don't take a shower or a bath during an electrical storm.

What should you do?

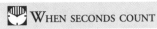 WHEN SECONDS COUNT

When you arrive at the scene of a lightning strike, check to see how many people have been hurt. Then send someone to call for emergency medical help.

If several people have been injured, first attend to anyone who isn't breathing. Check to see if this person has a pulse. If not, start CPR if you know how. (See *Performing CPR on an adult,* page 579, *Performing CPR on a child,* page 585, or *Performing CPR on an infant,* page 590.)

If the person *does* have a pulse, start rescue breathing (mouth-to-mouth resuscitation). Keep giving rescue breaths until emergency personnel arrive.

> Don't extend the person's head back too far to open the airway. Doing so could worsen any neck or spinal injury. Instead, raise the chin with the person's head flat on the ground.

What to do if the storm continues

If the electrical storm is still raging, get the person to a safe place, preferably indoors. Don't worry — touching the person won't harm you. After moving the person, help him or her to lie down and raise the feet and legs 8 to 12 inches.

Conserve body heat by wrapping the person with a coat or blanket, if possible. Then call for medical help immediately. Even a person who is conscious and talking could have massive internal injuries.

How is a lightning strike treated?

Emergency rescuers give the person oxygen and continue rescue breathing, if necessary. Some people require these treatments for several hours after their heartbeats have been restored.

The medical team continues to monitor the person's heart rhythm. They start intravenous lines to administer fluids and medicines, dress any burns, and splint any broken bones. They also check carefully for internal bleeding, abdominal injuries, and hidden fractures and closely monitor the function of the person's nervous system.

What else should you know?

Lightning can carry 100 million volts of electricity at a peak current of about 200,000 amps. So what explains the fact that most lightning victims survive the strike, even though they may have appeared to be dead afterward?

Unlike the alternating current in your house, lightning is a direct current and therefore less dangerous. Also, a lightning strike lasts only milliseconds; this usually limits internal damage to short-circuiting of the body's electrical systems. Many victims of lightning can be revived after they stop breathing.

If the electrical storm is still raging, get the person to a safe place, preferably indoors. Don't worry — touching the person won't harm you.

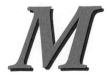

MEMORY LAPSE

We all forget things occasionally, especially as we get older. Many people over age 65 have trouble remembering names and absorbing new information.

But some people suffer memory lapses that aren't age-related. Even children can have memory lapses. (See *Seizures and memory lapses in children,* page 353.)

Doctors separate memory problems that aren't age-related into organic amnesia, hysterical amnesia, and treatment-caused amnesia.

Organic, or true, amnesia

This form of memory lapse results from a dysfunction in the brain. Typically, the person retains patches of memory. Causes of organic amnesia include:

■ head injury
■ seizures
■ Alzheimer's disease
■ herpes simplex encephalitis, a brain inflammation
■ Wernicke-Korsakoff syndrome, a behavior disorder caused by thiamine deficiency that is most common in alcoholics
■ shortage of oxygen to the brain
■ problems in the arteries of the neck or at the base of the skull.

Hysterical amnesia

This form of memory lapse has no underlying physical cause. Usually, the memory loss is complete. It starts and ends abruptly.

Treatment-induced amnesia

This form of memory lapse can come from:
■ drugs, such as general anesthetics (used for surgery), barbiturates (like Seconal), and some sedative-hypnotic medications (especially Halcion)
■ surgery on one of the brain's temporal lobes, which usually causes brief, slight memory loss.

> *Organic (true) amnesia results from a dysfunction in the brain. Typically, the person retains patches of memory.*

What are the symptoms?

Depending on the cause, memory lapse can come on suddenly or gradually. It may be partial or complete, temporary or permanent.

Some people have what doctors call *anterograde amnesia*, meaning they can't form new memories or remember events that have occurred since the memory loss started. Others have *retrograde amnesia* — loss of memory for past events or trouble remembering events that happened before the onset of amnesia.

Other symptoms to watch for

Depending on the cause, the person may have any of these other symptoms:

- agitation
- confusion
- inability to concentrate
- disorientation
- headache
- vision changes
- tingling sensations.

What should you do?

If the memory lapse is sudden or follows an injury, get emergency medical assistance.

For a more gradual memory lapse, call the doctor to report the problem and any other symptoms, and make an appointment for an exam.

If the memory lapse is sudden or follows an injury, get emergency medical assistance. For a more gradual memory lapse, call the doctor.

How is memory lapse treated?

To determine the right treatment, the doctor evaluates the person to find out the type of memory loss and identify the cause. To check the person's *recent memory*, the doctor asks questions like "How did you get here?" and "What was the day before yesterday?" To test *intermediate memory*, the doctor asks questions like "Who was the president before this one?" or "What was the last car you bought?" Asking "How old are you?" or "Where were you born?" helps the doctor evaluate the person's *remote memory*.

The doctor also performs a physical exam, including a check of the pupils, level of consciousness, movements, and sensory function.

Performing diagnostic tests

Depending on what the exam reveals, the doctor may recommend diagnostic tests to pinpoint the cause of the memory lapse. These tests may include:

- computed tomography (commonly called a CAT scan)
- recordings of brain wave activity (commonly called EEG)
- special X-rays of the brain's blood vessels (called cerebral angiography).

Treating the underlying cause

If the memory loss stems from an injury, the doctor may prescribe steroids and Osmitrol, a diuretic, to reduce brain swelling.

Helping the person cope

A person who can't remember events before the amnesia started may benefit from frequent orientations to reality — say, being shown familiar photos or objects by family members and friends.

If the person can't remember new information, you can help by writing down important information like drug dosages and locations of important documents in the home so he or she won't have to rely on memory.

What else should you know?

Depression, difficulty sleeping, and drug use can impair memory — especially in the elderly. In fact, depression may make an older person appear senile. Suspect depression in an older person with these symptoms:

- apathy
- lack of energy
- trouble sleeping
- poor appetite
- poor hygiene
- inability to find pleasure in life.

Drug-related memory lapse

Older adults who take many medicines are at particular risk for memory impairment. The problem may come from drug interactions or from overmedication (people become more sensitive to drug effects as they age). If the person incorrectly assumes that the memory lapses stem from aging, he or she might not suspect that the drugs are the problem.

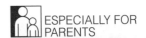

ESPECIALLY FOR PARENTS

Seizures and memory lapses in children

A child who gets seizures may suffer memory lapses. Sometimes, the memory lapses lead to the child mistakenly being classified as "learning disabled."

Talk to the doctor

If this has happened to your child, talk with the doctor about ways you and your child's teachers can cope with the problem.

Other tips

- Be sure your child follows the prescribed schedule for anti-seizure medicine.
- Continually review events the child has forgotten.
- Remind your child that he or she isn't to blame for the memory lapses or the seizures.

MIGRAINE

Everyone gets headaches once in a while. Most ordinary headaches succumb to simple measures, such as over-the-counter medications like aspirin, acetaminophen (Tylenol), or ibuprofen (Advil or Motrin).

But some headaches are so severe that they disrupt the person's life. Migraine is an example. More than 10% of Americans get migraines — more women than men. Often, migraine runs in families. Typically, the person first gets migraine as a child or teenager and then has recurrences throughout adulthood.

Biochemical abnormality?

Migraines are called *vascular headaches* because they're linked to contractions of blood vessels in the head. Medical scientists don't know exactly what causes them, but they suspect that certain biochemical abnormalities occur during a migraine. These abnormalities may include:

■ leakage of a substance that widens blood vessels through already enlarged arteries in the head

■ a decrease in the level of serotonin, a crucial chemical messenger in the brain.

Types of migraine

Migraines occur in four basic types.

■ *Common migraine,* the most prevalent, tends to occur on weekends and holidays. The day before it starts, the person may experience fatigue, nausea, and vomiting.

■ *Classic migraine* typically strikes compulsive personalities and runs in families.

■ *Basilar artery migraine* tends to afflict young women before their menstrual periods.

■ *Hemiplegic and ophthalmoplegic migraine,* the rarest type, usually occurs in young adults. Even after this headache goes away, the person may have nervous system problems, such as partial or complete paralysis of half of the body.

What are the symptoms?

Migraines cause intense, throbbing pain. The pain may begin on one side, then spread throughout the head.

Migraines cause intense, throbbing pain. The pain may begin on one side, then spread throughout the head.

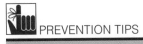

Beating migraines through diet

Changing your diet may help you avoid migraines and other vascular headaches. That's because chemicals in certain foods act directly on blood vessels to trigger headaches. Read this chart to learn which foods are safe and which foods you should avoid.

FOOD GROUP	FOODS TO AVOID	FOODS TO ENJOY
Bread and cereal	■ Hot, fresh homemade yeast bread, yeast coffee cake, sourdough bread, doughnuts ■ Bread or crackers containing cheese ■ Baked goods made with chocolate or nuts	■ Bagels; crackers; English muffins; French or Italian, rye, white, or whole-wheat bread; melba toast
Dairy products	■ Cultured dairy products, such as buttermilk and sour cream ■ Chocolate milk ■ Bleu, brick, Camembert, cheddar, Gouda, mozzarella, Parmesan, provolone, Romano, Roquefort, Stilton, and Swiss (Emmentaler) cheeses	■ Whole milk, 2% and 1% milk, skim milk ■ American, cottage, cream, farmer, and ricotta cheeses; processed and imitation cheeses ■ Yogurt (no more than $\frac{1}{2}$ cup per day)
Meat, fish, and poultry	■ Aged, canned, cured, or processed meat or fish, such as hot dogs, canned ham, pickled herring, cold cuts, and bacon ■ Meat prepared with meat tenderizer, soy sauce, or yeast extract	■ All fresh or frozen beef, lamb, pork, poultry, and veal ■ Fresh and frozen fish ■ Eggs (no more than three per week)
Fruits and vegetables	■ Apples, applesauce, apricots, avocados, cherries, figs, fruit cocktail, papaya, passion fruit, peaches, pears, raisins, and red plums ■ Broad, fava, lima, navy, pinto, or pole beans; garbanzos; lentils; olives; onions (except for seasoning); pickles; sauerkraut; snow peas	■ All fruits and vegetables except those listed unless instructed otherwise by the doctor ■ Citrus fruit (limit to $\frac{1}{2}$ cup per day)
Sweets and desserts	■ Mincemeat pie ■ Cake, candy, cookies, ice cream, or pudding containing carob or chocolate	■ Cake and cookies made without chocolate or yeast, gelatin, ice milk ■ Jam, jelly, hard candy, honey, sugar

(continued)

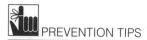

Beating migraines through diet *(continued)*

FOOD GROUP	FOODS TO AVOID	FOODS TO ENJOY
Miscellaneous	■ Bouillon cubes, canned soup, or soup base with monosodium glutamate (MSG) ■ Cheese sauce; snack foods and dishes containing cheese ■ Yeast and yeast extract, brewer's yeast ■ Meat tenderizer, MSG, seasoned salt, soy sauce (read labels) ■ Marinated, pickled, or preserved food ■ Nuts and seeds	■ Cream soups made with permissible ingredients, homemade broth ■ Salt (in moderation), lemon juice ■ Butter, margarine, cooking oil ■ Whipped cream ■ White vinegar, commercial salad dressing in small amounts

Aura: A common warning sign

Before a migraine starts, the person may experience a sensation called an aura. During the aura, the person may:

■ see spots, light flashes, or a luminous object with zigzag outlines
■ lack vision in half the visual field
■ smell peculiar odors.

Other symptoms to watch for

During a migraine, some people also experience:

■ irritability
■ appetite loss
■ nausea
■ vomiting
■ unusual sensitivity to light or noise
■ abnormal sensations, such as prickling or tingling, on one side of the body
■ speech disorders.

What should you do?

If the person already has been diagnosed with migraine, make sure he or she takes the prescribed migraine drug at the first sign of an attack. Have the person lie down in a quiet, dark room and rest until the pain subsides. Place ice packs over the forehead or a cold cloth over the eyes. Call the doctor and report all symptoms.

If the person has been vomiting, give plenty of fluids once the vomiting subsides to ward off dehydration.

How is migraine treated?
The doctor may prescribe a drug like Imitrex, Ergostat, or Cafergot. These drugs work by narrowing the arteries in the head. They're most effective when taken as soon as the migraine starts. People who can't take Ergostat or Cafergot by mouth because of nausea and vomiting should ask the doctor to prescribe the rectal suppositories.

To help *prevent* migraine, the doctor may prescribe a drug like Inderal, Tenormin, Catapres, or Elavil.

What else should you know?
Some migraine sufferers find that modifying their diet helps to prevent migraine. (See *Beating migraines through diet,* page 355.)

MOUTH SORES

Mouth sores can take the form of ulcers (most common), cysts, blisters, or lesions. The sores may occur anywhere on the lips, cheeks, inside of the mouth, tongue, gums, salivary glands, or mucous membranes.

Most mouth sores aren't serious. But some may indicate a potentially serious problem and should be examined by a doctor right away.

Understanding the causes
Mouth sores most commonly come from:
- a virus
- an infection
- ill-fitting dentures
- uneven teeth.

Less commonly, mouth sores result from an injury, a body-wide illness, drugs, or radiation therapy.

Most mouth sores aren't serious. But some may indicate a potentially serious problem and should be examined by a doctor right away.

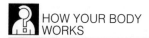

HOW YOUR BODY
WORKS

A look at an aphthous ulcer

With aphthous stomatitis, numerous small
round blisters, or ulcers, erupt in the mouth.
The blisters soon break, leaving shallow,
red-ringed ulcers.

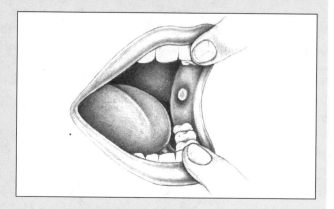

What are the symptoms?

Many mouth sores cause pain. But some cause no symptoms; if
they're deep in the mouth, they may be discovered only through a
complete mouth exam.

Besides mouth pain, the person may experience:
- bleeding or swollen gums
- extreme tenderness of the mouth
- fever.

Other symptoms depend on what is causing the mouth sores.

Symptoms of a herpes infection

The person with herpes simplex virus may have sores on any part of
the mouth or throat — especially the tongue, gums, and inside of
the cheeks. Eventually, the sores resemble blisters with reddened
edges. Pain usually disappears 2 to 4 days before the sores heal completely. If a child with oral herpes simplex sucks his or her thumb,
the sores can spread to the hands.

Symptoms of aphthous stomatitis

This recurring condition typically causes burning, tingling, or slight
mouth swelling, plus shallow ulcers (canker sores) with white centers and red borders. (See *A look at an aphthous ulcer.*)

Symptoms of candidiasis

Also called *oral thrush,* this condition may cause cream-colored or bluish-white patches on the tongue, mouth, or throat. Although seldom painful, the patches may cause a burning sensation.

What should you do?

If the mouth sores don't heal within 2 weeks, have the person see a doctor or dentist. To prevent further irritation, he or she should avoid highly seasoned foods, citrus fruits, alcohol, and tobacco.

Emphasize good oral hygiene

Proper oral hygiene is important, too. If the sores make brushing the teeth difficult or painful, the person should rinse the mouth in salt water or a solution of one part water to one part hydrogen peroxide.

> ✖ Don't use commercial mouthwashes that contain alcohol; the alcohol could irritate the mouth sores.

How are mouth sores treated?

Treatment depends on the cause of the mouth sores. The doctor usually prescribes therapy to relieve pain and other symptoms — for instance, a topical anesthetic, such as lidocaine, or an anesthetic mouthwash, such as liquid Xylocaine.

Treating an oral infection

Treatment may include oral surgery, antibiotic drug therapy, or improved oral hygiene.

Treating herpes

During an initial outbreak of herpes simplex, the doctor may prescribe aspirin or acetaminophen (Tylenol) to reduce fever and relieve pain. Anesthetic mouthwashes help ease pain from mouth sores. (See *How to soothe a cold sore.*)

Treating candidiasis

The doctor recommends ways to make the person less vulnerable to the infection, such as controlling diabetes or discontinuing antibiotic drugs. The doctor may also prescribe an antifungal medicine, such as Diflucan, Monistat, Mycelex, or Nizoral.

What else should you know?

In children, mouth sores typically result from:

How to soothe a cold sore

Although there's no cure for a cold sore caused by herpes simplex, you can take steps to relieve the discomfort.

Use cold treatments and pain medicine

- Try applying cool compresses to the sore. As the doctor directs, take aspirin, acetaminophen (Tylenol), or other pain relievers.
- Also consider using an over-the-counter cold sore remedy recommended by your doctor, such as Campho-Phenique or Blistex.

Other instructions

- Avoid irritating foods and beverages. For instance, stay away from grapefruit juice, which has a high citric acid content.
- Call your doctor if the cold sore doesn't heal in 10 days or if you get frequent recurrences.

- herpes simplex virus
- chickenpox
- measles
- scarlet fever
- diphtheria
- hand-foot-and-mouth disease.

In newborns, candidiasis or congenital syphilis are common causes of mouth sores.

NAUSEA AND VOMITING

Nausea is a feeling of profound revulsion to food. It often leads to vomiting, or regurgitating.

Both nausea and vomiting are responses to a message from the brain. The message causes muscles in the abdomen to contract and the ring of muscle between the stomach and the esophagus, called the *esophageal sphincter*, to open. As a result, the stomach contents, which normally flow down through the digestive tract, push upward and out of the mouth by reverse contractions of the esophagus.

Understanding the causes
Nausea and vomiting can be early symptoms of pregnancy or can result from many other conditions. These conditions include:
- a peptic ulcer
- liver inflammation (hepatitis)
- inflammation of the appendix (appendicitis)
- acute inflammation of the stomach lining (gastritis); for instance, from aspirin or aspirin-related drugs, steroids, alcohol, or infectious bacteria
- gallbladder disease
- a digestive tract infection such as the flu
- a central nervous system problem
- food poisoning
- anxiety
- pain
- overeating
- alcohol intoxication
- surgery
- migraine
- radiation therapy.

What are the symptoms?
Nausea and vomiting are often accompanied by:
- increased salivation

Nausea and vomiting are responses to a message from the brain. The message triggers a series of events that causes the stomach contents, which normally flow down through the digestive tract, to push upward and out of the mouth.

- sweating
- fast pulse
- pale skin
- rapid breathing.

What should you do?

Get medical help right away if the person has blood in the vomit or severe stomach pain or if he or she has suffered a head injury. Also call for immediate help for an infant who is experiencing forceful vomiting. (See *What to do when your child vomits.*)

Get prompt medical attention for someone who is experiencing severe nausea or frequent vomiting or has been vomiting for more than 24 hours.

What to do if the person is unconscious

If the person is unconscious and vomiting, place him or her on the side with the neck extended (unless you suspect a head, neck, or back injury). This will prevent the person from choking on the vomit.

If the person has a head injury, roll him or her to a side-lying position. This position drains the vomit and keeps the airway open. While rolling the person, be sure to stabilize the neck against movement.

What to do for simple nausea and vomiting

For simple nausea and vomiting accompanied by an upset stomach, try to make the person comfortable. After the vomiting has stopped, replace lost fluids. For instance, give a teaspoonful of clear liquid every 15 minutes until the person can keep it down. Safe liquids include:
- flat ginger ale
- flat cola (unless the person has diarrhea)
- gelatin that is not gelled (any color except red, which can irritate the stomach).

Then progress to small sips of clear liquids every 15 minutes. Make sure the liquids you give are at room temperature.

How are nausea and vomiting treated?

For severe nausea and vomiting, the doctor orders treatments to relieve symptoms, replace lost fluids, and correct the underlying condition. Depending on the cause of the nausea and vomiting, the person may need drugs or even surgery.

If the person is unconscious and vomiting, place him or her on the side with the neck extended (unless you suspect a head, neck, or back injury). This will prevent the person from choking on the vomit.

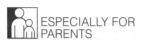

ESPECIALLY FOR
PARENTS

What to do when your child vomits

A common childhood symptom, vomiting usually comes from having an upset stomach. Often, it's not serious. But sometimes vomiting calls for immediate medical attention. Read what follows to learn how to respond to either situation.

When to call the doctor
Get medical help immediately if your *infant* experiences *projectile vomiting.* In this type of vomiting, the child expels the vomited material with such force that it shoots out of the mouth 1 or 2 feet across the room. Projectile vomiting could indicate a partially or completely blocked intestine.

Other urgent situations
Call the doctor immediately if:
- your child's vomit contains blood
- your child vomits several hours after a fall or a head injury
- vomiting is accompanied by a headache or stomachache

How to deal with prolonged vomiting
Prolonged vomiting, especially when coupled with diarrhea, warrants a prompt call to the doctor. This problem can lead to dehydration, or loss of body fluids, which is particularly dangerous in a child.

How to cope with simple vomiting
For simple vomiting without other worrisome symptoms, try to keep your child comfortable. Support his or her forehead with your hand during vomiting. Afterward, offer water to rinse out the mouth and sponge off your child's face.

To replace your child's lost body fluids and help prevent repeated vomiting, follow these suggestions.

Replace lost fluids
- Start by giving very small sips (1 teaspoon) of flat soda, tea, or juice (not orange), every 10 to 20 minutes until your child keeps it down. Or have your child suck on lollipops or ice pops.
- Gradually increase the amount of liquid you offer your child.

Add solid foods
- If your child goes 4 hours without vomiting, offer dry toast or plain crackers. Progress to a bland, light diet.
- Slowly reintroduce your child's regular diet after the stomach has settled.

For simple nausea and vomiting, treatment includes comfort measures, fluid replacement, and a gradual return to a regular diet.

What else should you know?
During recovery from a bout of nausea and vomiting, the person may begin to consume progressively larger amounts of beverages and foods. For instance, if he or she goes 4 hours without vomiting, you can give increasingly large sips of clear liquid at room temperature, plus dry toast or plain crackers.

If these foods don't upset the person's stomach, advance to bland, light foods like soft-boiled eggs, boiled chicken, and clear — not cream — soups. After 24 hours without vomiting, the person can start to eat regular foods but must avoid spices and overeating.

NEAR DROWNING

In near drowning, a person survives an episode of inhaling water. (See *What happens when someone drowns.*)

How near drowning occurs
Many drowning and near-drowning victims find themselves in water unexpectedly; for example, after a boating accident or a fall from a dock or bridge. Others are swimmers who can't stay afloat for reasons ranging from poor swimming skills and fatigue to poisonous stings from aquatic animals, heavy drinking, or a medical emergency like a heart attack.

Unattended toddlers have drowned after falling into toilets. An adult can drown in a bathtub that contains only a few inches of water or in a bucket left in the backyard. (See *How to prevent drowning,* page 366.)

Unattended toddlers have drowned after falling into toilets. An adult can drown in a bathtub that contains only a few inches of water or in a bucket left in the backyard.

What are the symptoms?
No matter how expert a swimmer a person may be, he or she can run into trouble in the water. Stay alert for the following symptoms of distress in a swimmer:
- difficulty breathing
- signaling for help (although some drowning people aren't able to)
- struggling or making little or no forward progress.

Symptoms after rescue
After rescue, the person may be unconscious or have a decreased level of consciousness (such as stupor). Or he or she may seem apprehensive, irritable, restless, or sluggish. Other symptoms at this time may include:
- rapid, slow, or absent pulse
- irregular heartbeats

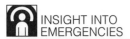

What happens when someone drowns

Being submerged in water is obviously life-threatening but not precisely for the reason you might assume — inhaling water. Although inhaling water does trigger a chain of dangerous events, the real peril is shortage of oxygen in the body.

Path to peril
Here's what happens: While submerged in water, the person inhales or swallows water. In response, he or she starts to hold the breath. This increases the amount of carbon dioxide in the bloodstream.

The drive to breathe
After a certain point, the increased carbon dioxide level stimulates the brain's respiratory center. This in turn forces the person to breathe. While breathing, the person swallows or inhales even more water. Then the person vomits and may inhale some of the vomit. After this, he or she may lose con-

sciousness, have seizures, and inhale even more water.

What happens if the throat closes
In some people, the throat closes up after they inhale water. This blocks the airway and prevents inhalation of more water. The person then asphyxiates — stops breathing from lack of oxygen — and loses consciousness.

Surviving a cold-water near drowning
Some people — especially young children — who have been submerged in cold water (below 70° F [21.1° C]) survive near drowning without brain damage. Rescue breathing, CPR, or both must begin immediately and continue until the person warms up and starts to breathe unassisted. This can take several hours.

- shallow or gasping breathing, or no breathing
- vomiting
- low body temperature (if the near drowning took place in cold water)
- cough that produces pink, frothy phlegm
- swollen abdomen
- pale or bluish skin
- chest pain
- stoppage of the heart.

What should you do?
If you decide to try to rescue a drowning person, keep in mind that poor judgment or poor technique could cause *both* of you to drown. For instance, the drowning person could pull you under in a desperate, flailing panic.

For this reason, it's best to attempt a rescue by reaching out to the person or throwing the person a life preserver. Read what fol-

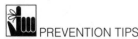
PREVENTION TIPS

How to prevent drowning

The best way to prevent drowning is to obey water safety measures when swimming. Also, if you spend time near the water, consider taking a water safety course sponsored by the Red Cross, YMCA, or YWCA.

Follow water safety guidelines
■ Never swim alone. Remember the buddy system: If everyone is responsible for one other person, no one can slip away unnoticed into the water.
■ Don't dive into shallow water. If you're not sure how deep the water is, don't dive.

Stay sober and alert
■ Avoid drinking alcohol or taking drugs before swimming or boating.

■ Don't steer a boat after using prescription drugs that can cause drowsiness.

Take precautions in winter
■ Don't walk on ice unless you're certain it's frozen solid.
■ Don't sled on frozen ponds if the ice isn't solid.

Be careful during a flood
■ Never try to navigate a road that's been closed because of small-stream flooding.
■ Keep children away from streams that have suddenly risen. Children may not understand that the trickle they waded in last August is now a raging torrent that could sweep them away. Better yet, never leave a child unattended near water.

lows to learn about the reaching assist, the throwing assist, and several other rescue methods.

Reaching assist
While staying on dry land, reach out your hand to the person or offer a paddle, tree limb, chair, board, rope, or pole.

Throwing assist
Toss the person a life preserver that's tied to your boat, the dock, or the side of the pool.

Wading assist
Wade out to the person who is struggling in shallow water, but don't go in deeper than waist-high water. Extend a pole, stick, life preserver, or rope. Then pull the person to safety.

Rowing assist
If you have a boat, you can row out to the person. Have the person hang on to the back of the boat, if he or she is able, while you row to

shore. If the person can't do this, try to lift him or her carefully into the boat without tipping it over.

> ⊗ Be sure not to attempt a swimming rescue unless you've been trained to do so. You could drown if the person pulls you under.
>
> ⊗ Never overestimate your strength when attempting a rescue. Know your physical limitations.

⊞ WHEN SECONDS COUNT

When you reach the person, look, listen, and feel for breathing. If breathing is absent, start rescue (mouth-to-mouth) breathing immediately — even before you've pulled the person completely out of the water, if necessary. Have someone call for emergency medical help. Continue rescue breathing while supporting the person, such as in a boat or in shallow water. Once the person is out of the water, place him or her on a firm surface and continue rescue breathing. Then start CPR, if you know how. (See *Performing CPR on an adult,* page 579, *Performing CPR on a child,* page 585, or *Performing CPR on an infant,* page 590.)

> ⊗ Don't waste time trying to drain water from the person's lungs. Instead, begin rescue breathing at once if the person isn't breathing.
>
> ⊗ Be sure you don't stop rescue breathing too early; this method may take some time to restore the person's breathing. Continue it until the emergency rescue team arrives. If you get tired, ask someone to relieve you.
>
> ⊗ Never move the person if you suspect a neck injury, unless the person's life or your own is in danger. If you must move the person to save his or her life, first place a board under the person for support. If the person is face down in the water, gently roll him or her over, keeping the head, neck, and body aligned. (See *Protecting the person's neck,* page 368.)

If the person isn't breathing, start rescue breathing immediately, even before you've pulled the person completely out of the water, if necessary.

How is near drowning treated?

Emergency treatment for near drowning begins with CPR, oxygen administration, and neck stabilization in case of spinal injury. When the person arrives at the hospital, the medical team establishes an open airway, if necessary, while continuing to perform CPR. The person may need to have a breathing tube inserted as well as breathing assistance from a mechanical ventilator.

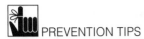 PREVENTION TIPS

Protecting the person's neck

Every year, many people dive into shallow water or injure themselves while surfing. Tragically, some suffer neck or spinal injuries that paralyze them for life.

That's why it's important to learn what to do — and what *not* to do — if you come across someone who has just had a diving or surfboard accident. Your first actions may help the person avoid permanent injury. Here's how to proceed.

Call for help

■ Have someone call for emergency medical help immediately.

■ If a rescue team is expected soon, wait for them to arrive. They'll have the proper equipment for handling a suspected neck injury.

Keep the head, neck, and body aligned

■ If emergency help isn't available, you may have to move the person. Try to enlist the aid of another rescuer to do this. And remember the cardinal rule of moving someone with a possible neck or spinal injury: *Keep the person's head, neck, and body aligned at all times.*

■ If you find the person face down, gently turn him or her over.

■ While the person is still in the water, place a surfboard, other board, or table leaf under the head, neck, and torso. Make sure the board extends under the buttocks. Then use the board to lift the person out of the water.

■ If a board isn't available, tow the person by gently lifting him or her under the armpits.

Other important precautions

■ Don't pull the person sideways. Whether you push or pull, always keep the person's head in line with the body.

■ Keep the person on the board after rescue. Don't rush to move him or her unless you're sure the person is in danger.

■ If you must perform rescue breathing or CPR, move the person as little as possible. For example, lift the chin only as much as necessary to open the airway.

Drug treatments

Drugs used to treat a near-drowning victim may include:
■ high concentrations of oxygen
■ steroids to reduce swelling within the brain
■ antibiotics to prevent infection
■ bronchodilators to widen the airways.

Observation

Because of the possibility that breathing distress will recur, the person is usually observed in the hospital for 24 to 48 hours.

What else should you know?

Respiratory distress may suddenly arise several minutes or even several days after a near drowning. For instance, the person may suffer pulmonary edema (leakage of fluid into the lungs) or aspiration pneumonia, caused by inhaling water. That's why even if the person seems to have completely recovered, he or she requires 24 hours of observation to detect late-developing symptoms.

NECK PAIN

Ranging from mild to severe, neck pain usually results from an injury. But it can also be a symptom of a wide range of diseases. (See *What causes neck pain?*)

Neck pain can arise from any part of the neck — from the membranes that enclose the spinal cord to the neck bones (vertebrae) to the blood vessels, muscles, or lymphatic tissue.

When is neck pain serious?
Sometimes, neck pain reflects a serious condition. For example, a person whose neck is injured in a car accident may have suffered damage to the brain or spinal cord.

What are the symptoms?
Neck pain may be:
- mild, moderate, or severe
- persistent or changing
- recurrent or limited to one episode.

The pain may be aggravated by movement, or it may restrict the person's movement. Pain location can vary too. It may be centered in the back or front of the neck, may affect the entire neck, or spread to the shoulders or arms.

Other symptoms to watch for
Neck swelling, stiffness, and rigidity often go along with neck pain. Other symptoms vary with the underlying cause. They may include:
- headache
- numbness or tingling in the arms and legs
- weakness of the arms or legs
- pain on moving the arms or legs
- deformity of the back or neck

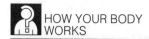
HOW YOUR BODY WORKS

What causes neck pain?

Many different diseases and injuries can cause neck pain. Here's a partial list.

Bone and joint diseases
- ankylosing spondylitis, a chronic inflammatory disease of the spine
- arthritis
- Paget's disease, a bone disorder
- stiffness of the neck joints
- thinning bones (osteoporosis)

Cancers
- cancer of the voicebox (larynx)
- Hodgkin's disease, a cancer of the lymphatic system
- spinal tumor

Other diseases
- infection of the neck portion of the spine
- inflamed lymph nodes in the neck
- inflammation or infection of the brain and spinal cord membranes (meningitis)

Injuries
- broken neck
- injury to the food tube (esophagus), thyroid gland, or windpipe
- "slipped" (herniated) disk in the neck
- sprained neck

Stabilizing the neck with a Philadelphia collar

To stabilize a person's neck after a neck injury, the medical team may apply a Philadelphia collar. This device immobilizes the neck, eases muscle spasms, and reduces pain. It also prevents further injury and promotes healing.

How the collar keeps the neck straight

Made of lightweight, molded polyethylene, the collar keeps the neck straight while keeping the person's chin slightly elevated and tucked in. It prevents the person from moving the neck too far backward or forward but allows slight neck rotation and sideways movement. (However, depending on the person's condition, the doctor may not want the person to move the neck at all.)

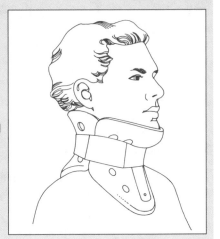

- tenderness along the back of the neck or spine
- complete or partial paralysis
- loss of bladder or bowel control
- inability to breathe.

What should you do?

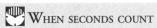 **WHEN SECONDS COUNT**

Get medical help immediately for a person who has suffered a neck injury.

What to do if the person is unconscious

- Assume that the neck and spine are injured. To prevent further injury to the neck, you must immobilize the person's neck and back. You can make a neck collar from fabric, folded newspaper, towels, or a blanket that has been folded to a width of about 4 inches. Without interfering with the person's breathing, fasten the collar and tie it loosely. Support the person's shoulders and back. (See *Stabilizing the neck with a Philadelphia collar.*)

- Next, check for an open airway, feel for a pulse, and look, listen, and feel for breathing. If the person isn't breathing, don't tilt the head back to try to open the airway. Instead, kneel behind the person's head. Then grasp the person's lower jaw by placing your thumbs on the jaw near the corner of the mouth; make sure your thumbs point toward the person's feet. With your fingertips at the angles of the jaw, lift the lower jaw upward with your index fingers while pushing your thumbs down. This action will make the person's jaw jut forward without tilting the neck.

■ After you've opened the airway, give rescue breaths (mouth-to-mouth resuscitation) if necessary to restore breathing. (See *Performing CPR on an adult,* page 579, *Performing CPR on a child,* page 585, or *Performing CPR on an infant,* page 590.)

 Never move the person unnecessarily. Movement could cause serious injury, paralysis, or even death.

 Don't give the person anything to eat or drink.

What to do if the neck hasn't been injured

If the person is experiencing neck pain but hasn't been in an accident, call the doctor as soon as possible for an evaluation.

How is neck pain treated?

The doctor tries to make the person as comfortable as possible, such as by prescribing anti-inflammatory drugs and pain relievers, as needed. To find out what is causing the neck pain or to evaluate the extent of neck injury, the person may undergo diagnostic tests, such as X-rays, computed tomography (commonly called a CAT scan), blood tests, and a spinal tap.

Other treatments

If arthritis or a neck sprain is the cause of the neck pain, helpful treatments may include:

■ heat application (hot packs or a heating pad)
■ anti-inflammatory drugs
■ massage.

If neck pain stems from Hodgkin's disease or another cancer, the person may need to undergo chemotherapy or radiation. For information on treatment of a broken neck, see "Spinal injuries," page 475.

What else should you know?

Injuries to the neck and spine are among the most serious because they can lead to paralysis or death. Always suspect a neck or spinal injury if a person complains of neck pain after:

■ a diving accident
■ a fall from a height greater than the person's height

To treat neck pain, the doctor tries to make the person as comfortable as possible, such as by prescribing anti-inflammatory drugs and pain relievers.

- an injury involving severe, blunt force to the head or trunk
- an injury that penetrates the person's head or trunk
- a motor vehicle accident in which the person wasn't wearing a seat belt
- an accident in which the person was thrown from a motor vehicle
- an accident in which the person's helmet was broken
- a lightning strike.

NECK STIFFNESS

When your neck is stiff, you can't flex it or move it from side to side without experiencing pain or muscle spasms. When a stiff neck comes from muscle sprain or strain (as it typically does), the condition usually is brief, relatively mild, and resolves quickly.

Understanding other causes
A severe, persistent stiff neck can herald a dangerous condition, such as:
- bleeding within the membranes covering the brain or spinal cord
- infection of these membranes (meningitis)
- severe brain inflammation and swelling (encephalitis).

Sometimes a stiff neck is a late sign of neck arthritis. In this disorder, the neck gradually becomes less mobile and flexible.

A severe, persistent stiff neck can herald a dangerous condition, such as bleeding within the brain, meningitis, or severe brain inflammation and swelling.

What are the symptoms?
A stiff neck causes varying degrees of neck pain and muscle spasms that worsen with movement. The stiffness may develop gradually or abruptly. It may be worse in the morning or after a period of inactivity.

Other symptoms to watch for
A person with a stiff neck also may have:
- neck tenderness
- headache
- fever (possibly with chills)
- nausea.

A stiff neck caused by muscle sprain or strain may be coupled with muscle aches, tension, or spasms in the neck.

Symptoms of a life-threatening problem
Suspect inflammation or infection of the brain and spinal cord membranes if the person has severe neck pain and muscle spasms when he or she tries to flex the neck. The stiff neck usually starts abruptly and is coupled with a severe headache. The person may also experience:
- nausea and vomiting
- sagging eyelids
- difficulty swallowing
- confusion
- lethargy
- coma.

What should you do?
For mild neck stiffness accompanied by muscle tension, spasms, and pain, the person should call the doctor to arrange for an appointment.

When SECONDS COUNT
Get medical help immediately if the person:
- has severe neck stiffness
- has neck stiffness that starts abruptly
- also has a severe headache, fever, nausea and vomiting, sagging eyelids, difficulty swallowing, confusion, lethargy, or loss of consciousness.

These symptoms could indicate encephalitis, meningitis, or bleeding with the brain or spinal cord membranes. (See *Danger in a child's stiff neck,* page 374.)

Get medical help immediately if the person has severe neck stiffness or neck stiffness that starts abruptly.

How is neck stiffness treated?
The person with a simple stiff neck receives treatments to relieve pain, inflammation, and other symptoms. The doctor typically recommends rest and pain relievers, such as aspirin, ibuprofen (Advil or Motrin), or acetaminophen (Tylenol).

Treating severe stiff neck
The doctor tries to pinpoint the underlying cause by performing a physical exam and ordering diagnostic tests, such as computed tomography (commonly called a CAT scan) and neck X-rays. To find

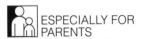

Danger in a child's stiff neck

If your child suddenly develops a severely stiff neck along with fever and irritability, get medical help immediately. These are symptoms of meningitis — a serious nervous system disease.

What causes meningitis?

In recent years, meningitis has been occurring among children in day care centers. The disease typically results from bacterial infection. Even an ear or sinus infection can lead to this life-threatening disease.

Other worrisome symptoms

Be aware that an infant aged 3 months to 2 years may have meningitis *without* a stiff neck. Call the doctor at once if your infant has any of these symptoms:

- fever
- vomiting
- irritability
- seizures
- a high-pitched cry
- bulging of the head.

out if the stiff neck results from brain or spinal cord inflammation, the doctor may do a spinal tap.

After identifying the cause of the stiff neck, the doctor orders appropriate treatments and takes steps to prevent complications.

What else should you know?

For a stiff neck caused by muscle strain or sprain, the person may benefit from self-treatments such as:

- gentle stretching exercises
- heat application
- massage.

NOSEBLEED

A severe nosebleed can come from an allergy, a cold, overusing nose drops, or blowing your nose too hard. But the most common reason for nosebleed is injury to the nose.

Dangerous situations

Sometimes a nosebleed results from a serious condition — for instance, high blood pressure. (See *Nosebleeds and high blood pressure: What is the link?*) Two other potentially dangerous situations are:

- when nosebleed results from a blow to the head
- when the bleeding is severe.

Nosebleeds in children

Nosebleeds are twice as common in children as in adults. In a child, a nosebleed tends to be mild and to originate in the front of the nasal septum — the partition that divides the two nostrils. (See *Stopping your child's nosebleed,* page 376.) In adults, nosebleed is more likely to be severe and to start in the back of the septum.

What are the symptoms?

A person with a nosebleed may have active bleeding from the nose or dried blood in the nostrils. Some people have no obvious bleeding but feel a sensation of blood trickling down the back of the throat.

What should you do?

Get medical help right away if the bleeding is severe or uncontrollable or if you suspect a broken nose or a serious head or neck injury.

What to do if the bleeding is moderate

Take these steps to stop the bleeding:

- Have the person pinch the nostrils firmly, unless you suspect the nose is broken. (See *Pinching to stop a nosebleed,* page 377.)
- Tell the person to sit up and lean slightly forward so blood won't drip down the back of the throat and be swallowed. Then instruct the person to spit out the blood into a bowl or other receptacle instead of swallowing it. Swallowing blood from a nosebleed can upset the stomach and cause vomiting.
- Instruct the person to pinch the nostrils with the thumb or forefinger for about 10 minutes while breathing through the mouth. At the same time, apply cold compresses to the nose.
- If bleeding continues after 10 or 15 minutes of direct pressure, call the doctor.
- Tell the person to keep breathing through the mouth for about 1 hour after the bleeding stops.

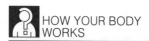

HOW YOUR BODY WORKS

Nosebleeds and high blood pressure: What is the link?

People with high blood pressure have a higher risk for nosebleeds. Here's why.

Arteries in the nose harden

High blood pressure tends to harden the arteries. The hardening causes blood vessels in the nose to degenerate. Blood vessels in poor condition are more likely to bleed.

More serious nosebleeds occur

The story doesn't end there. Nosebleeds tend to be more serious in people with high blood pressure because of the increased pressure on blood vessels. As a result, these people often require medical treatment to stop the bleeding.

How to ward off problems

If you have high blood pressure, consult your doctor to identify the exact cause of your nosebleeds. Then follow the doctor's recommendations to stop the nosebleeds from recurring.

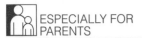

ESPECIALLY FOR
PARENTS

Stopping your child's nosebleed

Nosebleeds are common — and sometimes frightening — in kids. You can help prevent panic from setting in by teaching your child how to stop the bleeding. Follow these guidelines.

Apply pressure to the nose

■ Show your child how to use the thumb and fingers to pinch the lower half of the nose tightly shut. Tell him or her to breathe through the mouth while holding the nose like this for about 10 minutes.

■ If your child gets tired before the bleeding stops, show him or her how to switch hands by placing the thumb and fingers of the rested hand above the thumb and fingers of the tired hand. Tell the child to start pinching with the rested hand just before letting go with the tired one. Then the child can slide the fingers down the nose until they're pinching the lower half of the nose as before.

Practice on each other

■ If your child gets frequent nosebleeds, teach the pinching technique when the nose isn't bleeding. This will prepare your child to pinch properly the next time a nosebleed occurs.

■ Practice pinching each other's noses. This way, you'll both learn how much pressure to apply, and you'll know how your fingers feel when they're in the right position.

■ Watch to be sure your child compresses the entire lower half of the nose, not just the tip.

Sit still, don't panic — and other tips

■ Teach your child to sit down quietly and calmly whenever the nose starts to bleed. Demonstrate how to tilt the head slightly forward to avoid swallowing or choking on blood.

■ Warn the child not to tilt the head backward, not to lie down, and not to stuff a tissue in the nose.

■ Instruct your child to spit out — not swallow — any blood that gets in the mouth or throat. Spitting into a container is best because it will allow you or another adult to estimate the blood loss.

■ Let your child know that he or she can resume playing after the bleeding stops, as long as the play is quiet, not vigorous, to keep the bleeding from starting again.

■ Remind your child not to pick or blow the nose after a nosebleed because the bleeding may recur.

Get help

■ Tell your child to ask an adult for help if a nosebleed doesn't stop after 10 minutes or if bleeding starts again. Remind him or her to stay calm and to walk (not run) to find help.

■ Tell the child to hold the head straight or bent slightly downward and to keep applying pressure on the nose until help arrives.

⊗ Never let the person sit up if you suspect a serious head or neck injury.

⊗ Don't give the person anything to drink if he or she has blood in the mouth, throat, or stomach. Drinking at this time may cause vomiting.

Pinching to stop a nosebleed

Pinching the nostrils is one way to stop a nosebleed. Have the person sit up, lean forward, and pinch the nostrils together, as you see here.

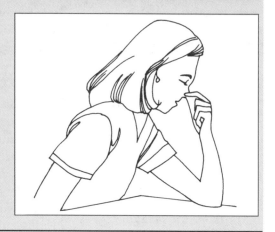

✖ Don't pack the nostrils with gauze if there is a chance the person has a broken nose.

How is a nosebleed treated?
Treatment depends on what part of the nose the bleeding is coming from. The doctor uses a bright light and an instrument called a nasal speculum to locate the bleeding site. Sometimes the doctor orders blood tests to evaluate the person's blood count and blood clotting ability as well as other tests to check for an underlying disorder.

Treating bleeding from the front of the nose
The doctor usually applies a cotton ball soaked with cocaine to the bleeding site and then presses on the nose. (Cocaine slows the bleeding by shrinking the blood vessels.) Then he or she may use a hot instrument or caustic substance to deaden the bleeding site. If bleeding continues, gauze packing is inserted into the nose.

Treating bleeding from the back of the nose
The doctor inserts gauze packing through the nose or inserts postnasal packing through the mouth. In some cases, the doctor inserts a tube with a balloon tip. Once inserted and inflated, the balloon compresses blood vessels to halt bleeding.

Gauze packing generally remains in place 24 to 48 hours; postnasal packing, for 3 to 5 days. If packing must stay in the nose longer than 24 hours, the doctor may prescribe antibiotics to help prevent infection.

Treating continued bleeding

If the bleeding persists, the person may need to take vitamin K supplements to help the blood clot. Severe bleeding may call for blood transfusions and surgery to close off the bleeding artery.

What else should you know?

After a nosebleed stops, the person can avoid a recurrence by taking these precautions:

- Don't pick or rub your nose or insert foreign objects into it.
- Sneeze with your mouth open.
- Avoid bending, lifting, or too much physical exertion.
- Elevate your head with two pillows when lying down.
- Keep your nostrils moist by applying a small dab of petroleum jelly inside your nose.
- For a week after the nosebleed, avoid aspirin, hot beverages, alcohol, and smoking.

Humidify the air

Be aware that a seasonal allergy may trigger springtime nosebleeds, especially if your home is heated with circulating hot air during the winter. Breathing hot, dry air can leave your nasal cavity irritated and prone to bleeding.

To avoid this problem, consider using a cold-mist humidifier to add moisture to the air you breathe. Discuss with your doctor the possibility that you may have allergies.

To help stop the nosebleed from recurring, the person should avoid bending, lifting, or too much physical exertion. Also, the person should sneeze with the mouth open.

*N*UMBNESS

Numbness is a sensation of having diminished feeling or no feeling. Most common in the arm or leg, numbness is often accompanied by tingling or prickling sensations. Sudden numbness that occurs for no apparent reason is cause for concern.

"Pins and needles"

Most of us are familiar with the "pins-and-needles" sensation that comes from cutting off circulation to an arm or a leg. If you sit on your hand, for instance, it may "go to sleep" from pressure that blocks the blood vessels or nerves. In this case, the numbness and tingling disappear when circulation returns to normal and aren't worrisome.

Understanding other causes

Other common causes of sudden numbness include:

■ deep, fast breathing (hyperventilation), which can lead to numbness by lowering the amount of carbon dioxide in the blood
■ irritation of the nerve roots in the neck or back
■ viral infection of the nerve roots (shingles)
■ frostbite, which causes numbness and tingling as the tissues thaw
■ carpal tunnel syndrome — pinching of the hand nerve inside the wrist opening.

What are the symptoms?

Numbness may be brief or lasting. Depending on the underlying condition, the person may have other symptoms, too. Here are some examples.

■ When an artery is blocked, numbness may be accompanied by pale, cool skin.
■ During an episode of extremely high blood pressure, the person may have a headache, drowsiness, and vomiting.
■ With carpal tunnel syndrome, the person typically has pain, weakness, or burning in one or both hands.

What should you do?

Get medical help immediately for a person who experiences sudden numbness and tingling and has pale, cool skin. These symptoms warn of a blocked artery.

Also get medical attention right away for someone who experiences sudden numbness along with symptoms of extremely high blood pressure — headache, drowsiness, and vomiting.

What to do if the person is hyperventilating

If the numbness comes from breathing rapidly, have the person breathe slowly into a paper (not plastic) bag held tightly against the face for 10 minutes or longer. This should restore normal carbon

Get medical help immediately for a person who experiences sudden numbness and tingling and has pale, cool skin. These symptoms warn of a blocked artery.

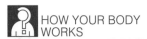
HOW YOUR BODY WORKS

Understanding carpal tunnel syndrome

You've probably heard of carpal tunnel syndrome, and if you use a computer a lot, you may worry about getting the ailment. But unless you've experienced the condition yourself, you may not know exactly what it is. Here are the facts.

The price of repetitive use
A common, painful disorder of the wrist and hand, carpal tunnel syndrome comes from repetitive, rapid use of the fingers, as when you punch the buttons on a keyboard, cash register, or calculator.

From repetition to pinched nerve
The repeated trauma causes pinching or compression of the hand's median nerve inside the carpal tunnel — an opening inside the wrist formed by the carpal bones and a ligament called the transverse carpal ligament. In the hand shown on the opposite page, you can see how the median nerve and flexor tendons of the fingers pass through the tunnel.

From numbness to crippling pain
In some people, nerve compression causes mild numbness and tingling of the hand and wrist. In others, it leads to crippling pain in one or both hands, which may be felt in the forearm or shoulder. The hands may become weak and clumsy, unable to perform simple tasks like opening a jar.

Who is at risk?
You don't have to work at a keyboard to get carpal tunnel syndrome. The condition is common among musicians, factory workers, and people exposed to steady, wrist-shaking vibrations — for instance, those who work with chain saws. You're also at high risk if you have some condition that makes the wrists swell, such as arthritis, obesity, or pregnancy.

Wrist relief
To ease discomfort, try taking aspirin or another mild anti-inflammatory medication. If possible, rest your hands for a few days to avoid the motions that stress the carpal tunnel.

dioxide levels in the blood. If the numbness and tingling don't disappear, get medical attention for the person at once.

What to do if the person is numb from frostbite
If numbness results from frostbite, warm the affected areas in tepid water (104° to 106° F [40° to 41.1° C]). Get medical attention to prevent possible complications.

⊠ Don't rub the skin when trying to thaw a frostbitten area. (See "Frostbite," page 257.)

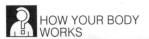

HOW YOUR BODY WORKS

Understanding carpal tunnel syndrome *(continued)*

Use wrist splints

Your doctor may suggest using wrist splints — cloth-covered metal braces that attach to the forearm with Velcro straps. You can get the splints at a drug store or medical supply company, or you can have splints custom made. The splint holds your wrist in about the same position it is in when you hold a pen — cocked slightly back, with the thumb parallel to the forearm.

Massage the wrists

Another treatment option is massage. Recently, massage therapists have reported good results with specific massage routines.

Consider surgery

If your symptoms persist despite treatment, the doctor may recommend surgery to remove pressure on the median nerve.

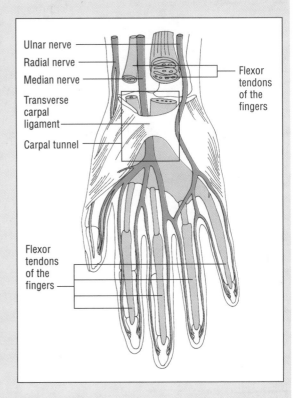

How is numbness treated?

Treatment focuses on correcting the underlying cause of numbness. For someone with high blood pressure, for example, the doctor may prescribe drugs to control blood pressure, may change the dosage of current drugs, or may add new drugs to the regimen.

Treating carpal tunnel syndrome

The doctor may recommend conservative measures to start — for instance, splinting the wrists in a neutral position for 1 to 2 weeks to rest them. (See *Understanding carpal tunnel syndrome.*)

What else should you know?

In an otherwise healthy person, numbness or tingling in the hand or arm may come from pressure on the spinal nerve roots that pass through the bones of the spinal column (vertebrae). Muscle spasms or a slightly displaced vertebra can cause this. Treatment can correct this condition.

PAINFUL URINATION

Sometimes urinating can be an uncomfortable experience. Most often, painful urination results from a urinary tract infection.

How an infection occurs

Usually, bacteria are washed out of the urethra (the structure that drains urine from the bladder) when a person urinates. But the urinary tract can become infected when a bacterium works its way up the urethra and begins to grow in the bladder.

An infection in the urinary tract can involve the urethra; this condition is called *urethritis*. Or it can irritate the bladder or cause it to have spasms; this is known as *cystitis*. If the infection spreads further upward, through tubes called ureters and toward the kidneys, the person may get a condition known as *acute pyelonephritis*.

Danger zone

The closer the infection gets to the kidneys, the more dangerous it becomes. Most urinary tract infections stay in the urethra and bladder, which are in the lower part of the urinary tract. That's why doctors call urethral or bladder infections *lower urinary tract infections*.

Why women are at greater risk

Urinary tract infections affect nearly 10 times as many women as men — probably because a woman's urethra is much shorter than a man's. (See *Learning about your urinary system,* page 384.) The risk of these infections increases dramatically when a young woman begins having sexual intercourse.

Urinary tract infections are also fairly common in children. In men and children, they may stem from an anatomic problem.

Understanding other causes

Painful urination sometimes comes from irritation of the urethra

Painful urination usually results from a urinary tract infection. This tract can become infected when a bacterium works its way up the urethra into the bladder.

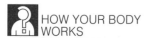

Learning about your urinary system

The kidneys, shaped like lima beans, are the production center of the urinary system. The kidneys purify blood as it passes through them; urine is a byproduct of this process.

Path of urine

After urine is produced by the kidneys, it travels down the ureters — tubes about 12 inches (30 centimeters) long — to be stored in a collapsible bag called the urinary bladder.

Urge to urinate

When the bladder reaches a certain level of fullness, the person feels the urge to urinate. Finally, urine travels down a small tube called the urethra and leaves the body.

Infections and the female urethra

The urethra is much longer in a man (about 8 inches [20 centimeters]) than in a woman (less than 2 inches [5 centimeters]). So in a woman, bacteria don't have nearly as far to travel before they can start multiplying in the bladder. Doctors suspect that's why women get so many more urinary tract infections than men.

caused by the following:

- bubble baths
- feminine deodorants
- scented sanitary products
- certain detergents
- other chemicals that come in contact with the urethral opening.

(See *How to avoid a urinary tract infection*.)

What are the symptoms?

A person with a lower urinary tract infection usually experiences:

- a more intense urge to urinate (urinary urgency)
- a more frequent need to urinate (urinary frequency)
- pain or burning during urination.
  Some people also experience these symptoms:
- blood in the urine
- discharge from the penis
- itching sensation when urinating
- pain in the low back, abdomen, or over the bladder area
- nausea
- vomiting
- fever
- chills
- a general feeling of discomfort.

What should you do?

Have the person see the doctor as soon as possible. In the meantime, place a warm heating pad on the lower abdomen to help relieve the pain.

How is painful urination treated?

For a lower urinary tract infection, the doctor prescribes an antibiotic that's known to work against the bacteria involved. The person usually has to take the antibiotic for 7 to 10 days. Or the doctor may prescribe only 3 to 5 days of treatment or a single dose of an antibiotic.

During antibiotic therapy, the doctor tests the person's urine to determine how well the infection is clearing up. Depending on the cause of the infection, the person's sexual partner may need to be treated, too.

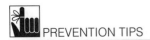

PREVENTION TIPS

How to avoid a urinary tract infection

A woman's anatomy makes her more susceptible to urinary tract infections than men. But that doesn't necessarily doom a woman to recurrent infections. Read what follows to learn how to prevent urinary tract infections.

Wear the right clothes
- Put on fresh underpants each day.
- Wear cotton underpants, not nylon.
- Avoid tight jeans and slacks; they don't allow enough air to circulate.

Avoid irritation
- Take showers instead of baths. Bath water contains bacteria that could enter your urethra. If you do take a bath, don't use bubble bath or bath oil.
- Avoid perfumed vaginal sprays.

- Don't use strong bleaches or laundry detergents.
- Limit your intake of caffeine, carbonated beverages, and alcohol. These beverages can irritate your bladder.

Other instructions
- Wipe from front to back when you go to the bathroom. This reduces the chance that bacteria from your rectum will enter your urinary tract.
- Drink lots of water — enough so that you urinate about every 3 hours.
- Urinate as soon as you feel the urge, and empty your bladder completely. Any urine that's left in your bladder helps bacteria to grow.
- Urinate before — and especially after — you have sex.

What else should you know?
Here's some advice that will help speed recovery from a urinary tract infection.

Take medicine properly
- Take your medicine exactly as prescribed, for as long as prescribed.
- Don't stop taking the medicine too soon — say, if you start to feel better. The infection may still be in your system and could come on strong again in the absence of the antibiotic.

Watch what you drink and eat
- Drink about 3 quarts (3 liters) of fluid a day, preferably water. This will help you urinate often enough and forcefully enough to flush out the bacteria in your lower urinary tract.
- Eat foods with a high acid content. This makes your urine more acidic, which helps to inhibit bacterial growth. Acidic foods include meats, nuts, plums, prunes, whole-grain breads and cereals, and cranberry and other fruit juices.

However, if you're taking a sulfonamide drug, such as Gantrisin or Gantanol, *don't* drink cranberry juice. Its high acid content can interfere with the way the drug works.

■ Limit your intake of milk and other high-calcium foods and beverages.

PALPITATIONS

Some people can feel their heart racing — beating too fast. For some, the racing comes in short spurts called *palpitations*. For others, the heart beats rapidly nearly all the time. A heartbeat above 100 beats a minute is considered abnormally fast. (See *Is your heart rate normal for your age?*)

Understanding the causes
Common causes of a constantly racing heartbeat include:
■ anxiety or fear
■ diet pills or other over-the-counter drugs (cold preparations, for example)
■ excessive use of caffeine or other stimulants (see *Racing with caffeine*, page 388)
■ fever (see *How to deal with a child's palpitations,* page 389)
■ food allergies
■ anemia
■ shortage of oxygen in the blood
■ overactive thyroid gland
■ heart disease.

Palpitations can warn of a serious problem — for example, an irregular heartbeat, tetany, or a severely overactive thyroid gland.

When palpitations are serious
Palpitations sometimes warn of a serious problem. One such problem is an *irregular heartbeat*. The heart has a built-in system, called a natural pacemaker, that regulates the timing of heartbeats. But in some people, this natural pacemaker misfires, causing the heart to beat erratically or perhaps even to stop beating.

Tetany is another serious problem that may trigger palpitations. This condition is caused by a shortage of calcium in the bloodstream.

In a third serious condition, *thyroid storm,* a severely overactive thyroid gland can lead to palpitations, then severe heart abnormalities and even death.

What are the symptoms?

Many people describe palpitations as a pounding, jumping, turning, fluttering, or flapping sensation in the chest, throat, or neck. A person whose heart beats fast almost all the time may not be aware of individual beats but may feel irritable, overenergized, and then tired.

Other symptoms of a racing heartbeat include:

- sweating
- light-headedness
- dizziness
- shortness of breath
- headache.

What should you do?

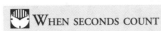 **WHEN SECONDS COUNT**

If someone complains of palpitations, check for pale or clammy skin and find out if the person feels dizzy or short of breath. If the symptoms are present, the person could have an irregular heart beat, thyroid storm, or another condition that requires immediate medical care. Call for emergency medical assistance at once.

Take the person's pulse

If the person isn't pale and doesn't feel dizzy or short of breath, take the pulse. Chances are, this person's palpitations aren't from an underlying medical condition, so simple lifestyle changes may put an end to them.

Help the person make lifestyle changes

Lifestyle changes that may ease palpitations include:
- stopping or reducing the use of caffeine, alcohol, nicotine, marijuana, or amphetamines
- avoiding diet pills or other over-the-counter drugs known to cause palpitations
- reducing everyday stress.

If these remedies don't help, the person should consult a doctor and report any episodes of palpitations or a racing heartbeat. He or she should tell the doctor whether the palpitations occur only under specific conditions, such as after taking certain medicines or eating certain foods.

Is your heart rate normal for your age?

Your age determines how fast your heart should beat, as you can see in the chart below.

Athletes may be exceptions

If you're an athlete, you may have a heart rate slower than 60 beats a minute. Don't worry, though. Chances are, the slow rate is normal for you.

AGE	HEART RATE (beats per minutes)
Under age 1	80 to 160
Age 2	80 to 120
Age 6	75 to 115
Age 10	70 to 110
Age 14	65 to 100
Over age 14	50 to 100

Racing with caffeine

If your heart feels like it's racing, ask yourself whether you're consuming too much caffeine. By stimulating the central nervous system, caffeine can make your heart race. The table below shows the caffeine content of several different beverages.

Just a cup or two can do it

Although the effects of caffeine vary from person to person, one or two cups of coffee usually have a stimulant effect. Very large amounts of caffeine (three to five cups or more a day) can lead to palpitations and other problems — restlessness, difficulty sleeping, and trembling. People who are very sensitive to caffeine may develop mild symptoms after just a cup or two of coffee.

BEVERAGE	SERVING	CAFFEINE CONTENT
Drip coffee	6 ounces	108 milligrams (mg)
Tea, brewed 5 minutes	6 ounces	36 mg
Coca-Cola	12 ounces	43 mg

How are palpitations treated?

If the person isn't in distress, the doctor asks about habits and recent events that could have affected the heartbeat. For instance, he or she may ask whether the person drinks a lot of coffee, uses other stimulants, or takes any prescription or over-the-counter drugs.

The doctor checks for all of the usual causes of palpitations or a racing heartbeat and asks if the person has related symptoms, such as weakness, light-headedness, or shortness of breath.

Discerning a pattern

To find out the pattern of the palpitations or racing heartbeat, the doctor may ask the person to drum out the beats on the table. A skipped beat may point to one type of irregular heart rhythm, whereas clusters of fast beats that stop abruptly suggest another type.

Finding and treating the cause

The person's health history, results of diagnostic tests (such as an electrocardiogram or chest X-rays), and a physical exam can show if the fast heartbeat comes from a heart problem, a disruption in the heart's electrical system, or some other cause (like stress or a chemical imbalance).

Once the underlying cause is discovered, the doctor orders treatments aimed at correcting it.

Correcting a misfiring heart

If the cause of the racing heartbeat is misfiring of the heart's natural pacemaker, the doctor may use an artificial pacemaker to deliver timed electrical impulses directly into the heart. Pacemakers have enabled hundreds of thousands of people to lead normal lives.

Most pacemakers work on demand — that is, only when the person's natural heartbeat slows to less than 60 beats a minute. Usually, the pacemaker is surgically inserted under the skin of the upper chest or the abdomen.

What else should you know?

Everyday stresses can speed the heartbeat, even in a person with no underlying heart problem. In fact, anyone can get palpitations — especially after a day that includes, say, several cups of coffee, not enough sleep, work pressure, and, say, an unwelcome visitor.

Palpitations often result from:
- physical or psychological stress
- certain medicines (for example, those used to treat seizures, arthritis, heart disease, colds, and allergies)
- marijuana, amphetamines, or diet pills
- excessive use of caffeine or other stimulants.

ESPECIALLY FOR PARENTS

How to deal with a child's palpitations

In a child, a fast heartbeat or palpitations can come from a fever or a heart defect present at birth.

What to do

If your child complains of pounding in the chest or other symptoms that sound like palpitations, don't panic. Make an appointment with the doctor to have your child examined.

What to expect at the doctor's office

Children usually can't describe palpitations adequately, so the doctor will investigate your child's problem through heart monitoring, a physical exam, and laboratory tests.

PANIC ATTACK

A panic attack is a feeling of terror so severe that the person can't function normally. It may start as moderate to severe anxiety — a sense of apprehension or tension when the person anticipates danger. Then the anxiety progresses and balloons out of control, resulting in a panic attack.

What are the symptoms?

A panic attack may occur suddenly, get worse, and then subside in a few minutes. The person may feel as if he or she is having a heart attack because of such symptoms as heart pounding, shortness of

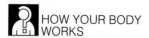

HOW YOUR BODY WORKS

How your body responds to anxiety

When you're anxious, your heart beats faster, your breathing becomes fast and shallow, and your face may become flushed. You may also feel faint or nauseated.

This illustration shows these changes as well as your body's other reactions to anxiety.

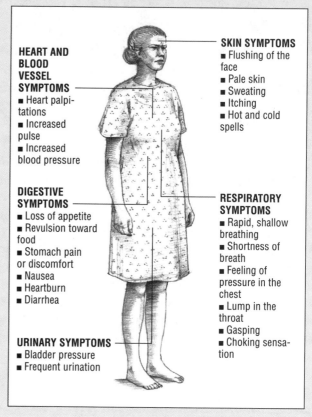

HEART AND BLOOD VESSEL SYMPTOMS
- Heart palpitations
- Increased pulse
- Increased blood pressure

DIGESTIVE SYMPTOMS
- Loss of appetite
- Revulsion toward food
- Stomach pain or discomfort
- Nausea
- Heartburn
- Diarrhea

URINARY SYMPTOMS
- Bladder pressure
- Frequent urination

SKIN SYMPTOMS
- Flushing of the face
- Pale skin
- Sweating
- Itching
- Hot and cold spells

RESPIRATORY SYMPTOMS
- Rapid, shallow breathing
- Shortness of breath
- Feeling of pressure in the chest
- Lump in the throat
- Gasping
- Choking sensation

breath, dizziness, and light-headedness. (See *How your body responds to anxiety.*)

Defense mechanisms to watch for
During a panic attack, a person also may use more defense mechanisms, such as:

- projection — attributing his or her own ideas and feelings to other people
- denial — refusing to accept the truth
- rationalization — providing plausible but untrue reasons for his or her behavior).

Communication patterns to watch for

The person may show certain communication patterns, too, including:

- pressured speech
- shutting out certain thoughts
- talking excessively
- stammering
- dwelling on a certain topic.

Questioning of beliefs and values

Some people prone to panic attacks question previously held beliefs and values. This tends to happen as increasing anxiety interferes with the person's ability to think clearly and make decisions. He or she may then feel hopeless, which only deepens the anxiety.

What should you do?

Get medical help immediately. A panic attack is an emergency. So is a heart attack, which can cause similar symptoms.

In the meantime, try to keep the person calm, quiet, and free from physical danger. Stay with the person at all times to help decrease the sense of isolation.

What to do if the person is hyperventilating

If the person is breathing fast and deep, you must take immediate steps to get more carbon dioxide into the bloodstream before the person loses consciousness. Have the person breathe into a paper (not plastic) bag while you coach him or her to take slow, deep, controlled breaths. Reassure and calm the person often.

> ✖ Don't leave the person alone during a panic attack. Feeling isolated could worsen the anxiety.

How is a panic attack treated?

Treatment for a panic attack typically includes:

- correcting any continuing hyperventilation
- therapeutic communication — a specific way of communicating that helps the person identify and deal with the cause of the anxiety
- reducing stimulation in the environment
- drugs, such as tranquilizers and antianxiety agents
- relaxation techniques to reduce anxiety. (See *Warding off a panic attack,* page 392.)

Get medical help immediately; a panic attack is an emergency. In the meantime, try to keep the person calm, quiet, and free from physical danger.

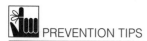

PREVENTION TIPS

Warding off a panic attack

To keep anxiety from mounting, try using one of the relaxation techniques described below — separately or in combination — when you feel tense. The following instructions tell how to perform each technique.

Deep breathing

Inhale slowly through your mouth, then exhale slowly. Focus on controlling your breathing. This should increase your overall sense of control, which in turn reduces anxiety.

Abdominal breathing

Sit or lie comfortably with one hand on your lower abdomen. Slowly inhale while counting to four, hold your breath to the count of four, then exhale to the count of four. Repeat the process several times.

Once you've established a regular breathing pattern, switch from counting to silently repeating a message — for example, "I'm breathing in quiet, calm energy. As I exhale, I release tension and anxiety."

Progressive muscle relaxation

Sit or lie comfortably, using pillows or cushions for support, if necessary. Slowly tense each muscle group for 5 to 7 seconds; then relax them for 20 to 30 seconds. Focus on the sensations of tension and relaxation.

Repeat this pattern several times, as you work your way through your body's major muscle groups. Start with your hands and arms, progress to your head, neck, and shoulders, and from there to your chest, abdomen and lower back. Finish with your thighs, buttocks, legs, and feet.

Focused relaxation

Rest comfortably in a quiet room with minimal distractions. Empty your mind of all thoughts. Constantly repeat a chosen sound, word, or phrase while you focus on your normal breathing rhythm. Gently but immediately dismiss any distracting thoughts that arise during this exercise.

Visualization

Sit or lie comfortably in a quiet room with your eyes closed. Breathe slowly, deeply, and rhythmically as you relax tense portions of your body.

At the same time, visualize a peaceful place where you would normally feel calm and relaxed. Or see yourself successfully resolving the cause of your anxiety. After a specified time, count to four and open your eyes.

Giving drugs

For some people, a brief course of drug therapy is an important part of treatment. Commonly prescribed drugs include Ativan, Atarax, Buspar, Centrax, Librium, Novoxapam, Paxipam, Valium, and Xanax.

What else should you know?

If the panic attack results from chronic anxiety, the person may benefit from long-term treatment, such as behavior modification and other methods.

Behavior modification
With this therapy, the person receives positive or negative reinforcement from others. This helps the person learn how to modify his or her behavior and adopt new ways to cope with stress.

Desensitization
Based on relaxation techniques, desensitization gradually makes the person less vulnerable to the condition that causes the anxiety. This therapy is useful only when the person's anxiety stems from a specific fear.

Extended drug therapy
When anxiety interferes with a person's ability to engage in a relationship with a therapist, extended drug therapy may be necessary.

Cognitive therapy
This therapy uses such techniques as stopping or restructuring certain thoughts. The goal is to help the anxious person adopt new thought patterns that support rational beliefs and appropriate behaviors.

PARALYSIS

Paralysis is a loss of voluntary movement. Stroke and injuries to the head, neck, and spine are the most common causes of paralysis.

Understanding other causes
Paralysis also may result from:
- a degenerative disease of the nerves and muscles, such as multiple sclerosis, myasthenia gravis, polio, Parkinson's disease, or Lou Gehrig's disease
- a tumor of the brain or spinal cord
- an infection of the nervous system, such as botulism or encephalitis.
  Temporary paralysis may result from Guillain-Barre syndrome, migraines, and seizures.

Paralysis is a loss of voluntary movement. Stroke and injuries to the head, neck, and spine are the most common causes.

Types of paralysis

Doctors classify paralysis according to its location and severity.

■ *Paraplegia* — paralysis of the legs.

■ *Quadriplegia* — paralysis of the arms, legs, and the body below the level of the spinal injury or abnormality.

■ *Hemiplegia* — paralysis of only one side of the body.

What are the symptoms?

A paralyzed person can't willingly move or control the affected part of the body. Depending on the cause and type, paralysis can be widespread or limited to one limb. Also, it can be temporary or permanent.

Other symptoms to watch for

Some paralyzed people suffer uncontrolled muscle spasms, a condition called *spastic paralysis,* or completely limp muscles, called *flaccid paralysis.* Other symptoms that sometimes occur with paralysis include:

■ fever

■ headache

■ vision disturbances

■ difficulty swallowing

■ nausea and vomiting

■ loss of bowel or bladder control

■ muscle pain or weakness

■ fatigue.

What should you do?

WHEN SECONDS COUNT

Get medical help immediately for a person who suddenly develops paralysis. If you suspect a head, back, or neck injury, don't move the person unless his or her life is in immediate danger — say, from a fire or an explosion. Instead, wait for professional rescuers to arrive.

In the meantime, to prevent further damage, immobilize the person's spine, keeping the head in line with the rest of the body. To do this, place folded blankets, towels, or clothing at the person's sides, head, and neck.

 Don't give the person anything to drink.

Get medical help immediately for a person who suddenly develops paralysis. If you suspect a head, back, or neck injury, don't move the person unless his or her life is in immediate danger.

How is paralysis treated?

The emergency rescue team immobilizes the person's spine, takes steps to decrease pressure within the skull, and administers oxygen. To aid breathing, they may insert an artificial airway.

Ensuring breathing

In the hospital, the person may be connected to a mechanical ventilator to maintain breathing. He or she usually undergoes tests to find the underlying cause of paralysis.

Helping the person to swallow

If the person has paralysis of the cranial nerves — the nerves that control eye and tongue movements, facial expressions, swallowing, and other important functions — he or she will have trouble swallowing. To prevent malnutrition, the doctor may prescribe a liquid or soft diet, tube feedings, or intravenous feeding.

What else should you know?

Long-term paralysis may cause complications from immobility, such as muscle, joint, skin, and lung problems. The person may need daily care to prevent or minimize these problems.

Maintaining muscle tone and joint function

To maintain muscle tone in paralyzed limbs, the person's arms and legs may be exercised in a routine called *passive range-of-motion exercises.*

To prevent abnormal joint positions called *contractures,* splints may be applied to paralyzed limbs. Footboards or other devices may be used to prevent footdrop, a condition in which the person can't bend the foot upward.

Minimizing bedsores

Bed sores can be minimized by changing the person's position often and providing meticulous skin care.

Preventing lung problems

The doctor may prescribe frequent *chest physiotherapy.* This therapy consists of techniques such as chest tapping, chest vibration, and special positioning as well as coughing and deep-breathing maneuvers. Chest physiotherapy helps the person to:
- cough up lung secretions

Chest physiotherapy may prevent lung problems in a paralyzed person. This therapy involves such techniques as chest tapping, chest vibration, special positioning, coughing and deep-breathing maneuvers.

■ expand the lungs
■ use respiratory muscles more efficiently.

Promoting rehabilitation
As the person recuperates, physical, speech, or occupational therapy may help the person meet specific challenges.

PELVIC PAIN

Pelvic pain is discomfort, cramping, or tenderness in the pelvis, or lower abdomen. In women, pelvic pain may come from painful menstruation or pelvic inflammatory disease (PID).

Painful menstruation may result from an underlying gynecologic disorder, a hormonal imbalance, or psychological factors. Gynecologic disorders that can cause pelvic pain include:
■ endometriosis — when endometrial tissue occurs outside of its customary location, the lining of the uterine cavity
■ narrowing of the cervix
■ uterine fibroids — smooth-muscle tumors of the uterus
■ uterus misplaced from its normal position
■ pelvic tumors.

PID is an infection of the reproductive organs, such as the cervix, uterus, fallopian tubes, and ovaries. The disorder can spread throughout the entire reproductive system and cause lasting damage. (See *Facts about pelvic inflammatory disease.*)

What are the symptoms?
Symptoms depend on the underlying cause of pelvic pain.

Symptoms of painful menstruation
The woman may have irregular, sharp, cramping pain in the lower abdomen, similar to labor pains. The pain commonly spreads to the back, thighs, groin, and vulva. It typically starts with or just before the menstrual period and peaks within 24 hours. Accompanying symptoms may include:
■ frequent urination
■ nausea

A woman with painful menstruation may have irregular, sharp, cramping pain in the lower abdomen. The pain typically starts with or just before the menstrual period and peaks within 24 hours.

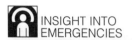

Facts about pelvic inflammatory disease

Every year, more than 1 million women in the United States get pelvic inflammatory disease (PID). Because PID doesn't have to be reported, the actual number of women infected may be as high as 3 million.

To protect yourself from PID, here are the facts you need to know.

Who gets PID?

PID usually affects women between ages 15 and 24, especially those who can't afford health care and who have a poor understanding of sexually transmitted diseases. Adolescents are the group hardest hit.

Other risk factors

The risk of getting PID also increases with:
- multiple sex partners
- a history of cervical inflammation from gonorrhea or chlamydial infection
- a previous bout of PID
- use of an intrauterine device (IUD)
- failure to use a barrier contraceptive, such as a condom, spermicide, or diaphragm, during sexual activity.

Where does it strike?

PID can spread throughout the reproductive system and damage the endometrium, uterus, fallopian tubes, and ovaries. In severe cases, it may involve the membrane that covers the abdominal wall, called the peritoneum.

What damage can it do?

Untreated, PID may cause infertility and can lead to potentially fatal blood infection, blood clots in the lungs, and shock.

What should you do if you have PID?

If you've been diagnosed with PID, be sure to comply with the prescribed treatment regimen. Tell your sexual partners to get examined and, if necessary, get treated for infection. Immediately report any fever, increased vaginal discharge, or pain.

PID may cause painful intercourse, so consult with your doctor before engaging in sexual activity.

- vomiting
- diarrhea
- headache
- chills
- a bloated abdomen
- painful breasts
- depression
- irritability (premenstrual syndrome, or PMS).

Symptoms of PID

PID may cause extreme pelvic pain when the cervix moves or during a gynecologic exam. The woman may have a discharge of pus from the vagina, plus a slight fever and an overall ill feeling.

What should you do?

A woman with pelvic pain should call her gynecologist or a nurse practitioner and make an appointment to discuss her symptoms.

How is pelvic pain treated?

Treatment varies with the cause of pelvic pain.

Treating painful menstruation

The doctor prescribes treatments to relieve the pain and correct the underlying cause. For instance, he or she may prescribe an over-the-counter pain reliever like aspirin or ibuprofen (Advil or Motrin) for mild to moderate pain. Occasionally, a woman needs a narcotic for severe pelvic pain.

Applying heat to the lower abdomen may ease pelvic pain, too. If conservative measures fail, the woman may need surgery to correct the underlying condition, such as endometriosis or fibroids.

For painful menstruation with no known underlying cause, sex hormones, such as oral contraceptives, may correct the condition.

Treating PID

The doctor prescribes antibiotics to eliminate the infection. If the woman also has a pelvic abscess (an accumulation of pus in the pelvis), the abscess is drained. If it ruptures, surgery may be done to remove the uterus, fallopian tubes, and ovaries.

What else should you know?

For menstrual cramps, the doctor may advise the woman to exercise several times a day. Helpful exercises include:
- bicycling movements with the legs up in the air
- modified sit-ups
- elbow-to-knee stretches.

The doctor prescribes antibiotics if the woman has PID. If she also has a pelvic abscess, the abscess is drained.

PENETRATING HEAD INJURIES

Penetrating head injuries break the skin of the head (scalp). Various instruments — including bullets, knives, and many tools — can cause such injuries.

Bullets: The most common cause

Bullets fired by handguns, shotguns, and rifles are the leading cause of penetrating head injuries. As the bullet passes through the brain, it destroys brain tissue in its path. And it creates a cavity that may be many times its size. Fragments of bone and other tissue may cause secondary damage. (See *How a bullet damages the brain,* page 400.)

What are the symptoms?

A person with a penetrating head injury may have:
- a scalp wound, which may bleed profusely
- a deformed skull
- vomiting
- blurred vision
- dizziness
- confusion
- loss of consciousness or a decreased level of consciousness
- changes in the pupils, such as tiny pupils, enlarged pupils, or one pupil bigger than the other
- changes in the pulse, blood pressure, and breathing rate.

The victim of a gunshot wound also has an entrance wound in the head.

What should you do?

WHEN SECONDS COUNT

- Ask someone to call for medical help immediately.
- Check the person's airway, breathing, and pulse. If the person isn't breathing and has no pulse, start CPR immediately, if you know how. (See *Performing CPR on an adult,* page 579, *Performing CPR on a child,* page 585, or *Performing CPR on an infant,* page 590.) But remember — a penetrating head injury may also injure the neck or spine. So **don't** open the airway by moving the head.

Stabilize the spine

- Place rolled blankets or similar materials on either side of the person's neck and torso.

> Don't let the person's body bend or twist at any time; this could worsen a possible neck or spinal injury.

Control bleeding

- Next, try to control severe bleeding by applying direct pressure.

To stabilize the spine, place rolled blankets or similar materials on either side of the person's neck and torso. Don't let the person's body bend or twist.

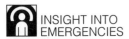

INSIGHT INTO
EMERGENCIES

How a bullet damages the brain

A bullet that enters the brain causes damage in two ways:

- by crushing tissue in its path
- by stretching the surrounding tissues.

Creating brain cavities

As the bullet penetrates the brain, it makes a *permanent cavity* of crushed tissue. This cavity may take the shape of a cylinder with the same diameter as the bullet.

At the same time, the energy created by the moving bullet, called *kinetic energy*, rapidly pushes tissues away from the bullet. This produces a large *temporary cavity*, which may be 30 times larger than the bullet itself.

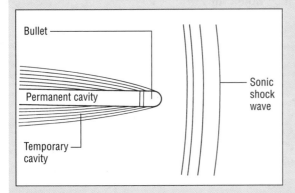

Creating a vacuum

Just after the bullet passes through the tissue, the temporary cavity collapses. But then it forms and collapses again, several more times. This process creates a vacuum along the bullet's path — a vacuum strong enough to suck bits of debris from the person's skin into the wound.

Bullet speed and brain injury

Bullets fired at high speed, or velocity, tend to cause more damage than those fired at low speed. Why? As bullet speed increases, the bullet becomes less stable in flight.

Expanding the destruction

Instead of traveling in a straight line, a fast-moving bullet rolls end over end or swings around its axis. This instability increases the size of the permanent cavity in the brain, widening the area of tissue destruction.

Tracing the bullet's path

The path a bullet takes in the brain depends on whether it leaves the brain or remains lodged there. A high-speed bullet that exits the brain creates a small entrance wound, a path of pulped tissue and bone and metal fragments, and a larger exit wound.

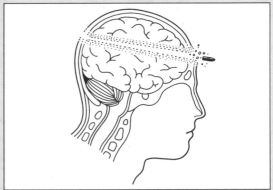

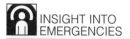

INSIGHT INTO
EMERGENCIES

How a bullet damages the brain *(continued)*

When the bullet lodges in the brain
Sometimes a bullet creates an initial path through
the brain, then ricochets off the inside of the skull.
This produces another path of pulped brain tissue. The bullet then lodges in the brain, so it
doesn't create an exit wound.

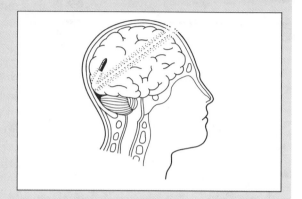

■ If you suspect a severe head injury, like a skull fracture, apply pressure around the wound edges by making a doughnut pad. To make
this pad, obtain a narrow bandage, such as a roller bandage. Wrap
one end of the bandage several times around four of your fingers to
form a loop. Next, pass the other end of the bandage through the
loop again and again until you've used the entire bandage.
Important: Use protective equipment whenever you're exposed to
another person's blood or other body fluids. It can protect you against
any blood-borne diseases, such as hepatitis and human immunodeficiency virus. Latex gloves offer the best protection. If they aren't
available, use any waterproof material — plastic bags or plastic wrap,
for instance — or several layers of gauze pads or clothing.

Place the person in the proper position
■ If the person has vomited, roll him or her into a side-lying position. This position drains the vomit and keeps the airway open. While
rolling the person, be sure to stabilize the neck against movement.
■ Stay with the person until professional help arrives.

✖ Don't raise the person's legs because this could cause pressure
within the skull to rise.

✖ Don't give the person anything to eat or drink.

What to do for a stab wound

To control scalp bleeding, apply direct pressure with a an elastic bandage or another bandage that exerts pressure. Keep the person's head and shoulders slightly raised to help control the bleeding.

> ⊗ Don't remove the weapon if it's impaled in the person's skull. Instead, leave it in place and stabilize it with bulky dressings. Apply a doughnut pad around the weapon.

If a weapon is impaled in the person's skull, don't remove it. Leave it in place and stabilize it with bulky dressings.

How are penetrating head injuries treated?

First, the medical team stabilizes the spine and establishes an open airway. Then, if the person isn't breathing, the team inserts an artificial airway or makes an opening through the neck into the windpipe (called a tracheotomy) so a breathing tube can be inserted. They also treat the person for shock and check the entire body quickly to find out the extent of injuries. Some people need emergency surgery to repair damage caused by the head injury.

Treating a scalp wound

The doctor inspects the scalp wound, removes any foreign matter in the wound, and evaluates the skull for signs of fracture. Stitches are used to close the wound. To help ward off infection, the person may receive antibiotics and a tetanus shot.

What else should you know?

Some of the damage inflicted by a gunshot wound comes from combustion burns caused by gunpowder. These burns may destroy internal tissues and bones.

POISONING

A swallowed poison enters the body by passing through the mouth and throat into the stomach. Children are the typical victims of accidental poisoning because of their natural curiosity. (See *Poison-proofing your home.*)

PREVENTION TIPS

Poison-proofing your home

Children are the most common victims of accidental poisoning, but adults can be poisoned too. You can reduce poisoning risks for everyone in your household by taking the precautions described below.

Store medicines safely

■ Store all medicines properly in child-proof containers and keep them out of reach of children.
■ Avoid taking medicine in front of young children. When giving medicine to a child, don't call it "candy" to get him or her to take it.

Take medicines with care

■ Read the label before taking any medicine.
■ Don't take more than the amount recommended or prescribed.

■ Don't take medicines prescribed for someone else.
■ Don't transfer medicines from their original bottles to other containers without labeling them properly.
■ Discard old or expired medications.

Use chemicals properly

■ Use toxic sprays only in well-ventilated areas and follow label instructions carefully.
■ Store chemicals properly; don't put unused portions in old food containers.
■ Keep household cleaning supplies in a locked cupboard.
■ Discard empty household chemical containers properly.
■ Use pesticides carefully.

Of course, adults can suffer accidental poisoning, too. And some people deliberately swallow poison in a suicide attempt.

Types of poisons

Swallowed poisons fall into three general categories.
■ *Corrosive (caustic) substances.* This category includes household bleaches, metal polishes, anti-rust solutions, paint and varnish removers, drain cleaners, refrigerants, fertilizers, and photographic developers.
■ *Petroleum-like substances.* Examples includes floor polish and wax, furniture polish and wax, gasoline, kerosene, and lighter fluid.
■ *Substances that are neither corrosive nor petroleum-like.* Most accidentally swallowed poisons fall into this category. The variety of these substances is enormous and isn't restricted to liquids.

With some substances — say, plants that irritate the skin — the part of the body that contacts the substance may be injured. But the main concern after a person swallows a poison is the possibility of body-wide effects.

What are the symptoms?

Symptoms of poisoning vary with the type and amount of poison swallowed. They may include:

- nausea and vomiting
- breathing changes or difficulty breathing
- diarrhea, possibly with stomach cramps
- enlarged or tiny pupils
- a dull, masklike facial expression
- facial twitching
- drooling or excessive salivation
- excessive sweating
- altered state of awareness, delirium, or mental disturbances
- changes in skin color, particularly around the lips or fingernails
- burning sensations in the mouth, throat, or stomach
- fast or slow pulse
- coughing
- abdominal gas
- headache
- muscle spasms
- seizures
- complete or partial paralysis
- loss of muscle control
- clumsiness
- burned or damaged skin
- unusual breath odor
- change in urine or stool color
- weakness or tiredness
- difficulty hearing
- vision disturbances.

If you didn't see the poisoning take place, you may find telltale signs that a poisoning has occurred, such as an open medicine or household chemical container.

Signs that a poisoning has occurred

If you didn't see the poisoning take place, you may find telltale signs that it has occurred, such as:

- an open medicine or household chemical container
- spilled liquid, powder, or pills
- liquid, powder, or pills in the person's mouth or on the teeth
- stains on the person's clothing
- burns or swelling on the person's hands or mouth
- a peculiar odor on the person's breath, body, or clothes. (See *What the victim's breath may reveal.*)

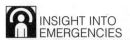
INSIGHT INTO
EMERGENCIES

What the victim's breath may reveal

Some swallowed poisons affect the person's breath. If you suspect a person has been poisoned, smell the breath and report any peculiar breath odor to the poison control center, doctor, or emergency personnel. The table at the right matches breath odors to possible poisons.

ODOR	POSSIBLE POISON
Alcoholic	Alcohol
Bitter almonds	Cyanide
Garlic-like	Phosphorus, arsenic
Gasoline-like	Petroleum-like products
Pear-like	Chloral hydrate
Shoe polish-like	Nitrobenzene
Stale tobacco	Nicotine
Sweet	Acetone
Violets	Turpentine

What should you do?

Most accidental poisonings involve nontoxic substances or substances taken in small amounts that are harmless. Most can be managed at home and require no first-aid. (See *What to do if someone has been poisoned,* page 564.)

When seconds count

If a person shows serious symptoms of poisoning, check to see if he or she is breathing. Open the person's airway and loosen any tight clothing. If the person has stopped breathing, start giving rescue breaths (mouth-to-mouth resuscitation) if you know how. (See *Performing CPR on an adult,* page 579, *Performing CPR on a child,* page 585, or *Performing CPR on an infant,* page 590.)

If the person is conscious and not having seizures, give 1 to 2 cups of water or milk. Have the person rest on the left side to slow absorption of the poison into the blood. (See *How to position the poisoning victim,* page 406.)

How to position the poisoning victim

Stopping a swallowed poison from being absorbed into the person's blood is crucial. You can help accomplish this by keeping the person on his or her left side, as you see in this picture.

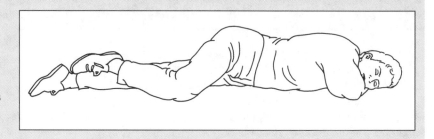

A desirable delay

Lying on the left side delays stomach contents from emptying into the small intestine, where poisons are absorbed more quickly into the blood. In this position, the end of the stomach (pylorus) points straight up, so stomach contents could take 2 hours longer to empty into the small intestine.

An added benefit

Another advantage to this position: If vomiting occurs, resting on the side will help prevent the person from choking.

Get immediate help

Immediately call the poison control center or the doctor. If you don't have access to these telephone numbers, dial 911 or the operator, explain what has happened, and ask for the number of the nearest hospital emergency department.

Have the following information ready when you call the poison control center, doctor, or emergency department.

- the person's age and weight
- the name of the poison and its ingredients (or if it's a plant, the type of plant)
- the amount of poison the person has swallowed
- the time the poisoning occurred
- the person's symptoms, such as vomiting
- any medical condition the person suffers from — for instance, diabetes, high blood pressure, or epilepsy
- what medicines, if any, the person takes regularly.

Follow the instructions of the poison control center, doctor, or emergency personnel exactly.

Give ipecac syrup, if directed

If you're instructed to give the person ipecac syrup to induce vomiting, do so. Save any vomit for examination. If the person doesn't

ESPECIALLY FOR
PARENTS

Ipecac to the rescue

You'll be prepared to deal with most accidental poisonings if you always keep a 1-ounce bottle of ipecac syrup on hand. Ipecac syrup saves lives — 150,000 every year, according to some estimates.

Understand how it works
Ipecac syrup is an emetic — a substance that makes people vomit. Vomiting is one of the most effective ways to get a toxic substance out of the stomach before it's absorbed into the person's blood.

Store it properly
Ipecac is available in most drug stores without a prescription. It will stay fresh for several years if you keep it tightly closed and stored at room temperature. Check the expiration date each time you check the products in your medicine cabinet (which should be at least every 6 months).

Give only as directed
Not all poisonings require removal of the poison from the stomach, and in some cases vomiting is dangerous. That's why you should never give anyone ipecac unless you're told to do so by the poison control center, doctor, or hospital emergency personnel. (Be sure to keep the phone number of the poison control center handy.)

Give the right amount
Dosages of ipecac differ for infants and older people. The poison control center, doctor, or hospital emergency personnel will give you complete instructions. Here are the normal doses:
- people under age 1: 2 teaspoons followed by at least two to three glasses of water
- people age 1 or older: 1 or 2 tablespoons followed by at least two to three glasses of water.

Give ipecac with water
Be sure to give ipecac with water, not milk. If possible, have the person drink more water after taking ipecac.

After the person takes ipecac, have him or her vomit into a large bowl or pot. Save the vomit; you may need to take it to the hospital for analysis.

Give a second dose, if necessary
If the person doesn't vomit within 20 minutes, you can repeat the dose of ipecac. If the person doesn't vomit after a second dose, call the poison control center, doctor, or hospital emergency department for further instructions.

Never give a third dose. Ipecac itself is a poison, and more than two doses may be toxic.

vomit after you've given ipecac syrup twice, call the poison control center, doctor, or emergency department for advice. (See *Ipecac to the rescue.*)

Take the person to the hospital
You may be instructed to take the person to a hospital emergency department immediately. If possible, take with you the following:
- the poison container and any of its remaining contents, or parts

of the poisonous plant. This will help the doctor identify the poison and estimate how much the person swallowed. Take enough of a poisonous plant for identification — for example, an entire mushroom or a branch with leaves, flowers, and berries.

■ a container of the person's vomit. The vomit can be tested to determine the nature of the poison. If the person has vomited undigested pills, the doctor may be able to estimate how many the person took by inspecting the vomit.

If possible, have another person drive while you keep the person comfortable. If the person is vomiting, have him or her lie on the side to keep the airway clear.

How is poisoning treated?

The medical team tries to resuscitate the person, if necessary, and takes steps to prevent further absorption of the poison. When possible, they give a specific antidote to the swallowed poison.

Removing the poison

A crucial goal of treatment is to remove the poison from the person's body or to negate its action before it's absorbed into the blood, where it can cause body-wide effects. With a substance that isn't corrosive or petroleum-like, the best way to do this is to make the person vomit. Ipecac syrup is a safe and sure way to induce vomiting. However, vomiting is effective only if done within several hours of poison ingestion.

With a corrosive or petroleum-like substance, specific treatment hinges on exactly what substance the person swallowed. Depending on how much poison was swallowed and when the accident occurred, the medical team may pump the person's stomach to get the poison out of the body. Stomach pumping is never done if the person swallowed a caustic substance.

What else should you know?

Never induce vomiting in someone who has swallowed a corrosive or petroleum-like substance. Vomiting could cause further damage or lead to other complications. For instance, an acid or alkaline substance burns the mouth and throat when swallowed and can cause more burning if vomited. A petroleum-like product gives off fumes that can cause a severe type of pneumonia if inhaled into the lungs during vomiting.

Make sure not to induce vomiting in a person who has swallowed a corrosive or petroleum-like substance. Vomiting could cause further damage or lead to other complications.

Other situations when you shouldn't induce vomiting
Make sure not to induce vomiting in a person who:
- is unconscious or losing consciousness
- is having or has just had a seizure
- complains of pain or a burning sensation in the mouth or throat
- has a serious heart condition (the strain of vomiting could aggravate the condition).

POISON INHALATION

Certain gases, vapors, fumes, and dusts may cause widespread effects throughout the body if they are absorbed from the lungs into the blood. Carbon monoxide gas, for example, can be fatal because it prevents the blood from carrying oxygen. (See *The perils of carbon monoxide,* page 410.)

What are the symptoms?
Typically, the person who inhales a toxic gas isn't even aware that the gas is present. Symptoms are often vague and may resemble those of the flu. For instance, the person may experience:
- headache
- ringing or tinkling in the ears
- chest pain
- muscle weakness
- nausea and vomiting
- dizziness
- vision changes, such as blurred or double vision
- eventual loss of consciousness, followed by stoppage of breathing and cardiac arrest.

Pattern of symptoms
Symptoms may come and go, and may get worse or improve at certain times of the day or when the person changes location. People or animals who share the person's home or workplace may also develop symptoms. (See *Pathway for poisons,* page 411.)

Symptoms of poison inhalation are often vague and may resemble those of the flu. They may include headache, ringing in the ears, chest pain, nausea, and vomiting.

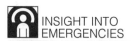

The perils of carbon monoxide

Carbon monoxide is a colorless, odorless gas — the product of incomplete combustion. Inhaling even a small amount can cause serious problems, such as coma or even death.

Squeezing out oxygen

What makes this gas so dangerous? Carbon monoxide displaces oxygen in the blood. As a result, the blood carries too little oxygen to nourish body tissues.

A dire oxygen shortage

Someone who inhales carbon monoxide requires the same emergency first aid measures as any victim of an inhaled poison. However, this person has an even more urgent need for prompt oxygen treatment because of the dire shortage of oxygen in the blood. If the person is pregnant, her fetus is endangered as well.

Read what follows to learn about the circumstances that can expose you to carbon monoxide poisoning and the symptoms to watch for.

Know when you are at risk

You can suffer carbon monoxide poisoning if you inhale smoke, are exposed to an improperly vented gas heater or other appliance, or breathe in exhaust fumes from a car.

Recognize the symptoms

The person's symptoms vary with the severity of the poisoning.

Mild carbon monoxide poisoning

The person may have:
- headache
- vision disturbances
- decreased mental function.

Moderate carbon monoxide poisoning

Symptoms include:
- continued headaches
- ringing or tinkling in the ears
- dizziness
- nausea
- drowsiness
- altered mental state, such as irritability, confusion, or stupor
- slow or irregular pulse
- dizziness and weakness (from low blood pressure)
- pale to reddish-purple skin.

Severe carbon monoxide poisoning

The person is likely to experience:
- seizures
- coma
- heart and lung problems leading to death.

What should you do?

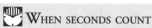
WHEN SECONDS COUNT

- Immediately move the person away from the source of the poison to fresh air. If the person is in an area filled with smoke, gas, or fumes, take several deep breaths of fresh air before entering. Then inhale deeply and hold your breath as you go in.
- Have someone call for medical help while you loosen the person's clothing and open the airway. Look, listen, and feel for breathing; if

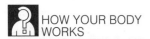

HOW YOUR BODY
WORKS

Pathways for poisons

Poisons can enter our bodies in four ways. These illustrations show how a poisonous substance can be ingested, inhaled, injected, or absorbed.

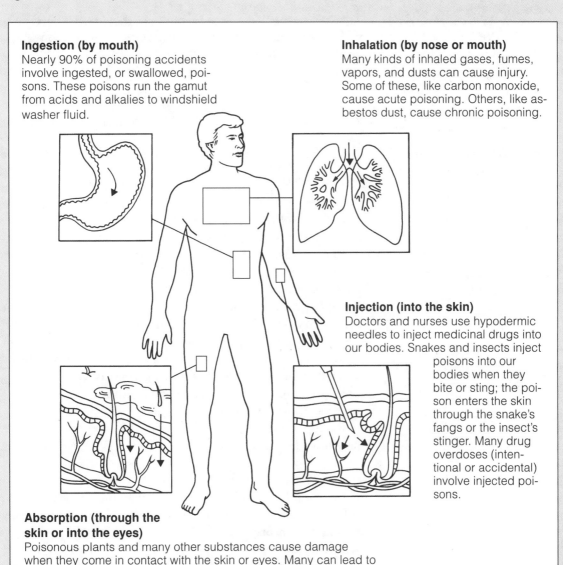

Ingestion (by mouth)
Nearly 90% of poisoning accidents involve ingested, or swallowed, poisons. These poisons run the gamut from acids and alkalies to windshield washer fluid.

Inhalation (by nose or mouth)
Many kinds of inhaled gases, fumes, vapors, and dusts can cause injury. Some of these, like carbon monoxide, cause acute poisoning. Others, like asbestos dust, cause chronic poisoning.

Injection (into the skin)
Doctors and nurses use hypodermic needles to inject medicinal drugs into our bodies. Snakes and insects inject poisons into our bodies when they bite or sting; the poison enters the skin through the snake's fangs or the insect's stinger. Many drug overdoses (intentional or accidental) involve injected poisons.

Absorption (through the skin or into the eyes)
Poisonous plants and many other substances cause damage when they come in contact with the skin or eyes. Many can lead to further damage if they're absorbed through the skin into the blood.

breathing is absent, start giving rescue breaths (mouth-to-mouth resuscitation) immediately. (See *Performing CPR on an adult,* page 579, *Performing CPR on a child,* page 585, or *Performing CPR on an infant,* page 590.)

■ If an ambulance isn't available, drive the person to the nearest hospital emergency department. He or she must receive oxygen treatment immediately.

> ⊗ Don't stop giving rescue breaths until the person is breathing well or help arrives. Don't worry about inhaling the poison while giving the rescue breaths; you're delivering air *to* the person.
>
> ⊗ Be sure not to light a match, turn on a light switch, or produce a flame or spark in the presence of gas or fumes.
>
> ⊗ Don't attempt first-aid measures until you're in fresh air.
>
> ⊗ Never try to rescue someone from smoke, gas, or fumes before you've called for help or if you're alone. Otherwise, you, too, may be overcome by the smoke, gas, or fumes.

Be sure not to light a match, turn on a light switch, or produce a flame or spark in the presence of gas or fumes. Also, don't attempt first-aid measures until you're in fresh air.

How is poison inhalation treated?

The emergency rescue team establishes an open airway and administers 100% oxygen to the person. At the hospital, the medical team may need to insert a breathing tube and place the person on a mechanical ventilator.

Diagnostic tests can help determine the extent of damage to the respiratory system. For instance, the doctor may perform a procedure called bronchoscopy by inserting an instrument called a bronchoscope into the person's airway. Also, a sample of the person's blood is taken to monitor the blood's ability to carry oxygen.

The doctor orders other treatments aimed at:
■ relieving respiratory problems
■ restoring a normal level of oxygen to the blood
■ preventing further complications.

Relieving respiratory problems
To help eliminate thick lung secretions, make breathing easier, and ward off pneumonia, the doctor may recommend the following breathing treatments:
■ aerosol treatments to deliver drugs that widen the airways
■ lung medicines to ease airway spasms and lessen the risk of airway obstruction
■ special coughing and deep breathing exercises

■ chest physiotherapy — a group of techniques that help expel lung secretions and expand the person's lungs.

Other treatments
The doctor also may prescribe antibiotics to fight off infection and steroids to decrease inflammation.

What else should you know?
Someone who has inhaled a poison may not show symptoms for up to 48 hours after exposure. But delaying treatment that long could have serious consequences.

As a safeguard, suspect inhalation injury in anyone who was exposed to a burning agent or fumes in an enclosed space or who has lost consciousness.

POISON IVY, OAK, AND SUMAC

Poison ivy, oak, and sumac are the best known of several plants that are poisonous to the touch. The sap of all three contains a resin called *urushiol.* Many people get an allergic reaction known as *contact dermatitis* when their skin comes in contact with urushiol.

Although the urushiols of the three plants aren't identical, they're so similar that a person who is allergic to one will probably react to all three. Seven of ten Americans are allergic to urushiol and will develop contact dermatitis if exposed to large enough doses. Five of ten Americans will develop dermatitis if exposed to much smaller doses.

Related offenders
If you're allergic to poison ivy, oak, or sumac, beware: You may also be allergic to related plants, including:
■ cashews
■ pistachios
■ mangos
■ Chinese or Japanese lacquer trees.

Some people experience outbreaks when exposure to the oil of

If you're allergic to poison ivy, oak, or sumac, you may also be allergic to cashews, pistachios, mangos, and Chinese or Japanese lacquer trees.

cashew shells; some get allergic reactions after handling wooden and lacquered items made in China or Japan. (*Urushiol* comes from a Japanese word meaning "lacquer.")

Dangerous smoke
Urushiol can also be carried in smoke from burning plants. Branches of these plants sometimes are accidentally gathered for firewood, and people trying to rid their yards of the plants may burn them. The smoke these plants give off is particularly dangerous because it can enter the nasal passages, throat, and lungs of anyone who breathes it.

What are the symptoms?
The allergic response to poison ivy, oak, or sumac varies from one person to the next. Some people experience only mild itching and slight inflammation of the affected area. Others suffer severe burning and itching, followed by formation of watery blisters that ooze and then crust over. The blisters may fill with pus or contaminated fluid. The rash is worst after about 5 days and gradually improves within a week or two, even without treatment.

Itching and burning usually develop within 24 to 48 hours after contact in a sensitized person. However, in some people, these symptoms don't show up for days.

Other symptoms to watch for
If a large area is affected and inflammation is severe, the person also may report fever, headache, and general weakness.

What should you do?
Get immediate medical help if you know the person is highly sensitive to poison ivy, oak, or sumac.

For anyone who comes in contact with a poisonous plant, immediately wash the affected area with soap and cold water. Use yellow laundry soap, if available, and lather several times. After each sudsing, rinse the area in running water.

If you're in the woods, rinse in a running stream. If soap isn't available, apply rubbing alcohol liberally and rinse with water. Also wash and rewash any clothing that might have come in contact with the urushiol.

After contact with a poisonous plant, immediately wash the affected area with soap and cold water. Use yellow laundry soap, if available.

 Don't scrub the affected area with a brush when washing.

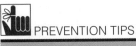

PREVENTION TIPS

How to identify poison ivy, oak, and sumac

Would you be able to identify poison ivy, oak, or sumac if you encountered one of these plants? Quick detection of these plants could spare you or a loved one a week or so of itchy, oozing misery. Fortunately, learning how to recognize a poisonous plant isn't difficult.

Poison ivy

The old saying "leaflets three, let it be" (or "leaves of three, quickly flee") is sound advice. Poison ivy has slightly glossy green leaves that grow in groups of three. The leaves may be notched or smooth, but they always grow in clusters of three — one at the end of the stalk, the other two opposite each other. In the early fall, the leaves may turn an attractive red.

Check for yellow-green berries

Although poison ivy usually grows as a vine, it can grow as a low shrub, especially along fences or stone walls or in fields. You may see waxy, yellow-green berries with markings that make them look like a peeled orange. Recognizing these berries can help you identify the plants in late fall, winter, and early spring when the leaves aren't present.

Poison ivy grows throughout the United States, although it is most common in the eastern and central states.

POISON IVY

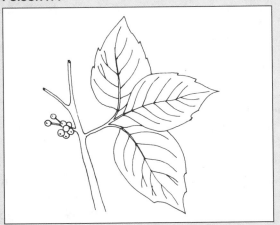

Poison oak

The leaves of poison oak also grow in groups of three. The resemblance of these leaves to oak leaves gives the plant its name.

Look for leaves with dark tops

Because the leaves are covered with fine hairs, their undersides are a much lighter green than the tops. You may see clusters of greenish or creamy white berries, but not all poison oak plants bear fruit.

Poison oak usually grows as a low shrub and is most common on the west coast from Mexico to British Columbia.

POISON OAK

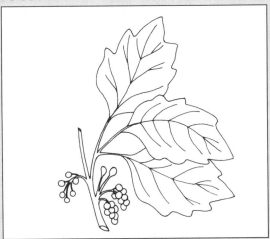

(continued)

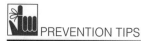

How to identify poison ivy, oak, and sumac *(continued)*

Poison sumac

Poison sumac has 7 to 13 leaves arranged in pairs, with a single leaf at the end of the stem. The leaves are long and smooth. In the spring, they're bright orange and velvety. Later, they become dark green and glossy on the upper surface and light green on the lower. Early in the fall, they turn reddish orange.

Beware of drooping, green berries

You can distinguish poison sumac from nonpoisonous sumac by its drooping clusters of green berries. Nonpoisonous sumac, in contrast, has red, upright berry clusters.

   Poison sumac grows as a tree, usually 5 or 6 feet high, although some plants grow to 25 feet. It is found in swampy areas throughout the eastern United States.

POISON SUMAC

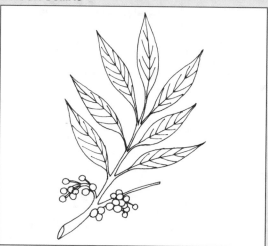

Be sure not to touch or scratch the blisters. Doing so can irritate the skin and introduce bacteria into the sores, causing infection. If traces of urushiol remain on the skin, touching the affected area and then another part of the body can transfer the urushiol and the rash.

How are poison ivy, oak, and sumac treated?

After washing off the urushiol, most people need little or no further treatment if the rash is mild. The sores heal on their own.

Relieving itching and burning

To ease itching and burning, the doctor may recommend applying compresses soaked in cool water or Burow's solution. To help dry the area, try using calamine lotion or another preparation with calamine in it, such as Caladryl. This preparation also relieves itching and burning.

   Bathing in lukewarm bath water sprinkled with one to two cups of a colloidal oatmeal preparation (such as Aveeno) can ease itching, too. You can buy these preparations at a drug store.

The same treatment is used for a moderate rash. Sometimes the doctor prescribes a topical steroid ointment to relieve itching.

Treating persistent itching

The doctor may suggest applying water hot enough to redden the skin, but not burn it. Doing this helps to release histamine, the substance that causes severe itching. Taking a hot shower or bath releases enough histamine to deplete the cells of this substance temporarily, giving the person up to 8 hours of relief from itching.

Treating frequent or severe outbreaks

For frequent or severe outbreaks of poison ivy, oak, or sumac, the doctor may recommend a series of injections to desensitize the person. This treatment may also benefit people who work outdoors in areas where these plants grow.

What else should you know?

The best way to prevent allergic reactions to poisonous plants is to learn how to recognize and avoid them. (See *How to identify poison ivy, oak, and sumac,* page 415.) The following tips can help you and your family avoid contact with these plants.

Keep covered

Always wear long sleeves, long pants, and gloves when working outdoors where these plants are known to exist or when hiking in unfamiliar woods. Thoroughly wash any article of clothing that comes in contact with one of these plants.

Beware of animals

Remember that although animals don't usually react to urushiol, they carry it on their fur. If you think your pet may have come into contact with a poisonous plant, give it a bath.

Eliminate poisonous plants

If you find a poisonous plant growing in your backyard, remove it with chemical weed killers or by digging up its roots when the ground is thoroughly wet.

If you use chemical weed killers, follow the directions carefully; these chemicals can harm people, animals, and vegetation. Store leftover weed killer in a locked cabinet and dispose of empty containers according to directions on the container. Bury uprooted plants; don't burn them or bundle them for garbage collection.

Always wear long sleeves, long pants, and gloves when working outdoors where these plants are known to exist or when hiking in unfamiliar woods. Wash any article of clothing that comes in contact with one of these plants.

PUNCTURE WOUNDS

Puncture wounds occur when the skin (and possibly the underlying tissue) is pierced by a relatively long, slender object that doesn't leave much of a visible wound. Objects that can cause puncture wounds include:

- nails
- knives
- pins
- splinters
- bullets
- wire.

Despite its minor appearance, a puncture wound can be dangerous, causing extensive internal damage or leading to infection.

No big deal?

At first glance, you may think a puncture wound is no big deal, especially if, like many such wounds, it creates just a small opening, bleeds very little, and seems to close up right away.

But a puncture wound *can* be dangerous despite its minor appearance. It can cause extensive internal damage or lead to infection. (See *Infection alert.*) In fact, because the puncturing object impales everything in its path, possibly including vital organs, the wound may be a life-threatening emergency.

The longer the puncturing object is and the further it penetrates the body, the more serious the injury. If the object damages vital organs, the person may go into shock and die unless treated.

What are the symptoms?

Depending on the severity of the wound, symptoms can range from a bloodless splinter to a large object lodged in the body. If vital organs have been injured, the person may show symptoms of shock, such as:

- restlessness
- weakness
- dizziness
- loss of consciousness
- pale skin.

Exit and entrance wounds

You may see only one hole in the skin, where the object went in and came back out. Or you may see both an entrance wound and an exit

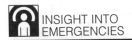

Infection alert

Puncture wounds don't bleed very much and the punctured skin tends to knit over the unhealed inner tissues. But don't let these facts fool you into thinking that puncture wounds aren't dangerous.

Why the risk is so high
Precisely because of the scant bleeding and the knitting over of unhealed tissues, puncture wounds carry a high risk of infection.

And if an infection occurs, it can considerably slow wound healing. Also, the dangerous bacteria could spread throughout the body.

Check for symptoms
After a puncture wound, check regularly for these symptoms of possible infection:
- swelling around the wound
- redness around the wound
- abnormally warm skin around the wound
- throbbing or increased wound pain
- fever
- pus, either collected under the skin or draining from the wound
- swollen lymph glands near the wound (in the groin for a leg wound, in the neck or armpit for a head or arm wound)
- red streaks leading away from the wound, which may mean the infection is spreading to the lymphatic circulation.

Take action — fast
Call your doctor at once if you detect any of these symptoms.

wound, as when a bullet travels through a leg and out the other side. In this case, the exit wound is larger than the entrance wound.

What should you do?
If the wound is obviously minor and the object hasn't penetrated too far into the skin, you can try to remove the object with tweezers that have been sterilized over an open flame or boiled in water. Or you can try soaking the wound in warm, soapy water for about 15 minutes to remove the object.

⊗ Don't touch the wound until you've thoroughly washed your hands.

⊗ Don't press so hard on the wound that you cause further injury.

Leave an impaled object in place
For a more serious puncture wound, as from stepping on a nail or

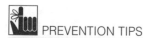

How to avoid puncture wounds

Following the common-sense guidelines below can help you and your family steer clear of puncture wounds.

Keep sharp objects at bay
■ Handle sharp objects carefully, and keep them away from children.
■ Don't use sharp objects for anything other than their intended purpose.
■ Don't let children run while holding sharp, elongated, or breakable objects.

Safeguard your home
■ Check your home frequently for objects that could cause a puncture wound.
■ Don't let kids play around potentially dangerous electrical appliances.
■ Remove all unused nails from lumber and other household items.
■ Keep your yard and storage areas free of trash and debris.

Practice firearm safety
■ Be especially careful with guns, even pellet and BB guns. Don't let kids play with them. And keep guns and ammunition locked in separate places.
■ Always assume a gun is loaded, but never load one until you're ready to shoot it.

falling on a stick, check to see if any part of the object has broken off in the wound. If you see something sticking out from the wound, don't try to remove it. It could break off deeper in the wound. Instead, take the person to the doctor.

 Don't put medication on the wound or try to clean it.

If the person has been impaled with a large object that's protruding from the body, *don't remove the object.* If necessary, cut it off a few inches from the skin surface and carefully secure it with a bandage to prevent further movement. If you have no choice but to move the victim yourself, place massive dressings around the protruding object and then get the person to the hospital immediately.

 WHEN SECONDS COUNT

The most serious puncture wounds come from injury to a vital organ that leaves a person impaled on a spike, a fence, or some other large stationary object. If you encounter someone in this situation, don't try to pull the person loose because you'll only make the injury worse — possibly fatal. Instead, call for emergency rescue help immediately.

How are puncture wounds treated?
The medical team first makes sure the victim is medically stable. They look for signs of internal bleeding and damage to internal organs. Then they clean and dress the wound and administer a tetanus booster if the person hasn't had one in the past 5 to 10 years.

What else should you know?
If the puncturing object is dirty, it could be carrying the germs that cause tetanus. This life-threatening nervous system infection may not show up for days or weeks after the accident. By then, the person could be having such symptoms as stiffness in the jaw (which is why tetanus is sometimes called "lockjaw"), painful muscle spasms, seizures, and inability to breathe.

Get a tetanus shot every 5 years
To avoid getting tetanus, be sure to keep your tetanus immunization up to date — don't wait until *after* you get injured. If you or your children haven't gotten a tetanus shot or booster in 5 years or more, see your doctor. And take steps to protect yourself and your children from injuries that can lead to tetanus. (See *How to avoid puncture wounds.*)

RADIATION EXPOSURE

Radiation is energy traveling in the form of particles or waves. During an average day, most people are exposed to minute amounts of naturally occurring radiation, such as from air, water, food, concrete or stone buildings, and watching color TV. This everyday exposure is harmless.

The dangers of ionizing radiation

In contrast, exposure to large amounts of *ionizing radiation* can cause serious, even fatal, effects. Sources of ionizing radiation include:
- nuclear reactors
- X-rays
- radioactive materials used in medicine and industry. (See *All about radiation,* page 422.)

How does such exposure occur? Here's a possible scenario: A train carrying radioactive waste collides with another freight train. The collision sets off an explosion or a fire, which releases the radioactive waste into the atmosphere and contaminates the surrounding area.

Effects of radiation exposure

Radiation may cause severe effects that arise within hours or days or long-term effects that don't show up for years or decades. Damage to the human body depends on the radiation dose. The dose, in turn, is determined by two things:
- the strength of the radiation (the amount of radiation per hour that the source emits)
- the duration of exposure.

The larger the radiation dose, the more acute the effects. A person who has been exposed to a very high dosage over a short period is likely to die within hours.

What are the symptoms?

A person whose entire body was exposed to radiation may have symp-

Radiation may cause severe effects that arise within hours or days or long-term effects that don't show up for years or decades.

All about radiation

When people talk about the dangers of radiation, they're usually referring to the potentially harmful type — *ionizing radiation.* When absorbed by living tissues, ionizing radiation splits atoms that lie in its path into free-floating ions.

Dissipation and disarray

These free-floating ions, in turn, bump into other atoms and ions. This sets off a process that continues until the ions' energy dissipates and body structures are left in disarray.

Alpha, beta, and gamma

Ionizing radiation comes in three forms: alpha particles, beta particles, and gamma rays.
- *Alpha particles* can be stopped by paper. Unless inhaled or swallowed, they're unlikely to damage the body.
- *Beta particles* can be stopped by heavy clothing. They rarely cause harm unless they enter the body though the nose, the mouth, or an open wound.
- *Gamma rays* can penetrate the entire thickness of the body. Only heavy lead shielding, concrete, and similar barriers can stop them.

How radiation exposure occurs

A person can be exposed to radiation by inhaling, swallowing, or coming in direct contact with a radioactive substance. Whether — and how much — tissue damage occurs depend on:
- the amount of body area exposed
- the length of exposure
- the radiation dosage absorbed
- the person's distance from the radiation source
- the presence of protective shielding.

Safe and unsafe exposure

The amount of radiation a person has absorbed is measured in radiation absorbed doses, or *rads.* A person can absorb up to 200 rads and survive. A dose of 450 rads is fatal in about half the cases; more than 600 rads is nearly always fatal.

Safety in controlled doses

When radiation is focused on a small area, the body can survive many thousands of rads, as long as they're administered in carefully controlled doses over a long time. This basic principle is the key to safe and successful radiation therapy.

---

toms of a whole-body illness, such as:
- nausea
- vomiting
- headache
- chest pain
- shortness of breath.

Exposure of just a part of the body may lead to localized symptoms like red, peeling skin and hair loss.

Clinical syndromes

Doctors sometimes speak of clinical syndromes caused by radiation exposure. For instance, *acute radiation syndromes* may involve the brain, digestive tract, and blood cells.

With the *brain syndrome,* caused by extremely high total body doses of radiation, the person suffers:

- nausea
- vomiting
- listlessness
- drowsiness
- tremors
- seizures
- staggering gait.

Death follows within hours.

The *digestive tract syndrome* leads to severe nausea, vomiting, and diarrhea. The person becomes severely dehydrated, suffers collapse of the heart and blood vessels, and usually dies within a few weeks.

The *blood-cell syndrome* causes apathy, nausea, vomiting, and appetite loss. These symptoms disappear within 24 to 36 hours after exposure. However, the lymphatic tissue, spleen, and bone marrow then start to shrink. As a result, the body can no longer make enough blood cells, and the person becomes extremely vulnerable to infection.

People who receive radiation therapy to treat cancer, especially of the abdomen, may suffer *acute radiation sickness.* Symptoms include nausea, vomiting, diarrhea, appetite loss, headache, and an overall ill feeling. Typically, these symptoms go away within hours or days.

Delayed and late symptoms

Radiation exposure can have *delayed symptoms.* Some of these include:

- stoppage of menstruation
- impaired fertility
- anemia
- shortages of certain types of blood cells
- cataracts
- hair loss
- skin ulcers
- skin cancer.

Late effects of radiation — say, years or decades after exposure — may include cancers of the blood (leukemia), bone, thyroid, and skin as well as cataracts and genetic defects.

What should you do?

Call for emergency medical help immediately if you believe a per-

Get emergency medical help immediately if you believe a person has suffered radiation exposure. Be sure to tell emergency personnel that the area may be contaminated by radioactive materials.

son has suffered radiation exposure. Be sure to tell emergency personnel that the area may be contaminated by radioactive materials. Remember — radiation can't be detected without special equipment, so it poses a hazard to both the victim and rescuers who must enter the radioactive area.

How is radiation exposure treated?

The person is removed from the area as soon as possible. Rescuers then establish an open airway, check to see if the person is breathing, and take steps to control any external bleeding.

Decontaminating the person

Next, the person is decontaminated. Depending on the radiation source, a special team may be called in to do this. Decontamination techniques include removing contaminated clothing and cleaning the person's skin with special solutions.

If the person swallowed radioactive material, the medical team may induce vomiting or pump the person's stomach. After decontamination, the person's radiation level is monitored closely.

Treating clinical syndromes

For a person with the acute *brain syndrome,* the doctor orders drugs and other therapies to combat shock, relieve pain and anxiety, and control seizures.

For *radiation sickness* caused by radiation therapy, the person may receive medication to reduce nausea and vomiting. (Some doctors prescribe this medication *before* each radiation session to prevent nausea and vomiting.)

To treat the acute *digestive tract syndrome,* the doctor typically prescribes sedatives and medications to stop the vomiting and nausea. Other treatments may include a bland diet and administration of fluids, electrolytes (salts), and plasma.

For the acute *blood-cell syndrome,* the doctor may order antibiotics and transfusions of blood and platelets to help prevent or treat infection, massive bleeding, and anemia. The person is kept in strict isolation to prevent exposure to harmful germs.

Someone who has suffered *chronic radiation exposure* may receive medications called chelating agents to help the body eliminate the radioactive substance.

What else should you know?

Ionizing radiation is by no means always a bad thing. In fact, many

To decontaminate the person, contaminated clothing is removed and the person's skin is cleaned with special solutions.

people owe their lives to it, at least in part. For instance, about half of all cancer patients undergo radiation therapy to destroy cancer cells or stop their growth. Radiation therapy can also relieve cancer pain and enhance the person's quality of life when hope for a cure no longer exists.

RAPE OR SEXUAL ASSAULT

Rape is legally defined as sexual intercourse without the person's consent, carried out by using force, threats, intimidation, or deception. Technically, rape requires penetration of the vagina by the penis. However, the legal definition of rape varies from state to state.

Sexual assault refers to penetration of any other orifice by the penis, other male appendage, or an object without the person's consent. Like rape, sexual assault is achieved through force, threats, intimidation, or deception.

Victims of rape and sexual assault range from very young children to elderly people. They include both males and females.

What are the symptoms?
Most physical symptoms of rape and sexual assault result from injuries inflicted during the attack. These vary with the nature of the attack, but may include:
- genital or rectal injuries
- genital or rectal pain or bleeding
- injuries to other parts of the body — typically, cuts, bruises, or burns.

Emotional and physical effects
The person may also suffer short- and long-term emotional and psychological effects. Immediately after the attack, for instance, she may be in shock and disbelief. She may cry, sob, or act restless and tense and may seem overcome with fear, anxiety, or depression.

What should you do?
If you're alone and have been raped, or if another person has been

Rape and sexual assault are carried out through the use of force, threats, intimidation, or deception. Victims range from very young children to elderly people.

raped, call the police immediately to report the crime. (The person can decide now or later whether to press charges.)

Next, call someone to help (a relative, a friend, or a rape hotline). Then call the doctor or the hospital emergency department to tell them that a rape has occurred and that you or the person will need medical treatment.

WHEN SECONDS COUNT

If the person is unconscious, call for medical help immediately. Check for and maintain an open airway. Feel for a pulse and look, listen, and feel for breathing. If the pulse and breathing are absent, start CPR if you know how. (See *Performing CPR on an adult,* page 579, *Performing CPR on a child,* page 585, or *Performing CPR on an infant,* page 590.)

Control bleeding

Stop any severe bleeding by applying direct pressure to the wound and keeping the injured area elevated. (See "Bleeding" on page 73.) Cover the person with a blanket or coat to prevent loss of body heat.

Don't let the person change clothes, wash or wipe the genitals, take a shower, or brush the teeth until after a medical exam. Doing these things could destroy evidence of a rape.

How is rape or sexual assault treated?

Typically, the person receives emergency care for physical injuries. However, extensive treatment is postponed to preserve evidence.

Collecting evidence

Physical evidence is obtained as soon as possible after the rape; otherwise, prosecution of the rapist is impossible. The person's clothing, fingernail scrapings, and pubic hair are examined for blood or skin fragments and foreign specimens. The doctor collects semen specimens from the person's vagina, rectum, urethra, mouth, or throat, as needed, to test for sperm.

Testing for disease

Specimens are also tested for sexually transmitted diseases (STDs). Not all STDs can be identified immediately, so tests may need to be repeated. A test for HIV infection should be repeated in 6 months. The doctor may order other lab tests, including a Pap test and a pregnancy test to determine prior pregnancy.

Don't let the person change clothes, wash or wipe the genitals, take a shower, or brush the teeth until after a medical exam. Doing these things could destroy evidence of a rape.

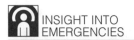
INSIGHT INTO
EMERGENCIES

Rape-trauma syndrome: Rape's agonizing aftermath

Many rape victims start to experience rape-trauma syndrome about 24 hours after the attack. Usually, the syndrome occurs in three phases, although a person won't necessarily experience them in sequence. Read the chart below to learn which symptoms occur during each phase.

PHASE	SYMPTOMS
Acute Victim may seek medical help or may keep the rape a secret.	■ Anger ■ Denial ■ Disbelief ■ Feelings of degradation, humiliation, guilt, and powerlessness ■ Vengefulness ■ Fear ■ Shock
Outward adjustment Victim may refuse emotional support and counseling.	■ Efforts to "take control," such as getting new door locks or buying a gun ■ Calm appearance ■ Denial of real feelings
Reorganization Victim wants to discuss feelings and work them out. She may seek counseling and support from others, or may continue to suffer silently.	■ Anxiety ■ Phobias ■ Sexual problems ■ Difficulty sleeping

Preventing and treating STDs and other infections

To treat STDs and prevent tetanus or infection of wounds, the doctor may give a tetanus shot and prescribe antibiotics. To help prevent STDs, the person may receive the drug Benemid along with penicillin or tetracycline.

If the person has delayed reporting the rape, she may undergo a simple exam for STDs and pregnancy.

Providing counseling

Professional counseling can help the person cope with *rape-trauma syndrome*. This syndrome, which starts just after the rape or sexual assault, refers to the person's short-term and long-term reactions to the rape. (See *Rape-trauma syndrome: Rape's agonizing aftermath*.)

What else should you know?

If the person chooses and the hospital allows, she may receive a post-coital contraceptive called diethylstilbestrol (DES) to prevent pregnancy. This 5-day therapy must begin within 72 hours (preferably within 24 hours) after the rape.

The risks of DES

DES could endanger the fetus if the person was pregnant before the rape or if the drug fails to stop a pregnancy caused by the rape. Also, it can cause such side effects as nausea and vomiting, vaginal spotting, rash, and difficulty sleeping.

RECTAL BLEEDING

Rectal bleeding is always significant because it can lead to serious loss of blood and fluids, possibly resulting in shock.

Rectal bleeding, or passage of bloody stools, usually comes from bleeding somewhere in the lower part of the digestive tract. Less often, it results from rapid loss of a quart or more of blood from the upper part of the digestive tract.

Rectal bleeding is always significant because it can lead to serious loss of blood and fluids, possibly resulting in shock.

Understanding the causes

Typically, the cause of rectal bleeding is a digestive tract disorder, such as inflammation of the colon (colitis) or colon cancer. But sometimes rectal bleeding stems from a bleeding disorder or a toxin. It can even result from a diagnostic test, such as colonoscopy (passage of a thin tube into the colon to check for abnormalities).

What are the symptoms?

Rectal bleeding ranges from passage of formed, blood-streaked stools to liquid bloody stools. The blood may be bright red, dark mahogany, or maroon. Usually, the bleeding starts abruptly and follows abdominal pain or cramping.

Depending on the amount of blood lost, the person may have symptoms of shock, such as:
- pale skin

- fast pulse
- dizziness and weakness (from decreased blood pressure)
- rapid breathing.

What should you do?

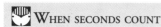 **WHEN SECONDS COUNT**

Get medical help immediately for a person with *severe* rectal bleeding. Help the person lie down and elevate the feet 8 to 12 inches.

How is rectal bleeding treated?

The medical team tries to restore a normal fluid balance and find the source of the rectal bleeding.

Identifying the bleeding source

Typically, the person undergoes endoscopy. In this procedure, the doctor inserts a thin tube into the digestive tract. Besides locating the bleeding source, endoscopy may help to stop the bleeding.

If endoscopy doesn't locate the bleeding site and if rapid rectal bleeding persists, the doctor may perform intestinal angiography. This procedure examines blood vessels in the abdomen by passing a catheter into an abdominal artery and then taking an X-ray.

Stopping the bleeding

Once the bleeding site is identified, a drug called vasopressin may be administered into the abdominal artery during angiography to halt the bleeding. If vasopressin doesn't work, the person may undergo a procedure called an *arterial embolization.* In this procedure, the doctor injects a blood-clotting material through the catheter into an artery to stop the bleeding.

Other treatments

Further treatments aim to rest and heal the bowel and correct the underlying cause of the rectal bleeding. To help reduce bleeding, the doctor may prescribe drugs that narrow the blood vessels. Some people need surgery to control bleeding or to remove the bleeding source.

What else should you know?

Sometimes, rectal bleeding is mistaken for bleeding caused by hemorrhoids. However, the two conditions are quite different. With rectal

To help ease rectal bleeding, the doctor may prescribe drugs that narrow the blood vessels. Some people need surgery.

bleeding, blood in the stools comes from the lower or upper digestive tract. With hemorrhoids, the person intermittently passes blood from enlarged, bleeding veins around the anus. (See "Hemorrhoids," page 301.)

RECTAL PAIN

Rectal pain is discomfort in and around the anus and rectum. Because this area contains many nerve fibers, sores, growths, and other abnormalities that occur there are especially painful.

Rectal pain may result from, or be aggravated by, diarrhea, constipation, or passing hard stools. The pain may be compounded by intense itching and continued scratching that irritates the skin and nerve endings.

Understanding the causes
Rectal pain usually comes from a disorder of the anus or rectum. Such disorders include:
- anal cancer
- anal fissure — a painful, lengthwise crack in the lining of the anus (see *What to do if your child has rectal pain*)
- anorectal abscess — a collection of pus in the anal or rectal area
- anal fistula — an abnormal opening onto the skin surface near the anus
- hemorrhoid
- spasms of the rectal and pelvic floor muscle.

Rectal pain may get worse during or after a bowel movement. Some people even avoid bowel movements because of the anticipated pain.

What are the symptoms?
Rectal pain may be sharp or dull, burning or knifelike. It may get worse during or after a bowel movement. Some people even avoid bowel movements because of the anticipated pain.

Other symptoms to watch for
Symptoms that may accompany rectal pain include:
- constipation or diarrhea

- itching
- rectal bleeding
- abnormal rectal discharge, such as pus
- a sensation of something protruding from the rectum, like a hemorrhoid.

What should you do?

Call the doctor to report symptoms and make an appointment.

How is rectal pain treated?

The doctor may perform tests called *anoscopy* and *proctosigmoidoscopy* to determine what is causing the rectal pain. In these tests, the doctor inserts a thin tube into the anus, rectum, or lower intestine to inspect the area and obtain a tissue specimen for analysis.

Relieving discomfort and treating the underlying cause

After determining the cause of rectal pain, the doctor orders treatments to relieve the discomfort and correct the underlying condition. For instance, applying hot, moist compresses and using sitz baths may ease discomfort by relieving the sphincter muscle spasms that rectal and anal disorders can trigger.

If rectal pain results from a protruding hemorrhoid, applying cold compresses may help shrink the hemorrhoid, prevent blood clots, and reduce pain. (See "Hemorrhoids," page 301.) Resting with the buttocks elevated (if the person's condition permits) may relieve rectal pain, too.

What else should you know?

A person with rectal pain should consult the doctor about using stool softeners, which make stools pass more easily, and applying an analgesic ointment or suppositories to relieve the pain. Eating a high-fiber diet is helpful, too, because it keeps the stools soft and avoids aggravating pain during bowel movements.

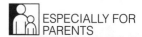 ESPECIALLY FOR PARENTS

What to do if your child has rectal pain

In children, an acute anal fissure is a common cause of rectal pain and bleeding. In this condition, a lengthwise crack forms in the lining of the anus.

From pressure to pain
During a bowel movement, pressure applied to this crack causes sharp rectal pain. In fact, the child may be so afraid of provoking this pain that he or she fears bowel movements and then becomes constipated.

When to consult the doctor
If your child complains of rectal pain, call the doctor. Stay alert for rectal bleeding, drainage, or symptoms of infection (such as fever and irritability). Report such symptoms to the doctor.

Rectal pain in infants
An infant may have rectal pain from a birth defect of the rectum. If your infant seems to be in pain when passing stools, call the doctor to arrange for an exam.

RESPIRATORY ARREST

Respiratory arrest occurs when a person stops breathing. This life-threatening emergency prevents the body's organs from getting the blood and oxygen they need to function. Without oxygen, brain cells start to die within 4 to 6 minutes; irreversible brain damage and death follow quickly. However, if a rescuer starts artificial respiration within a few minutes, the person has a good chance of surviving.

The most common cause of respiratory arrest is a blocked airway. Other conditions that can halt breathing include depression of the brain's breathing center and cardiac arrest.

Blocked airway
When a person loses consciousness, the muscles get slack. The base of the tongue may fall backward, cutting off the airway. In a conscious person, a blocked airway can come from:
- choking on food
- throat swelling
- throat spasms
- injury to the airway.

Depression of the breathing center
The brain controls breathing through the respiratory center, located in the base of the brain. A stroke, a head injury, or an overdose of certain drugs (such as narcotics) can depress the respiratory center. This causes breathing to slow down or even stop completely. An electrical shock can stun the respiratory center, halting breathing at least temporarily.

Cardiac arrest
When the heart stops beating — for example, from a massive heart attack — the brain and all other organs lose their blood supply and cease functioning. This means the brain's respiratory center can't send signals to the respiratory system telling it to keep breathing. About a minute after the heart stops beating, breathing ceases.

What are the symptoms?
The hallmark of respiratory arrest is absence of breathing. If you come upon someone who seems to be unconscious, check for signs

The hallmark of respiratory arrest is absence of breathing. If you come upon someone who seems to be unconscious, check for signs of breathing, taking no more than 5 seconds.

of breathing, taking no more than 5 seconds. Follow these steps:
■ Place your ear near the person's mouth and nose, and listen for air flowing in and out of the mouth or nose.
■ Look for the rise and fall of the chest.
■ Feel for exhaled air at the person's mouth or nose, and feel the chest wall for movement.

If you don't see the chest move or hear or feel the flow of air, assume the person isn't breathing.

Other symptoms to watch for
The person in respiratory arrest may have a bluish tinge to the lips, tongue, and nail beds. Or, if the person is dark-skinned, the mucous membranes inside the mouth and lips may be pale.

What should you do?

WHEN SECONDS COUNT

If the person is unconscious, have someone call for emergency medical help. Then place the person on his or her back. Next, open the person's airway. (For instructions on helping a conscious person who is choking, see *Clearing a blocked airway,* page 593.)

 Be sure not to delay your rescue efforts to warm the person or loosen the clothing.

 Don't take the time to move the person unless you're in a hazardous area — for example, at the scene of a fire or imminent gas explosion.

Open the airway
After you've verified that the person isn't breathing (by looking, listening, and feeling for the flow of air), use the *head-tilt, chin-lift method* to open the airway. To do this, follow these steps:
■ Place your hand that's closer to the person's head on his or her forehead. Then apply firm pressure. The pressure should be firm enough to tilt the person's head back.
■ Next place the fingertips of your other hand under the bony part of the person's lower jaw near the chin. Now lift the chin. At the same time, keep the person's mouth partially open.

 Don't place your fingertips on the soft tissue under the person's chin because doing so may obstruct the airway you're trying to open.

After you've verified that the person isn't breathing (by looking, listening, and feeling for the flow of air), use the head-tilt, chin-lift method to open the airway.

If you suspect a neck injury, use the *jaw-thrust maneuver* to open the airway instead of the head-tilt, chin-lift method. Here's how:

■ Kneel at the victim's head with your elbows on the ground. Rest your thumbs on the lower jaw near the corners of the mouth, pointing your thumbs toward the person's feet.

■ Place your fingertips around the lower jaw. To open the airway, lift the lower jaw with your fingertips.

If the person doesn't start breathing after you've opened the airway, you must begin rescue breathing.

Give rescue breaths

Rescue breathing (also called artificial respiration) forces air in and out of the person's lungs until he or she resumes breathing spontaneously. In most cases, you'll use *mouth-to-mouth* resuscitation, the most effective method. But for some people, you may need to use a different technique. (See *When mouth-to-mouth isn't the right method.*)

 Never give rescue breaths to someone who is breathing.

To prepare for rescue breaths, place the person on his or her back and loosen any tight clothing, if possible. If you suspect a neck or back injury, carefully logroll the person so he or she is lying on the back. Then follow these steps:

■ Place one hand on the person's forehead. Pinch his or her nostrils shut with the thumb and index finger of the hand you've had on the forehead. (See *Giving rescue breaths,* page 436.)

■ Take a deep breath and place your mouth over the person's mouth, creating a tight seal. Give two full breaths, taking a deep breath after each to allow enough time for the person's chest to expand and relax. Each breath you give should last 1½ to 2 seconds.

■ After giving each breath, break contact with the person's mouth and let the air escape as you turn your head to watch the chest fall. Look, listen, and feel for air movement.

■ If you don't detect air movement after the first two rescue breaths, reposition the person's head and give another rescue breath.

Remove an airway obstruction

■ If you still don't see, hear, or feel air movement after giving this rescue breath, check for and remove any foreign body that is blocking the airway, such as loose dentures.

■ Then give another rescue breath. If this isn't effective, you'll need to give *abdominal thrusts*. To do this, straddle the person's thighs. Then place your hands in the center of the person's abdomen, be-

To give abdominal thrusts, straddle the person's thighs and place your hands in the center of the abdomen. Using the heel of your hand, forcefully push upward.

When mouth-to-mouth isn't the right method

Although you'll give mouth-to-mouth resuscitation to most victims of respiratory arrest, this method isn't right for everyone. Read on to learn about alternative methods for giving rescue breaths, or artificial respiration.

Mouth-to-nose resuscitation

You'll need to give mouth-to-nose resuscitation if:
- the victim is an infant
- you can't get the person's mouth open
- the person's mouth has been badly injured
- you can't create an effective seal around the person's mouth — say, because of loose dentures or lack of teeth.

To give mouth-to-nose respiration, follow these steps.

Create a seal around the nose
- Tilt the person's head back by pressing one hand on the forehead.
- Using your other hand, lift the person's lower jaw and close his or her mouth.
- Take a deep breath.
- Next, seal your mouth around the person's nose, as shown below.

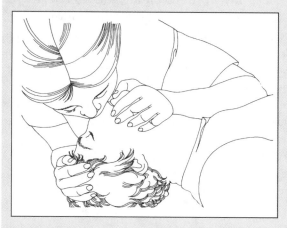

Continue giving breaths
- Exhale until you see the person's chest rise and feel the air flow.
- Remove your mouth from the person's nose. If possible, open the person's mouth to let the air out.

Mouth-to-stoma resuscitation

A person who has had the voicebox (larynx) removed breathes through a hole called a stoma in the front of the neck. The stoma may be a large, round opening in the skin; some people have a breathing tube in the stoma.

Giving mouth-to-mouth or mouth-to-nose resuscitation to someone with a stoma won't be effective because the air won't reach the lower airway. Instead, you must deliver breaths directly into the stoma. Here are the steps to use.

Uncover the stoma
- Remove any clothing and jewelry covering the stoma.
- Clear any foreign matter from the stoma.
- If the person has a breathing tube, make sure it isn't clogged. If it is clear, leave it in place. Otherwise, remove it.

Create a seal around the stoma
- Take a deep breath.
- Seal your mouth over the stoma.
- Blow into the stoma the same way you would give breaths at the mouth.

tween the ribs and navel. Using the heel of your hand, forcefully push upward to try to dislodge any object blocking the airway.
- Repeat the abdominal thrust four times. Then place your finger in the person's mouth and check for a dislodged object.

Giving rescue breaths

While pinching the person's nostrils shut, place your mouth over the person's mouth, forming a tight seal. Then breathe into the person's mouth, as you see here. Watch for the chest to rise.

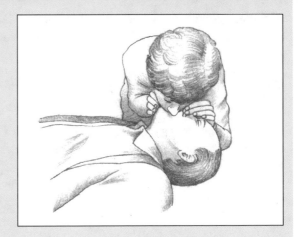

■ Even if you don't feel an object in the person's mouth, give another rescue breath (your finger sweep of the mouth may have moved a dislodged object enough to get air into the person's lungs). If this rescue breath does enter the person's lungs, give two more breaths. Between breaths, allow time for the air to leave the person's lungs.
■ On the other hand, if your rescue breaths still fail to enter the person's lungs, alternate between giving five abdominal thrusts, sweeping the mouth with your finger, and giving rescue breaths until air reaches the person's lungs.

Continue rescue breathing

After you've confirmed that your rescue breaths are entering the person's lungs, take a deep breath and repeat the cycle: Form a tight seal over the person's mouth, breathe into his or her lungs, then break contact and let air escape from the lungs. Deliver about 12 rescue breaths each minute (or one every 5 seconds). Repeat until the person is breathing regularly or until help arrives.

How is respiratory arrest treated?

If the person still isn't breathing by the time professional rescuers arrive, the emergency rescue team continues to give rescue breaths. As a stopgap measure until the person gets to the hospital, they may insert an artificial airway. Or, as a last resort, they may perform an emergency technique called a *cricothyrotomy*. In this procedure, they

Protection in a pocket mask

Most paramedics, emergency medical technicians, and other professional rescuers carry a pocket mask. This device diverts the person's exhaled air away from the rescuer's mouth during artificial respiration. The result: It eliminates direct contact with the person's mouth or nose and greatly reduces the risk of contact with the person's secretions.

Other advantages

Besides virtually eliminating the risk of catching a disease while giving artificial respiration, the pocket mask has other advantages:

- If appropriately equipped, the mask can be connected to an oxygen cylinder, which means the person can receive a high flow of oxygen to help support body tissues as the rescue effort continues.
- It can be strapped to the face and used as a simple face mask to deliver oxygen once the person starts breathing again.

How to use the mask

The rescuer fits the mask over the person's nose and mouth, clamps it to the face, and exhales into it until he or she sees the person's chest rises, as this picture shows.

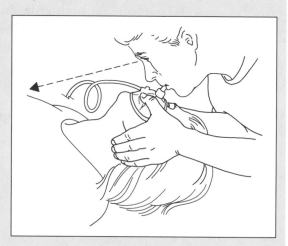

cut into the person's windpipe and insert a hollow object to keep the airway open.

Restoring breathing

At the hospital, the medical team may put a breathing tube in the person's airway or may perform a tracheotomy to establish breathing. In this procedure, they cut into the windpipe and insert a breathing tube. Sometimes, the person must be placed on a mechanical ventilator to aid breathing.

Other treatments

Other treatments depend on the cause of respiratory arrest. For information on treatment of drug overdose, electrical shock, head injuries, or heart attack, read "Drug overdose," page 198, "Burns caused by electricity," page 109, "Blunt head injuries," page 83, "Penetrating head injuries," page 398, or "Heart attack," page 283, respectively.

What else should you know?

Some people are afraid they might catch AIDS by giving mouth-to-mouth resuscitation. Is this a realistic fear? Probably not. Although a small percentage of people with AIDS carry HIV in their saliva, there are no documented cases in which HIV has been transmitted this way — not even among rescuers who've given mouth-to-mouth respiration to people with AIDS.

Doctors estimate that the chance of getting infected with HIV while giving mouth-to-mouth resuscitation is extremely small. To help eliminate even this tiny risk, most professional rescuers use a pocket mask to resuscitate people. (See *Protection in a pocket mask,* page 437.)

S

SCRAPES, ABRASIONS, AND BRUSH BURNS

A scrape is an injury caused by contact with a rough surface. An abrasion is rubbing away of the skin, as in a skinned knee. A brush burn (also called a friction burn) comes from rubbing or friction; think of a rope being pulled through your hand.

Paving the way for infection

Although seldom deep, scrapes, abrasions, and brush burns damage the skin's outer protective layer, leaving a raw surface with minor bleeding. Usually the injury heals within a few days. In the meantime, though, the wound becomes a path for germs to enter the body and start an infection.

What are the symptoms?

Typically, scrapes, abrasions, and brush burns leave a rough, reddened patch of skin, sometimes with minor bleeding. The wound may contain bits of dirt. After 1 or 2 days, the person may have symptoms of a localized infection, such as:

- pus
- pain
- redness
- swelling
- tenderness
- a sensation of heat
- red streaks leading away from the wound toward the center of the body.

What should you do?

As with any wound, your main goals are to stop the bleeding and prevent infection. If the wound is small, bleeding will probably stop on its own.

Scrapes, abrasions, and brush burns damage the skin's outer protective layer. The wound becomes a path for germs to enter the body and start an infection.

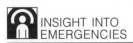

INSIGHT INTO
EMERGENCIES

When to get medical attention for a wound

Seek medical attention for the person with a scrape, abrasion, or brush burn if:
- the wound is deep
- the wound is jagged or irregular
- blood is spurting from the wound
- bleeding continues despite efforts to control it
- skin or tissue is ripped away
- a foreign object is embedded in the wound
- the person hasn't had a tetanus shot within 7 to 10 years.

Controlling bleeding

If the wound doesn't stop bleeding on its own or if it is large, take the following steps.

■ Put on disposable latex gloves to guard against blood-borne diseases. If gloves aren't available, use a waterproof material, such as a plastic bag, plastic wrap, or several layers of gauze pads.

Don't touch the wound with your unwashed hands, clothing, or anything else that might not be clean. Doing so could increase the risk of infection.

■ Remove or carefully cut away any clothing covering the wound so you can see where the blood is coming from.

■ If dirt, gravel, or other foreign objects are embedded in the wound, wipe them away with clean material. Always wipe *away* from the wound, not toward it.

■ Rinse the area by running clean, clear water directly into the wound and allowing it to run out. Gently pat the wound dry with a clean cloth.

■ If the wound is large, cover it with a sterile pad or clean cloth, and bandage it in place.

■ If the wound is very large or keeps bleeding, call the doctor. (See *When to get medical attention for a wound.*)

How are scrapes, abrasions, and brush burns treated?

The doctor orders treatments that promote skin healing and prevent infection. To help prevent infection, the person may need a tetanus shot if he or she hasn't had one in the past 7 to 10 years.

What else should you know?

Keep an eye on the scrape, abrasion, or brush burn as it heals. If it heals slowly or if the person develops symptoms of infection (such as pain, redness, swelling, or tenderness), call the doctor promptly.

If you suspect an infection, keep the person lying down with the injured area elevated and immobilized. Apply warm wet cloths over the area until you can get medical help.

SCROTAL LUMP OR SWELLING

The scrotum is the pouch of skin that contains the testicles and the spermatic cord (which consists of blood vessels, nerves, and other structures). This pouch can swell up suddenly, causing pain. Or a boy or man may feel a painless lump in the scrotum.

Common causes
Here are some common causes of scrotal swelling:
■ bacterial inflammation of the epididymis, a structure at the back of the testicle
■ torsion (twisting) of the testicle
■ a mass somewhere in the scrotum; it may contain blood, sperm, or fluid
■ hernia — a protrusion of part of the intestine into the scrotum
■ injury to the scrotum.

Less common causes
Less often, a swollen scrotum comes from cancer of the testicle. Although rare, testicular cancer is the most common cancer in men between ages 20 and 35. The cause of testicular cancer isn't known, but the incidence peaks between ages 20 and 40. It's most common in men whose testicles fail to descend or whose mothers took the drug diethylstilbestrol (known as DES) during pregnancy.

What are the symptoms?
Besides the swelling, the boy or man may have other symptoms. These vary with the underlying cause.

Symptoms of inflammation of the epididymis
This disorder causes a hot, tender, sausage-shaped swelling in the back of a testicle. Other symptoms may include:
■ severe pain that comes on gradually over hours or days
■ waddling gait (to avoid pressure on the groin and scrotum)
■ high fever
■ an overall ill feeling
■ cloudy urine
■ discharge from the penis
■ lower abdominal pain on the affected side
■ hot, red, dry, flaky, thin skin on the scrotum.

Inflammation of the epididymis causes a hot, tender, sausage-shaped swelling in the back of a testicle, along with severe pain, a waddling gait, and a high fever.

How to examine your testicles

To help detect abnormal changes early, you should examine your testicles once a month. Schedule this exam for the same date every month, perhaps the first of the month.

What's the best time to perform the exam?

The best time to examine your testicles is during or after a hot bath or shower. The heat will make your testicles descend and will relax your scrotum. This makes any abnormalities easier to find.

Now, follow these simple instructions, using the illustration below to locate anatomic landmarks.

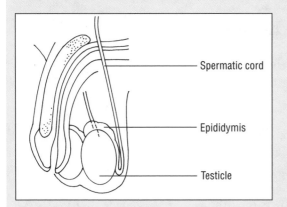

Spermatic cord

Epididymis

Testicle

First check your scrotum

With one hand, lift your penis and check your scrotum (the pouch of skin containing your testicles and parts of the spermatic cords). Feel for any change in shape or size. Also look for reddened, enlarged veins. Expect the scrotum's left side to hang slightly lower than the right.

Check each testicle

Next, place your left thumb on the front of your left testicle and your index and middle fingers behind it, as you see in the picture below. Gently but firmly roll the testicle between your thumb and fingers. Then, use your right hand to examine your right testicle in the same way.

Your testicles should feel smooth, rubbery, and slightly tender. They should move freely.

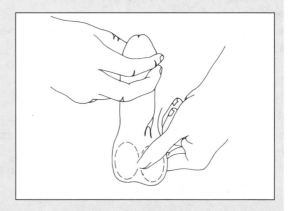

Check each spermatic cord

Locate the cordlike structure called the epididymis at the back of your testicle. Then locate the spermatic cord extending upward from it, as shown on the opposite page.

Symptoms of testicular torsion

This medical emergency causes:

- sudden, excruciating pain in or around the testicle, which may spread to the lower abdomen; the pain may get worse when the person stands
- swelling and rising of the affected testicle

How to examine your testicles *(continued)*

Check for lumps and masses
Gently squeeze the spermatic cord above your left testicle between your thumb and the first two fingers of your left hand. Then repeat on the right side, using your right hand. Check for lumps and masses along the entire length of the cords.

Consult your doctor
If you notice any lumps, masses, or other changes during the exam, call your doctor.

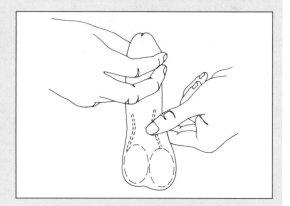

- nausea
- vomiting
- fever
- fainting or light-headedness.

Symptoms of a mass in the scrotum
A *cyst in the epididymis* produces painless scrotal swelling. A *tumor in the testicle* is usually painless.

Symptoms of a hernia
Protrusion of the intestine into the scrotum can cause swelling with either a soft or unusually firm scrotum.

Symptoms of injury to the scrotum
A blow to the scrotum can cause:
- swelling of the scrotum
- severe pain
- dark or bluish discoloration of the scrotum.

What should you do?
Anyone who discovers a lump or swelling anywhere in the scrotum should see the doctor right away. No matter how small or painless it may seem, this condition warrants immediate medical attention.

Anyone who discovers a lump or swelling in the scrotum should see the doctor right away. No matter how small or painless it may seem, this condition warrants immediate medical attention.

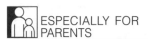

ESPECIALLY FOR
PARENTS

Checking for scrotal problems in your son

When your son is young, you'll be the one to spot any scrotal problems. Of course, as he matures, he'll be able to tell you if he's in pain or if he notices swelling.

Your infant
Your infant can't tell you when his scrotum has a problem, but you'll be able to spot problems when changing his diaper.

Scrotal symptoms in an infant may come from:
■ diapers that aren't changed often enough
■ abnormal fetal development, which can produce fluid accumulation in the scrotum (called a *hydrocele*) or cause part of the intestine to protrude into the scrotum (a condition called a *hernia*).

Your young son
In boys who are within a year or two of puberty, scrotal swelling most commonly results from twisting (torsion) of the spermatic cord. This extremely painful condition is an emergency.

Important: If your child has excruciating scrotal pain with a fever, call the doctor immediately. Don't give him anything to eat or drink or any medicine to relieve pain. He may need to undergo surgery.

Your teenager
After age 10, your son may be at risk for the same scrotal disorders that affect adult men:
■ epididymitis — inflammation of the cordlike structure at the back of the testicle
■ injury to the scrotum from contact sports
■ inflammation of the scrotum from mumps.

After puberty, mumps can cause scrotal swelling and sterility in teenage boys and men.

Have your son vaccinated against mumps
The mumps vaccination is given with the vaccine for measles and rubella. A single shot — generally to 15-month-old infants, with a booster at age 11 or 12 years — has almost eradicated these formerly common childhood disorders in North America.

 Never ignore a lump — in the scrotum or anywhere else. Call your doctor right away.

Don't mistake *painlessness* for *harmlessness.*

How is a scrotal lump or swelling treated?

To relieve symptoms, the doctor may prescribe bed rest. Placing a rolled towel beneath the scrotum may help reduce severe swelling. For mild or moderate swelling, a loose-fitting athletic supporter lined with soft cotton dressings is useful. Aspirin or ibuprofen (such as

Advil or Motrin) relieves pain and inflammation. Heat or ice packs also decrease inflammation.

Ruling out testicular cancer

Before more specific treatment can begin, the doctor must find out what's causing the scrotal swelling. To rule out a testicular tumor, the doctor usually uses *transillumination*. In this method, he or she shines a bright light through the scrotum to find out if the mass is a fluid-filled cyst or a solid mass. (A solid mass can't be transilluminated.) Lab tests, such as ultrasound and isotope scanning, can help confirm the diagnosis.

Once the underlying cause of scrotal swelling is diagnosed, the doctor orders appropriate treatments. For instance, a hernia may call for surgery. (To learn how inflammation of the epididymis and testicular torsion are treated, see "Testicle pain," page 524.)

Treating cancer of the testicle

The man may require surgery, radiation, or chemotherapy, or some combination. Surgery includes removal of the affected testicle and lymph nodes. Most surgeons remove the testicle, not the entire scrotum. The man may need to take hormones if both testicles are removed. After surgery, an athletic supporter helps to reduce pain.

Removal of one testicle doesn't mean the man will be sterile and impotent. Synthetic hormones can restore hormonal balance, if needed. In many cases, the doctor can insert a gel-filled artificial testicle that feels like a normal testicle.

What else should you know?

If you have a painless lump in your scrotum, don't panic. Lumps can have many causes. However, be sure to call your doctor at once. Only an exam can rule out testicular cancer.

Regular examination of the testicles and scrotum can help detect testicular cancer early. Boys and men should do this exam at least once a month. (See *How to examine your testicles,* pages 442 and 443, and *Checking for scrotal problems in your son.*)

A painless lump in the scrotum is no reason to panic. But it does call for a prompt visit to the doctor.

SEIZURES

Seizures are sudden bouts of uncontrolled electrical energy in the brain — a kind of short circuit. Some seizures are dramatic: The person collapses onto the floor, with arms and legs flailing and mouth frothing. Others are so fleeting and subtle that they go virtually unnoticed — even by the people experiencing them.

How seizures are classified
Seizures fall into two broad categories:
- *Partial seizures.* These come from abnormal electrical activity in a specific area of the brain.
- *Generalized seizures.* These are caused by abnormal electrical activity by nerve cells scattered throughout the brain.

Understanding the causes
Sometimes a seizure has no known cause. Other seizures can be linked to such conditions as:
- head injury
- a brain tumor
- infection
- stroke
- a metabolic or hormone problem, such as diabetes
- alcohol withdrawal.

What are the symptoms?
Symptoms of a seizure depend on the seizure type. *Note:* If possible, try to remember the person's symptoms. (See *Observing a person during a seizure.*)

Symptoms of a grand mal seizure
This generalized seizure is the most severe type of seizure. Just before it starts, the person may experience mood changes plus what doctors call an *aura.* During the aura, the person may smell, taste, feel, hear, or see peculiar things. Typically, the following things then occur:
- The person loses consciousness.
- Muscles of the trunk, arm, and legs contract and extend stiffly.
- The person falls to the ground and stops breathing. He or she may bite the tongue and lose bladder and bowel control.
- The muscles start to contract rhythmically.

Just before a grand mal seizure starts, the person may experience mood changes. Then he or she typically loses consciousness and the muscles contract and extend stiffly.

Observing a person during a seizure

To help the doctor later determine what type of seizure the person has had, watch the person closely during and after the seizure. Then, if possible, write down answers to the following questions.

How long did the seizure last?
- What time did the seizure start?
- What time did it end?

What happened just before the seizure?
- Did the person complain of odd feelings or a strange mood just before the seizure began?
- Did he or she smell, taste, feel, see, or hear anything unusual?

What happened during the seizure?
- Did the person lose consciousness or fall down?
- What type of muscle movements did the person make? Were they jerky or rhythmic? Constant or intermittent?

- Did the person laugh? Cry out? Snore? Make other noises?
- Did the person drool? Lose bowel or bladder control? Stop breathing? Breathe rapidly and deeply? Froth at the mouth?
- Did the person make repetitive movements, such as smacking the lips, grimacing, chewing, or rubbing or plucking at clothes?

What happened after the seizure?
- Did the person seem confused or groggy?
- Did the person fall asleep?
- Did he or she complain of a headache, muscle ache, or fatigue?
- Did he or she remember having had the seizure?

- The person begins to sweat, breathes rapidly and deeply, has a fast pulse, and may start frothing at the mouth.
- Muscles then relax and breathing gets deeper.
- The seizure ends, and the person awakens disoriented and confused, complaining of headache, muscle ache, and fatigue.

Typically, the person doesn't remember the episode. He or she may sleep for several hours afterward.

Symptoms of a myoclonic seizure
In this type of generalized seizure, the person experiences jerking of one or more muscle groups. The muscle jerking lasts a few seconds.

Symptoms of an atonic seizure
Also called a *drop attack,* this seizure also causes the person to jerk the muscles. Then the muscles fall slack.

Symptoms of an akinetic seizure
The person has a brief, complete loss of muscle tone and consciousness. He or she falls to the ground, possibly suffering a head injury.

Symptoms of an absence seizure

Also called *petit mal* seizure, this seizure causes the person to stop all activity and to stare into space, usually for less than 15 seconds. During this time, the person isn't aware of the surroundings. Others may notice nothing unusual about the person's behavior, although over time an observer may notice the staring episodes. Petit mal seizures are most common in children.

Symptoms of a simple partial seizure

The person with this type of partial seizure may have odd movements in one part of the body. Or the unusual movements may spread in an orderly fashion to surrounding body parts. Some people also have tingling or numbness of a body part, but their state of mind remains relatively normal.

Symptoms of a complex partial seizure

The person usually has an aura and then loses consciousness. He or she may also experience a twilight state, with time seeming to stand still. Or he or she may have a déjà vu ("I've been here before") experience. Some people laugh inappropriately.

If the abnormal brain activity is in the part of the brain called the temporal lobe, the person will have *automatisms*. These are involuntary repetitive movements like chewing, lip-smacking, facial grimacing, and rubbing one's clothes.

Symptoms of status epilepticus

This is a seizure that doesn't stop. It may be one prolonged seizure or many consecutive ones without the person fully recovering in between.

If the seizure is generalized, it can threaten the person's life by jeopardizing heart function and breathing. Status epilepticus can also cause brain damage.

What should you do?

Most seizures stop on their own within 30 seconds to a few minutes. Your main goal is to prevent the person from being harmed during the seizure. Follow these guidelines.

Prevent injury

- Try to catch the person as he or she is falling, and then lay him or her down.
- Move sharp objects, furniture, and other items out of the way.
- If the person falls to the ground before you have a chance to catch

Most seizures stop on their own. Your main goal is to prevent the person from being injured during the seizure.

him or her, protect the person's neck. Immediately support the head and neck using rolled-up clothing or other handy materials.

> ❌ Don't move the person's neck. If you must turn the head to one side — say, to clear vomit from the throat — use the logroll technique. You'll need an assistant for this maneuver: One person holds the head and neck in a fixed position as the other person rolls the victim's legs and trunk.

- Place pillows or rolled blankets around the person.
- Loosen clothing from around the person's neck.
- Keep the person lying on the side to prevent choking.
- If the person vomits, clear the mouth and nose of vomit, but don't use your fingers.

> ❌ Never force anything between the person's teeth during a seizure if the teeth are clenched. You could injure the teeth or get bitten. Also, if you try to push an object into the mouth, you might end up pushing the tongue back, blocking the person's airway.
>
> ❌ Don't try to stop the seizure — for instance, by throwing a liquid on the person's face or into the mouth.
>
> ❌ Don't restrain the person's movements unless they jeopardize his or her safety. (See *"My little Jared is having a seizure!"* pages 450 and 451.)
>
> ❌ Be sure not to give the person anything to eat or drink.

Get help

Seek medical help for the person as soon as possible. (See *When to get emergency medical care,* page 452.) Someone who's had a relatively minor seizure should consult the doctor promptly.

How are seizures treated?

If the seizure is still in progress, the medical team tries to maintain an open airway. They may need to insert an artificial airway to keep the person breathing.

They also loosen any tight clothing and place the person on his or her side to ease breathing. They take steps to ensure the person's safety and prevent injury from violent movements.

To stop the seizure, the doctor may order intravenous antiseizure drugs, such as Dilantin or Valium.

If the seizure is still in progress, the medical team tries to keep the airway open. To stop the seizure, the doctor may order intravenous antiseizure drugs.

STORIES OF SURVIVAL

"My little Jared is having a seizure!"

How I love visits from little Jared, my 6-year-old grandson. He's a handful for everyone but his doting grandmother. If you ask me, he takes after his father, who was just as rambunctious at that age. I dearly look forward to our time together.

Scared me half to death
One visit, though, Jared scared me half to death. He was taking his afternoon nap on the couch, curled on his side like a baby, his wavy hair matted to the cushion. I was sitting at the kitchen table, cutting out coupons and watching my favorite soap opera on the TV.

Just as Erica announced she was about to divorce yet another husband, I heard a rustling sound in the living room. I looked over and saw Jared in a spasm, his little body jerking up and down on the cushions.

I'll never forget it
Now, normally I can't move too fast on account of my hip, but I think I must have *flown* to the couch. White froth was bubbling from the corner of Jared's mouth, his eyes were rolled back in his head, and his teeth were clenched just as tight as can be.

I knew right away it was a seizure. Several years ago, I saw a child in an emergency room have one. She was right next to me, flailing around on the next bed. I'll never forget it.

I held his hands by his side
I knew enough not to stick anything in Jared's mouth — that much I knew. Trouble was, I didn't know what I was *supposed* to do.

Jared's arms kept jerking upward, like he was trying to grab his throat. I was so afraid he'd hurt himself, punch himself, or whatever. So I held his hands by his side as best I could. I'll tell you, he was stronger than you'd think a 6-year-old could be, but I held him tight.

Help me, please!
I wanted desperately to call 911, but I couldn't reach the phone. Plus, I didn't want to let go of Jared. I hollered for Millie, my next-door neighbor, but got no answer.

Just as I began to panic, Jared's seizure stopped. He began to breathe deeply, like he was sleeping, and his eyes stared straight ahead without really seeing.

As soon as I sensed that Jared wasn't going to have another seizure, I rushed to the phone and called an ambulance. Trying not to sound as scared as I felt, I told the operator, "My little Jared is having a seizure!"

The EMTs came right away and took Jared to the hospital. The doctor ran some tests and said Jared has a mild form of epilepsy. But if he takes his medicine right, he might never have another seizure.

I hope he doesn't. I hope he grows up never knowing another one.

Anything for Jared
When Jared visits me now, I make sure he takes his medicine the way he's supposed to. And I've enrolled in a first-aid course at the local Red Cross, so if Jared *does* have another seizure, I'll know more about how to help.

I'm the oldest person in the class, you know, which can be a bit embarrassing. But I'm a grandmother, and I'll do anything for my little Jared.

AfterWords
Jared's grandmother recognized his seizure immediately — something many people might not have been able to do. And she knew not to put anything in his mouth.

STORIES OF SURVIVAL

"My little Jared is having a seizure!" *(continued)*

Perhaps most important, she later signed up for a first-aid course to correct her lack of knowledge about how to help someone during a seizure. In that course, she'll surely learn that it's crucial to keep Jared's airway open, such as by holding the chin up. She'll also learn to keep Jared on his side throughout a seizure.

Another point the Red Cross instructor is sure to stress: Never forcibly hold down a person's arms or legs during a seizure. Doing so can lead to broken bones or dislocations.

Staying calm

Jared's grandmother will also learn how important it is to stay calm. No matter what kind of emergency she might face in the future, staying calm will help her keep her mind clear and her actions purposeful. Both are essential when someone's life is in jeopardy.

Treating status epilepticus

The medical team establishes an open airway, administers oxygen, and gives intravenous Valium or another antiseizure drug to help stop the seizure. To track the heart's functioning, they attach the person to a heart monitor. If all else fails, the doctor may use general anesthesia to bring the seizure under control.

What else should you know?

After the person is medically stable, the doctor may order a test to record brain-wave activity (commonly called an EEG). This test helps to pinpoint the site of the abnormal brain activity. Other helpful diagnostic tests may include:

- computed tomography (commonly called a CAT scan) to detect abnormalities in the brain
- magnetic resonance imaging (commonly called an MRI) to see brain areas that are hidden by bone on other tests
- blood tests to measure sugar and calcium levels.

Long-term care

A person who's diagnosed with a seizure will probably need to take antiseizure drugs, such as Dilantin, Tegretol, Depakene, or phenobarbital.

Self-care can play an important role, too. Like asthma, seizures

When to get emergency medical care

Seizures pose a more serious danger to some people than to others. Get medical help *immediately* for a person who:

- is pregnant
- has never had a seizure before
- recovers slowly from the seizure
- has a seizure that lasts more than 5 minutes
- is injured during the seizure.

often are triggered by conditions such as fatigue, stress, and drug or alcohol use.

To try to find the person's triggers, the doctor may advise him or her to keep a seizure diary. The person writes down information about daily diet, stress level, and other life-style factors. Then, if the person has a seizure, the doctor reviews the diary to try to link the seizure to a specific trigger.

Some people find that regular physical exercise and relaxation techniques help to control stress and, in turn, reduce the frequency of seizures.

Wear identification

A person who has had a seizure should wear medical identification, such as a Medic Alert necklace or bracelet. That way, if he or she loses consciousness, health care workers will know how to respond.

SHOCK

Shock is a state of extremely impaired circulation that reduces the flow of blood and oxygen to body cells. The body tries to compensate for the shortage through a series of complex responses. Unless treated promptly, these responses can eventually lead to death. (See *What happens in shock*.)

Shock can occur in just about anyone who suffers a medical emergency. Sometimes it is more dangerous than the condition that triggered it.

Forms of shock

Shock can take several forms. *Hypovolemic shock* occurs when an illness or injury leads to tremendous blood or fluid loss. Conditions capable of causing massive blood loss include:

- stab wounds
- gunshot wounds
- excessive vomiting or diarrhea
- burns.

Septic shock results from a widespread infection, which may have begun from a minor infection. Toxic substances are released from certain bacteria in the bloodstream, leading to massive infection. Septic shock is usually preceded by symptoms of severe infection.

Certain diseases and conditions can make a person more vulnerable to septic shock. They include:

- diabetes
- liver disease
- immune suppression, such as from AIDS or drug therapy for cancer
- invasive procedures, for example, insertion of a catheter or an intravenous line.

Anaphylactic shock is a severe allergic reaction. For more information, see "Allergic reaction to a bite or sting," page 23, "Allergic reaction to a drug," page 27, and "Allergic reaction to food," page 30.

What are the symptoms?

Early symptoms common to all types of shock include:

- anxiety
- restlessness
- fear
- a fast, weak pulse
- rapid, shallow breathing.

Later symptoms

If shock progresses, the person may show symptoms of decreased blood flow to the brain, such as confusion and sluggishness. Also look for enlarged pupils and either pale skin in a light-skinned person or pale mucous membranes in a dark-skinned person.

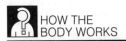

HOW THE BODY WORKS

What happens in shock

Normally, blood vessels open or close to control the amount of blood flowing to various parts of the body. In shock, blood flow regulation goes awry, and the mechanisms that the body uses to compensate can't keep up with the problem.

The result: Body tissues and organs don't get enough blood or oxygen.

Reasons for shock

Shock can result from:

- massive blood loss
- blood vessels that open but can't be filled because of a relative shortage of blood
- failure of the heart to pump and circulate enough blood.

Too little oxygen, too little time

Without sufficient blood flow to provide oxygen to body organs, cells begin to die. Brain cells in particular can't withstand an oxygen shortage for long without sustaining damage.

What should you do?

 WHEN SECONDS COUNT

Immediately call for emergency medical help if you suspect a person is in shock. Then check for a clear airway and look, listen, and feel for breathing. Open the person's airway if necessary. If you don't detect breathing, give two full rescue breaths if you know how. (See *Performing CPR on an adult,* page 579, *Performing CPR on a child,* page 585, or *Performing CPR on an infant,* page 590.)

Then feel for a pulse. If you can't detect a pulse, start chest compressions. If the person has medication (such as Adrenalin) for a severe allergic reaction, help him or her take it.

Don't hesitate to call 911 if you think someone is in shock.

Position the person correctly

Unless you suspect a neck or spine injury, keep the person lying down, preferably flat on the back. If injuries don't restrict the person's movement, elevate the feet 12 to 18 inches (30 to 45 centimeters). This will promote blood flow to the head and organs of the central body. If this position causes pain or difficulty breathing, lower the person's feet.

If vomiting seems likely, or if the person has suffered a jaw or mouth injury, place him or her on the side so fluids can drain out of the mouth.

Never move the victim if you suspect a head or neck injury, unless his or her life is in danger from a fire, an explosion, or some other threat. If the person has a head injury but not a neck injury, raise the head slightly.

Don't place the person on the back if he or she has trouble breathing or symptoms of heart attack (such as chest pain). Instead, raise the person to a half-sitting position to make breathing easier.

Control bleeding and splint broken bones

If the person is bleeding, try to stop the bleeding. (For instructions, see "Bleeding," page 73.) Be aware that bleeding may be internal. In that case, you won't see blood flowing from a wound, but you may notice other telltale symptoms. (See *When to suspect hidden bleeding.*)

Keep the person lying down, and elevate the feet 12 to 18 inches.

If you suspect the person has a broken bone, splint it as described in "Fractures (broken bones)," page 251.

Keep the person warm and comfortable
Wrap the person in blankets or other available materials. Be sure to cover the head, neck, and hands. If the person doesn't have a neck injury and is lying on cold, damp ground, put blankets underneath the body if you can safely do so.

 Be sure not to make the victim *too* warm.

Loosen any tight clothing at the victim's neck, chest, or waist that might restrict breathing or circulation.

Other steps to take
- Check the person's pulse at regular intervals, and continue to watch for changes in mental state. For instance, as shock worsens, the person may become confused or sluggish.
- If you know the person is diabetic and seems alert enough to swallow, give a small amount of sugar, orange juice, cake icing, milk, or candy to counteract low blood sugar.
- If the ambulance is several hours away and the person is awake and alert, offer water or a commercial electrolyte drink, such as Gatorade. Have the person sip the fluid slowly. Stop giving fluids if the person becomes nauseous or vomits.

Don't give fluids if the ambulance is on its way or if the person is unconscious, vomiting, or having seizures. Also withhold fluids if you think the person has a stomach wound, a brain injury, or rectal bleeding.

Be sure not to leave the person alone.

Don't let other people frighten the person by commenting on the injuries. Keep talking calmly and gently, and ask spectators for privacy.

How is shock treated?
The medical team takes emergency steps to restore normal circulation, such as:
- giving fluids and medicines through an intravenous line
- administering oxygen through a tube or by mask
- monitoring the person's heart function on a heart monitor.

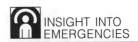
INSIGHT INTO EMERGENCIES

When to suspect hidden bleeding

You should suspect hidden (internal) bleeding in any person who has:
- suffered a hard blow
- fallen
- been in an accident
- had a stomach ulcer
- been a heavy drinker.

Look for clues
Some of the symptoms of hidden bleeding — anxiety, a fast pulse, and pale, cold, clammy skin — overlap with those of shock. However, hidden bleeding does produce some specific symptoms.

Watch for specific symptoms
Hidden bleeding may cause:
- vomit that is red or resembles coffee grounds
- vomiting of bright red blood
- black or bright red stools.

Take quick action
If the person has any of the above symptoms, suspect hidden bleeding and call for emergency medical help.

Other treatments
Other treatments depend on the specific type of shock. For example:
- A person with septic shock receives antibiotics.
- A person with shock caused by blood loss may receive blood transfusions.
- A person with anaphylactic shock receives medicine to reverse the severe allergic reaction.

What else should you know?
A person who's in *emotional* shock may have some of the same symptoms that occur with other types of shock. If you come upon someone who seems to be in this state, take the same actions described above. Keep the person calm and provide emotional support.

Shock in an infant
An infant can't tell you exactly how he or she is feeling. But you should seek prompt medical care if your infant suffers a burn or a serious fall.

Why? These injuries may lead to internal bleeding, which can trigger shock. Unfortunately, symptoms of internal bleeding aren't always evident. That's why you should always consider the possibility of shock if your infant has been injured or has pale, cold, or clammy skin. Call for medical help immediately. In the meantime, have the infant lie flat and wrap him or her in blankets to keep in body heat.

Shortness of breath may be a sign of a medical problem if the person wheezes or has trouble breathing even without exertion.

SHORTNESS OF BREATH

Normally, we're unaware of our breathing. Our brains regulate breathing to supply the body's demands for oxygen. These demands vary; they are greater when we're running, for instance, than when we're sleeping.

When breathing isn't easy
Many people experience shortness of breath after exertion, but it's usually relieved by rest. However, shortness of breath may result from a medical problem if the person also:

- wheezes (makes high-pitched or whistling sounds when breathing)
- feels a need to push or pull with the chest and neck muscles to breathe
- has difficulty breathing even without exertion.

Understanding the causes
Common causes of shortness of breath include:
- choking, usually from food or another object getting lodged in the windpipe
- asthma
- a respiratory infection, such as pneumonia or croup (in children) (see *What to do if your child becomes short of breath,* pages 458 and 459)
- a heart condition, such as congestive heart failure (see *"The day I almost lost Donald,"* page 460)
- chronic lung disease, such as chronic bronchitis or emphysema.
    Less often, shortness of breath comes from:
- an acute reaction to a drug or a toxin caused by an insect bite or sting
- a nervous system disease, such as multiple sclerosis or myasthenia gravis
- irregular heartbeats
- a lung tumor
- a blood clot in the lung
- a broken rib
- a heart defect present at birth.

What are the symptoms?
Shortness of breath can come on rapidly or slowly. Sometimes, the person also has some of these other symptoms:
- shoulders rising and falling with each breath
- gasping
- wheezing
- rapid breathing.

What should you do?

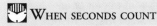 **WHEN SECONDS COUNT**

Get medical help immediately if the person:
- is choking
- breathes rapidly

Get medical help immediately if the person is choking, breathes rapidly, has bluish skin, seems restless, must struggle to breathe, or has chest pain.

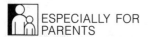

ESPECIALLY FOR
PARENTS

What to do if your child becomes short of breath

Watching a child struggle to breathe is a scary experience for any parent. Depending on the underlying cause of the problem, you may need to act immediately.

Read on to learn how to identify shortness of breath in a child, how to recognize the serious conditions that can cause this problem, and what steps to take if your child shows symptoms.

How to identify shortness of breath
Normally, an infant breathes by using the stomach muscles. By age 7, children breathe the way adults do — by using their chest muscles.

That's why you should suspect shortness of breath if your infant uses the chest muscles to breathe or if your older child uses the stomach muscles to breathe. Seek medical attention for *any* child who uses the neck or shoulder muscles to ease breathing.

Is your child choking?
More than 3,000 choking deaths occur every year. In a young child, choking typically occurs when a foreign object, such as a toy, a hot dog, or a coin, gets lodged in the airway.

How to identify symptoms
Suspect choking if your child:
■ turns blue, gray, or ashen
■ gasps, gets short of breath, or becomes unable to breathe, speak, or cough
■ looks panicked
■ clutches the neck with one or both hands.

Actions to take
Perform the Heimlich maneuver (see *Clearing a blocked airway,* page 593). Have someone call 911 immediately.

How to prevent this emergency
■ Don't let your infant eat hot dogs.

■ Keep toys labeled "Not for children under age 3" away from infants and toddlers.
■ Warn older siblings to keep their toys away from their younger brothers and sisters.

Does your child have croup?
Croup is a viral infection of the voice box and airway that causes severe shortness of breath and airway spasms. It can even lead to heart and lung collapse.

Croup is most common in children between ages 3 months and 3 years. It usually strikes during the winter and affects boys more often than girls.

How to identify symptoms
Suspect croup if your child has:
■ a barking cough
■ high-pitched, hoarse breathing sounds
■ severe shortness of breath.
Usually, symptoms develop slowly over a few days.

Actions to take
One of the best ways to relieve a croup attack is to turn your bathroom into a temporary steamroom. Take your child into the bathroom, close the door, and turn on the hot water in the shower. Then sit outside the shower with him or her while steam fills the room. Let your child breathe in the steam for a few minutes. *Important:* Don't let your child lie on his or her back, because this position may obstruct the airway.

You can also take your child out into the cool night air (weather permitting and with proper clothing). The cool air may relieve the breathing distress.

If these home treatments don't help your child to breathe more easily, call your doctor or take the child to the hospital emergency department.

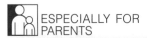

What to do if your child becomes short of breath *(continued)*

How the doctor treats croup
The doctor may prescribe:
- home care with rest
- a humidifier or vaporizer during sleep
- fever-reducing medicines such as Tylenol (or another drug containing acetaminophen) to relieve symptoms.

Stay alert for complications
Sometimes a child gets complications about 5 days after recovering from croup. Notify your doctor right away if your child develops:
- an earache
- a productive cough
- high fever
- increased shortness of breath.

Does your child have epiglottitis?
In a child between ages 2 and 8, shortness of breath may come from a disorder called *epiglottitis*. In this condition, a throat structure called the epiglottis becomes inflamed. In its acute form, epiglottitis is life-threatening.

How to identify symptoms
Suspect epiglottitis if your child has:
- high fever
- severe shortness of breath
- high-pitched breathing
- sore throat
- difficulty swallowing
- irritability
- restlessness
- drooling.

These symptoms come on quickly. Another clue to epiglottitis: The child stretches the neck way out, sits up, and leans forward with the mouth open, tongue sticking out, and nostrils flaring while struggling to breathe.

Actions to take
The swelling that accompanies this infection can obstruct your child's airway within 2 to 5 hours. Immediately call for emergency medical help.

How to prevent this emergency
Make sure your child gets vaccinated against *Haemophilus influenzae* type b (Hib), the most common cause of epiglottitis. The doctor usually recommends this as part of routine childhood immunization.

- has bluish skin
- seems restless
- must struggle to use the whole body to breathe
- also has chest pain.

If the person is choking, perform the Heimlich maneuver to help expel the object. (See *Clearing a blocked airway,* page 593.)

Make the person comfortable
If symptoms are less severe, help the person find the position that makes breathing easiest. Encourage the person to breathe more slowly. One way to do this is by saying "In through the nose, out

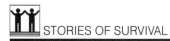

STORIES OF SURVIVAL

"The day I almost lost Donald"

I had taught with Donald for nearly 35 years, right here at Central High. He was a stubborn old coot. I can say that because I'm 2 years older and just as stubborn.

One day after school, I noticed that Donald was walking slowly down the corridor, much more slowly than usual. When I reached him, I could see that his face was almost gray and that he was struggling to breathe, almost like he was trying to blow out a candle. He looked horrible.

"Donald," I said. "What's wrong?"

"Nothing," he said. "I'm fine."

"Well, you don't look fine. Come with me."

No nurse is bad news

We went looking for the school nurse just a couple of doors down, but she had left for the day. I sat Donald on the chair next to the desk and took a good look at him.

He could hardly sit still. He was so short of breath that he was gasping for air. Sweat was beading up on his forehead, and his hands trembled. I had seen my mother look the same way years ago when she was in the hospital having heart trouble. She died from the attack, so I knew Donald was in trouble.

Been through this before

I found an oxygen tank and tubing in the first-aid closet, but I didn't know how to use it. Donald did, though, and took me through step by step. He had obviously been through this before.

"Donald, have you had an attack like this before?" I asked as I put the oxygen mask on him.

"Yes," he replied. "Once."

"Did you call the ambulance?"

Suddenly his eyes flared. "*No,* don't call the ambulance!" he commanded.

"My wife will get mad at me"

"Why not?" I asked.

"*Please,* don't call the ambulance," he gasped.

"My wife will get mad at me if I go to the hospital again."

I couldn't believe it. Here was a man struggling for breath — and he was worried about how his wife would react if he got help! Well, I was going to have no part of that, and I told him so.

"That's silly, Donald. I'm going to call the ambulance, and that's all there is to it." And I did.

Paramedics can be stubborn, too

The ambulance came right away and did their ambulance things. Even the paramedics had trouble persuading Donald to go to the hospital. But they took him there anyway. I was glad. I don't know what would have happened if he hadn't gone to the hospital, but I know it would have been bad.

Still stubborn, but healthier

Donald's little scare after school that day prompted his doctor to change his heart medicine, which worked well.

Donald looks much healthier when I pass him in the corridors these days. Of course, he's still stubborn. Thank goodness.

AfterWords

Donald's stubborn friend probably saved his life. Donald had become ashen and short of breath from congestive heart failure — a condition that, if left untreated, can cause death.

In congestive heart failure, the heart fails to pump enough blood to the body's tissues, which deprives those tissues of oxygen and causes the symptoms Donald experienced. Even Donald's "stubbornness" might have been caused in part by a lack of oxygen to the brain.

Donald's friend certainly did the right thing by calling 911. But she might have called *before* hunting for the oxygen tank, rather than afterward. In any case, her own stubbornness and clear thinking helped save her friend's life.

through the mouth" over and over until the person starts to breathe this way. Be sure to report the breathing problem to the doctor at once.

> ❌ Never delay seeking medical care for someone with shortness of breath.
>
> ❌ Don't wait until morning to consult a doctor about a child's shortness of breath.

How is shortness of breath treated?

To help diagnose the cause of shortness of breath, the doctor may order blood tests and chest X-rays. In an emergency, the person may need such treatments as oxygen administration and intravenous fluids and will be hooked up to a heart monitor to detect irregular heartbeats.

Drug therapy

Depending on the person's underlying condition, the doctor may order such drugs as:
- bronchodilators — medicines that ease breathing by widening the air passages
- drugs to regulate the heartbeat
- water pills (diuretics) to help rid the body of excess fluid
- nitroglycerin to lessen strain on the heart
- pain relievers.

What else should you know?

Here are some tips that may help you to prevent shortness of breath or relieve it once it starts:
- If you're exposed to irritating chemicals or gases at work, be sure to wear a protective mask.
- If you're a painter or an artist, wear a protective mask while you work — especially if you use an airbrush.
- If you're a smoker, stop smoking as soon as your breathing difficulty begins.
- If you have asthma, keep your prescribed asthma medicines with you at all times so you can take them as soon as an asthma attack starts.
- If you're with someone who has asthma and suddenly starts struggling to breathe, help the person retrieve the asthma inhaler and use it.

To help prevent shortness of breath or relieve it once it starts, wear a protective mask if you're exposed to irritating chemicals or gases.

SHOULDER INJURIES

At the shoulder, the body's most movable joint, these three bones come together:
- shoulder blade
- collarbone
- upper arm bone (called the *humerus*).

More mobile than stable
The shoulder is susceptible to injury because it is more mobile than it is stable. Anyone whose shoulder is subjected to stress may suffer any of these common injuries:
- shoulder dislocation
- shoulder separation
- swimmer's shoulder. (See *Comparing shoulder injuries.*)

Shoulder dislocation
This injury occurs when the upper arm bone comes out of the shoulder. The bone then sticks out on the front or top of the shoulder. In a severe dislocation, the bands of fibrous tissue that connect muscle to bone and bind joints together (called *tendons* and *ligaments*) are stretched; blood vessels and nerves in the shoulder area are injured, too.

Once a person has dislocated the shoulder a few times, he or she may find that less force is required to knock it out of joint.

A dislocated shoulder can come from:
- contact sports, such as football, hockey, rugby, soccer, and skiing
- a fall on the shoulder or on an outstretched arm or hand
- a blow to the shoulder
- a genetic tendency for the shoulder to "pop out" easily. (Shoulder dislocation seems to run in some families.)

Shoulder separation
This injury happens when the ligaments that attach the collarbone to the shoulder blade are torn. Sometimes, the collarbone becomes misaligned.

Separation of the shoulder results from an injury such as:
- a fall on the shoulder or on an outstretched arm or hand
- a blow to the shoulder
- contact sports, such as football, hockey, soccer, rugby, and skiing.

A shoulder separation can result from a fall on the shoulder or on an outstretched arm or hand, a blow to the shoulder, or contact sports.

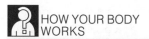 HOW YOUR BODY WORKS

Comparing shoulder injuries

The shoulder can sustain injury from a wide range of activities, not just sports.

Shoulder dislocation

In this injury, the humerus (upper arm bone) slips out of the shoulder. If severe, a shoulder dislocation may stretch tendons and ligaments and injure nearby nerves and blood vessels. The picture below shows a front view of a dislocated shoulder, along with the type of activity that can cause this injury.

SHOULDER DISLOCATION

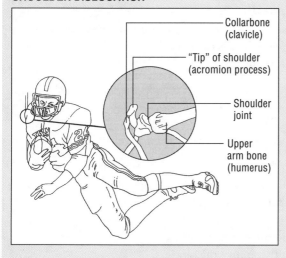

Shoulder separation

This injury occurs when the ligaments that attach the collarbone to the shoulder blade are torn. The collarbone may fall out of alignment.

Swimmer's shoulder

In this injury, the supraspinatus muscle (which lies atop the shoulder) or the rotator cuff (which surrounds the shoulder) is strained or torn. The picture below shows a front view of a torn supraspinatus muscle, along with the type of swimming movement that can cause this injury.

SWIMMER'S SHOULDER

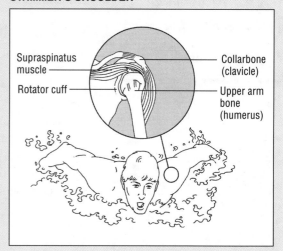

Swimmer's shoulder

In this injury, a strain or a tiny tear occurs in the muscle that lies atop the shoulder, between the neck and the top of the arm. Or the strain or tear may occur in the *rotator cuff* — a structure made up of intertwined muscles and tendons that surrounds the shoulder. An injured rotator cuff may swell and press against bone.

Usually, swimmer's shoulder comes from repetitive motion. A swimmer may experience it by using an improper stroke or after increasing swimming speed, distance, or both. Other sports that can cause swimmer's shoulder include:

- baseball (pitchers may get it from pitching the ball)
- football (quarterbacks may get it from throwing passes)
- tennis
- basketball
- golf
- weight lifting
- rock climbing
- racquetball.

Actually, anyone who raises the arm above the head repetitively can get swimmer's shoulder over time. That explains why it's sometimes seen in construction workers, painters, and plasterers.

What are the symptoms?

Shoulder dislocation and shoulder separation cause similar symptoms. Swimmer's shoulder is easier to distinguish because the injury tends to come on more gradually.

Symptoms of shoulder dislocation

This injury can cause:

- severe pain
- swelling
- bruising
- restricted shoulder movement
- shoulder deformity, with a bump sticking out.

Symptoms of shoulder separation

The person with this injury may have:

- severe pain
- swelling
- bruising
- restricted shoulder movement
- a malformed shoulder.

Symptoms of swimmer's shoulder

This injury can result in:

- pain on the top and in front of the shoulder
- pain and weakness when the person tries to extend the affected arm upward or forward

---

Shoulder dislocation can cause severe pain, swelling, bruising, restricted shoulder movement, and shoulder deformity.

- pain in the shoulder when the person lies on it
- sharp pain and restricted motion if the rotator cuff has been injured.

What should you do?
- If the person can't move the affected arm at all and the shoulder seems "frozen," seek immediate medical treatment.
- If the person has a sharp pain along with shoulder weakness, tell him or her to stop using the shoulder and call the doctor.

Here are some other steps to take.

What to do for shoulder dislocation or separation
If you suspect one of these injuries, apply an ice pack to reduce swelling. Support the person's arm in the position you found it in. Then apply a sling. (See *How to splint a broken bone or dislocated joint,* page 596.) Have the person seek prompt medical attention.

What to do for swimmer's shoulder
If the person can't raise the arm above his or her head or can't move it at all, call a doctor right away. In the meantime, apply ice to help prevent swelling and ease pain.

 Don't let the person try to work (or play) through the injury.

How are shoulder injuries treated?
Treatment varies with the specific injury.

Treating shoulder dislocation
The doctor restores the dislocated bone to its normal position. He or she prescribes ice or cold packs for the first few days, then may recommend heat to relieve the pain and increase blood flow to the injury. Medicines used to treat a dislocated shoulder may include:
- aspirin or acetaminophen combined with codeine for pain
- aspirin, ibuprofen (such as Advil or Motrin), or a similar drug, such as Naprosyn, to reduce inflammation and swelling and bring extra pain relief.

Wrapping or immobilizing the affected arm in a sling can promote healing. Some people need surgery to stabilize the shoulder, especially after repeated dislocations.

Healing may take 3 to 6 weeks. The doctor may recommend physical therapy once healing begins. A physical therapist or trainer can recommend the proper weight-training exercises to strengthen

Apply an ice pack to the injured shoulder to ease pain and swelling. Have the person see a doctor promptly.

shoulder muscles, ligaments, and tendons. The person should avoid sports until the shoulder has healed.

Treating shoulder separation

The doctor wraps or immobilizes the shoulder to promote healing. He or she recommends ice or cold packs for the first 2 days, then a heating pad.

A separated shoulder may take 2 to 10 weeks to heal. The doctor may recommend physical therapy once healing begins. In severe cases, surgery may be necessary to repair damaged ligaments.

The person should avoid participating in sports until the shoulder has fully healed. As with a dislocation, a trainer or physical therapist can advise the person on weight-training exercises to strengthen the shoulder.

Treating swimmer's shoulder

The doctor recommends ice or cold packs for the first 2 to 4 days. Some doctors recommend use of a heating pad later. Usually, he or she advises the person to avoid exercises that require pushing movements.

Swimmer's shoulder may take 4 to 8 weeks to heal. Once healing begins, the person may undergo physical therapy to strengthen the shoulder. He or she should avoid participating in sports until the shoulder has fully healed. To regain the previous level of activity, the person must progress very slowly at first.

A person who continues to have a limited range of motion in the shoulder should consult the doctor. In rare cases, surgery of the rotator cuff is required.

Treating recurrences

If swimmer's shoulder recurs, the person should apply ice for 2 to 4 days, then switch to a heating pad. When used consistently — not just when the shoulder hurts — anti-inflammatory drugs help prevent inflammation.

What else should you know?

The following advice can help you avoid a shoulder injury or prevent a recurrence if you've already had one:
- Avoid high-risk activities, such as contact sports, if possible.
- Strengthen your muscles and ligaments through supervised weight

To prevent a shoulder injury from recurring, avoid high-risk activities, such as contact sports. Also, strengthen your muscles and ligaments through supervised weight training.

training. A physical therapist or trainer can advise you on the correct exercises for your particular injury.

■ Wear several layers of clothing to help cushion your body during falls, even if you're not planning athletic activities.

SNAKEBITE

Snakebites can be poisonous and deadly. Most snakebites occur on the arms and come about when a person tries to capture, play with, or kill a snake. Fortunately, most snakebites are "dry," meaning no venom is injected. Consequently, deaths from snakebites are rare; they occur in only 3 of 5,000 cases.

Snakes are everywhere in the United States, so you should learn how to tell a poisonous snake from a harmless one. (See *Identifying poisonous snakes,* page 469.) In the United States, poisonous snakes include the coral snake and members of the pit viper group.

Most snakebites occur on the arms and come about when a person tries to capture, play with, or kill a snake.

Coral snake

This snake is found primarily in the southeastern part of the United States. With its relatively short fangs, the coral snake hangs onto and seemingly "chews" its victim. Although its venom is highly toxic to the human nervous system, this snake rarely bites people.

Pit vipers

Unlike the coral snake, pit vipers strike quickly and release. Their venom is toxic to humans.

Members of the pit viper group include:

■ rattlesnakes
■ water moccasins (cottonmouths)
■ copperheads.

Rattlesnakes are found in all parts of the United States, where they account for the majority of snakebite deaths. (To find out which poisonous snakes inhabit your area, see *Where the snakes are,* page 470.) Cottonmouths and copperheads are found mostly in the southeastern and south-central parts of the United States.

What are the symptoms?

Someone who's been bitten by a coral snake typically develops symptoms more gradually than does someone who's been bitten by a pit viper.

Symptoms of coral snake bites

The person may show the following symptoms (although some may not occur right away):

- slight pain
- local swelling
- droopy eyelids
- difficulty speaking
- drooling
- drowsiness
- heavy sweating
- nausea and vomiting
- breathing difficulty
- paralysis
- dizziness and weakness (from shock).

Symptoms of pit viper bites

A person who has been bitten by a rattlesnake, cottonmouth, or copperhead may experience:

- severe pain
- rapid swelling
- discoloration around the bite
- blurred vision
- nausea
- vomiting
- sweating
- weakness
- breathing difficulty
- seizures
- shock.

Get the victim away from the snake. Keep him or her calm, and seek medical attention immediately.

What should you do?

Although treatment at the scene varies somewhat depending on the type of snake, three general rules apply:

- Get the victim away from the snake without making yourself vulnerable to a snake bite.
- Keep the victim calm to help slow absorption of the venom.
- Get the victim to a medical facility as soon as possible.

Identifying poisonous snakes

If you can identify poisonous snakes, you'll have an easier time avoiding their bites. What's more, if you or someone you're with gets bitten, you'll be able to tell rescuers what kind of snake you think it was. That way, they'll be sure to prepare the right antivenin.

How to recognize pit vipers

This group includes rattlesnakes, water moccasins (cottonmouths), and copperheads. You can tell a pit viper by these traits:
■ a triangular head
■ a deep poison pit between the eyes and nostril
■ slitlike eyes, with oval "cat's eye" pupils
■ long fangs, whose bite leaves one or two punctures followed by a row of teeth marks.

Rattlesnake

The rattlesnake is named for the unique set of rattles at the end of its tail. When disturbed, it vibrates its tail, producing the characteristic rattling sound.

Water moccasin

You can recognize this snake if it opens its mouth: The white inside its mouth gives the snake its official name, cottonmouth. This snake is drawn to swamps.

Copperhead

This snake takes it name from its copper-colored head. Native to the southeastern and south-central parts of the United States, it's found mainly in dry, stony terrain.

How to spot a coral snake

Unlike pit vipers, the coral snake has round eyes and a black nose. Also, its fangs are shorter than those of pit vipers.

The body of this small, colorful snake is ringed with bright red, yellow, and black bands. Its pattern of rings distinguishes it from the nonpoisonous king snake: The coral snake's yellow rings *always* separate the red rings from the black rings.

Learn the snake rhyme

If you live in coral snake territory or plan a visit there, remember the following rhyme to help you identify this snake: "Red on yellow, kill a fellow. Red on black, a friend to Jack."

Move the person away from the snake

Snakes can bite more than once. That's why it's important to get the person to a safe place. Care in a medical facility is crucial because the person must receive the appropriate antivenin within 4 hours of the bite.

Call for help

As soon as possible, call or send someone else to call for immediate emergency help. Whoever calls should explain that the person has been bitten by a snake and mention which type of snake it is, if known. That way, the rescuers or medical team can prepare the right antivenin to neutralize the poisonous snake venom. If a telephone

Where the snakes are

This map shows the location of poisonous snakes in the United States. As you can see, rattlesnakes are found throughout most of the country.

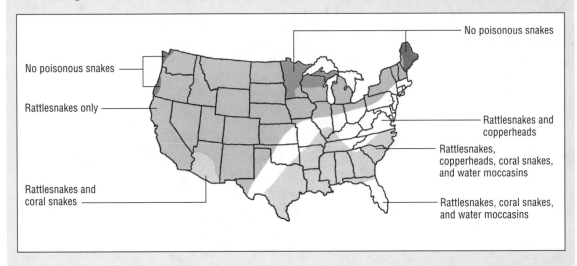

No poisonous snakes

No poisonous snakes

Rattlesnakes only

Rattlesnakes and
copperheads

Rattlesnakes,
copperheads, coral snakes,
and water moccasins

Rattlesnakes and
coral snakes

Rattlesnakes, coral snakes,
and water moccasins

or an ambulance isn't available, get the person to the nearest hospital emergency department or medical facility.

Avoid using a tourniquet.

Don't use the "cut-and-suck" method to release venom from a snakebite victim. This method could cause permanent damage to the person's nerves or sever blood vessels.

Never suck on the wound with your mouth. You could introduce harmful bacteria into the wound.

Avoid giving the victim water to drink if he or she is nauseous, vomiting, having seizures, or unconscious.

Don't let the victim walk. If walking can't be avoided — say, to get away from the snake — make sure the victim walks slowly.

Other steps to take depend on what type of snake bit the person.

What to do for a coral snake bite
■ First, wash the bite.

■ Next, apply ice.
■ Splint the affected arm or leg. (See *All about splints,* page 595.)
■ Call for emergency medical help or go directly to the nearest hospital emergency department or medical facility.

 Don't use a constrictive band.

 Don't suck out the venom.

What to do for a pit viper bite
■ Stay calm, and try to keep the snakebite victim calm and quiet. This slows the flow of venom through the bloodstream.
■ The American Medical Association recommends wrapping a light constrictive band, such as a belt or an elastic watchband, between the bitten area and the person's heart. For example, if the bite is on the person's arm, hand, leg, or foot, tie the belt or band 2 to 4 inches (5 to 10 centimeters) above the bite.

Make sure you tie the band tight enough so that it slows, but doesn't cut off, the blood flow to the bitten arm or leg. To test how tight the band is, try to slip your fingers under it; if you can get your fingers under it while meeting some resistance, the band is tied correctly.

Also, make sure you can feel a pulse below the band. If you can't, loosen the band. If the area around the band begins to swell, remove the band and refasten it 2 to 4 inches above the original location.

Be sure not to remove the band until the person reaches medical assistance.

■ Next, wash the bite with soap and warm water.
■ Apply ice packs to reduce pain and narrow the blood vessels (this slows the progression of the venom).
■ Use a splint to immobilize the injured arm or leg. Splint the arm so that the bite is below the level of the person's heart. You can improvise a splint by using a square piece of cloth and a straight piece of wood or plastic. (See *All about splints*, page 595.)
■ Offer sips of water if the person can swallow— but don't give water if he or she has been vomiting.
■ Call for emergency medical help or go directly to the nearest hospital emergency department or medical facility.

What to do for a nonpoisonous snakebite
Nonpoisonous snakes leave a horseshoe-shaped array of teeth marks.

For a pit viper bite, wrap a belt or an elastic watchband between the bitten area and the person's heart. Don't tie the belt or band too tightly; you should be able to slip your fingers under it with some resistance.

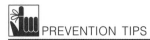

How to avoid a snakebite

Understanding snake behavior and staying alert for snakes can help you avoid becoming a snakebite victim. Read on for specific advice.

Learn about snake behavior

Snakes are cold-blooded. That means their body temperature and activity level are regulated by their environment. The upshot: They're likely to be sluggish in cold weather and most active in the middle of the day, when it's warmest. You'll typically find snakes sunning on rocks to warm themselves.

Take steps to protect yourself

Wear heavy, loose-fitting denim pants and high boots if you're going to spend time in a wooded area. When walking in such an area, step *on* to a downed tree before you step *over* it. Then, before you step over to the other side, look around for snakes.

When climbing on rock piles, be careful not to reach up on top without first checking to see if a snake is sunning up there.

Don't offend the snake

Most snakes strike only in self-defense. Given forewarning and a place to retreat, they're just as eager as you are to avoid a confrontation. Also, snakes sense vibrations. So when crossing an area that you think may harbor snakes, use a heavy walking stick to pound the ground with each step.

Back off slowly

If you come face to face with a snake, *slowly* back off and proceed in another direction. Although snakes are predators, they swallow their prey whole, so humans aren't on their regular menu.

Get a snakebite kit

If you're planning to spend time in a wilderness area that's more than an hour and a half from a medical facility, consider buying a snakebite kit with a suction device to keep with your supplies. This product can safely extract snake venom from a bite wound.

Be aware that some so-called nonpoisonous snakes, like garter and hognose snakes, have venom that can cause a limited reaction. However, these bites are not life-threatening emergencies.

If you're not sure whether the snake is poisonous, assume it is, and get immediate medical attention for a person who has been bitten.

If you're certain the snake is nonpoisonous, gently clean the bite with soap and warm water. Treat the bite as a minor wound, and get medical attention for the person.

How is a snakebite treated?

Rescuers inject antivenin into the victim as soon as possible to counteract the snake's poisonous venom. Then they clean and dress the wound.

If the person has been bitten by a nonpoisonous snake or if the bite appears to be "dry" (showing no signs of venom injection), treatment may consist only of a tetanus shot and wound care.

What else should you know?

The venom of young snakes is more poisonous than that of adult snakes. However, young snakes produce a smaller amount of venom, so their bites are usually less harmful.

Of course, most people can't tell how old a snake is, especially when running from one. And although running may be the instinctive reaction of many people, it's best to back off slowly when you encounter a snake. (See *How to avoid a snakebite*.)

SPEECH DIFFICULTY

When a person suddenly has difficulty speaking or understanding spoken language, the usual cause is disease of or damage to the brain's language centers. (See *Where language begins,* page 474.)

Understanding the causes

Many conditions can cause speech difficulty. *Sudden* speech difficulty may come from:

- a stroke
- use or abuse of alcohol or drugs (which can cause slurred speech)
- brain damage resulting from a head injury
- botulism, a severe type of food poisoning
- chemical poisoning, such as from mercury or manganese.

Alzheimer's disease and brain tumors can cause a *gradual* deterioration in speech. So can other nervous system diseases, namely:

- multiple sclerosis (caused by nerve damage)
- myasthenia gravis (a condition marked by slowly developing muscle weakness).

Common causes of sudden speech difficulty are stroke, use of alcohol or drugs, and brain damage resulting from a head injury.

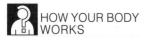

Where language begins

The brain has several language centers. Damage to one or more of these centers can cause difficulty speaking.

In most people, the language centers are found in the left side, or hemisphere, of the brain.

Broca's area

Broca's area lies next to the brain region that controls the muscles necessary for speech. Medical scientists think it's responsible for coordinating the movement of these muscles.

Wernicke's area

Wernicke's area helps control the content of speech. It also affects our comprehension of what we see and hear.

Crucial nerve bundle

A large nerve bundle that connects Wernicke's and Broca's areas also helps to control the content of speech. This cluster of nerves enables a person to echo sounds or words that he or she hears. Damage here can prevent the person from being able to repeat words or phrases.

What are the symptoms?

The key symptoms of speech difficulty are slurred or slowed speech or difficulty understanding speech. If the person has had a stroke, speech impairment may be either slight or dramatic (for instance, the person may be unable to speak at all).

Subtle symptoms

Sometimes, a person's symptoms are more subtle. That's why you should suspect speech difficulty in someone who has:
- difficulty finding words or naming things
- fluent speech that lacks meaningful content
- rapid but rambling speech.

Symptoms related to a stroke

A person whose speech difficulty stems from stroke may have any of these other symptoms:
- numbness around the lips or mouth
- impaired vision
- clumsiness
- weakness, paralysis, or numbness on one or both sides of the body
- confusion, disorientation, personality changes, or memory loss
- loss of bowel or bladder control.

What should you do?

Seek immediate medical attention for someone who suddenly begins to slur words. Be sure to tell the emergency rescuers or the doctor about any other symptoms, even if they seem unimportant or unrelated. This information can help the doctor determine what's causing the problem. Also, if possible, take all of the person's medicines to the doctor's office or hospital. Some drugs, such as tranquilizers, can produce speech problems.

 Don't interrupt the person who's struggling to communicate.

 Be sure not to cut off conversation attempts even if you get frustrated with the person.

How is speech difficulty treated?

A person with symptoms of a stroke is usually admitted to the hospital. The doctor performs a neurologic exam and may ask family members to recall any previous episodes of speech difficulty, impaired movement, or vision loss. After the immediate crisis has passed, the person can begin speech and physical therapy to help cope with diminished abilities.

What else should you know?
If the speech difficulty is permanent or follows a stroke, you can ease communication by being a patient listener. Here are some tips.

Show genuine interest
When you speak with the person, be sure to maintain eye contact to show that you're genuinely interested. Watch for nonverbal cues to help you decipher meaning. For instance, nodding, looking away, restlessness, and hand gestures can all give you insight into what the person is thinking or feeling.

Also, encourage the person to talk freely. If you interrupt or seem busy with other tasks, the person may stop trying to talk. The result? The person's communication attempts are likely to be less frequent. If the speech deficit is from a stroke but the person can still write, encourage the use of paper and pencil for communication.

SPINAL INJURIES

Like other parts of our bodies, our spines, or backbones, can get broken, bruised, or compressed. But an injury to the spine can be much more devastating than an injury to another part of the body. That's because a spinal injury can damage the spinal cord, causing permanent paralysis. (See *A look at your spinal column,* page 477.)

Understanding the causes
Spinal injuries usually result from trauma to the head or neck. Most serious spinal injuries result from:
■ motor vehicle accidents
■ falls
■ gunshot wounds
■ diving into shallow water (see *How to avoid spinal injuries,* page 478).
Less serious injuries result from lifting heavy objects and minor falls.

An injury to the spine can be much more devastating than an injury to another part of the body. If the spinal cord is damaged, permanent paralysis may result.

What happens when the back is broken
Fractures of the spine can affect the:

- bones of the neck, called *cervical vertebrae*
- bones of the upper back, called *thoracic vertebrae*
- bones of the lower back, called *lumbar vertebrae*
- sacrum, which consists of five fused vertebrae
- tailbone, or coccyx, which consists of four or five fused vertebrae.

A broken vertebra can injure spinal nerves, causing paralysis and loss of sensation.

What are the symptoms?

If a vertebra in the lower part of the spine is broken, the person may have pain that spreads to the legs and other parts of the body.

An injury to the spinal cord may cause:

- mild numbness
- tingling
- decreased sensation
- paralysis of all limbs, called *quadriplegia*
- paralysis of the legs only, called *paraplegia.*

Other symptoms to watch for
Stay alert for the following symptoms, which may mean the person has gone into a type of shock called *spinal shock:*

- restlessness or anxiety
- rapid breathing and pulse
- nausea and vomiting
- loss of bowel or bladder control
- loss of consciousness.

What should you do?

 WHEN SECONDS COUNT

Call for medical help immediately. Check the person for a clear airway. However, keep in mind that if the spine has been injured, any movement of the person's head, neck, or back can cause paralysis or make paralysis worse. It can even cause death.

This means that when you check the airway, you must not twist or rotate the person's head. Instead, *slightly* raise the chin, check for a foreign object in the mouth, and clear any object.

Next, feel the person for a pulse, and look, listen, and feel for breathing. If the person doesn't have a pulse and isn't breathing, be-

When checking for an open airway, don't twist or rotate the peson's head. Doing so could cause paralysis or make it worse.

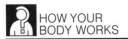

**HOW YOUR
BODY WORKS**

A look at your spinal column

Your spinal column extends from the bottom of your skull to the end of your tailbone. It consists of 26 bones called *vertebrae*, which are separated by disks that cushion the bones. Stacked on each other like building blocks, the vertebrae have a hollow center, through which the spinal cord passes.

The vulnerable cord
The spinal cord is actually many long sets of nerves that connect your brain to the rest of your body. These nerves govern sensation and movement.

Danger from a broken vertebra
Normally, the vertebrae protect the spinal cord. However, a broken vertebra can act as a dangerous weapon inside the body. If one pinches or cuts a spinal nerve, the person can become completely or partially paralyzed. The higher the injury is located on the spinal column, the more areas of the person's body it affects.

When to suspect a spinal injury
Always *assume* there's a spinal injury if you come upon someone who:
- is unconscious
- has fallen
- has had an accident while diving or traveling in a motor vehicle
- has suffered a head injury.

Act with caution
Never move a person if you suspect a spinal injury. Wait for professional rescue workers to arrive. Remember — it's better to do nothing than to risk causing permanent injury or death.

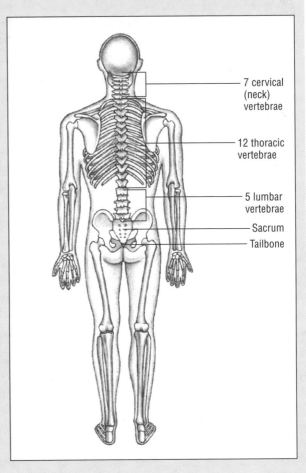

7 cervical (neck) vertebrae

12 thoracic vertebrae

5 lumbar vertebrae

Sacrum

Tailbone

gin CPR if you know how. (See *Performing CPR on an adult,* page 579, *Performing CPR on a child,* page 585, or *Performing CPR on an infant,* page 590.)

PREVENTION TIPS

How to avoid spinal injuries

A spinal injury can cause the worst kind of damage — permanent inability to move or to feel sensations. To help avoid these disabling injuries, follow these safety tips.

Be safe in the water

- Never dive into shallow water. Don't swim alone.
- Teach your children to respect water safety rules and to obey lifeguards.

Practice motor-vehicle safety

- Always wear your seat belt, even if your vehicle has an air bag. Make sure to fasten both the shoulder restraint and the lap belt.
- Teach your children to wear their seat belts.
- Strap infants and young children in appropriate car seats.

Safeguard your home

- Make sure your staircases have secure railings.
- Avoid throw rugs, especially if you have elderly persons in your home.

Protect your infant

- Fasten your infant in a high chair.
- Keep crib sides up.
- Lower the mattress when your infant learns to stand up.
- Don't let your child use an infant walker, especially near stairs.
- Install gates at the top and bottom of staircases.

Never move a person with a suspected back or neck injury unless his or her life is in immediate danger — for example, from a fire or an explosion.

How to help a conscious person

Ask the person about any numbness, tingling, weakness, or burning in the arms or legs. Ask whether he or she can move the arms, legs, feet, fingers, or toes.

Closely question the person about the injury. If you suspect spinal damage, don't move the person. Wait for emergency help to arrive.

 Don't give the person anything to drink.

How to help an unconscious person

Don't move the person. Place folded blankets, towels, or clothing at the person's sides, head, and neck to prevent movement and further spinal cord damage. Keep the person's body aligned at all times. (See *Supporting the person's head and neck*, page 480.)

Take care not to let the person's neck rotate.

How are spinal injuries treated?

The medical team immediately immobilizes the person to stabilize the spine and prevent spinal cord damage. For instance, they may apply a neck collar and place the person on a long backboard.

Maintaining vital functions

If the spinal injury damaged the nervous system, the person's breathing, blood pressure, heart rate, and temperature may be disrupted; the medical team must monitor closely for life-threatening changes. They place the person on a heart monitor and insert an intravenous line to administer drugs and fluids. To maintain breathing, they administer oxygen. The person may need special blankets or a warming mattress to keep warm.

Aiding breathing

If the top of the spinal cord has been injured, the victim won't be able to breathe and will need to use a mechanical ventilator to stay alive.

With an injury slightly lower in the neck, the person can still breathe but is in danger of lapsing into respiratory distress. The medical team checks the person's breathing status closely.

Checking for spinal shock

A spinal injury can cause spinal shock. In this condition, the person's blood pressure drops and the pulse slows. The medical team watches the person closely and administers fluids and drugs to raise the blood pressure.

Treating a minor spinal fracture

The person with a minor spinal fracture that's stable may need only a firm neck collar. He or she receives pain relievers and muscle relaxants until the fracture stabilizes (about 10 to 12 weeks). Exercises can help the person to strengthen the back muscles. A back brace or corset can provide support when the person walks.

Treating a broken neck

If the person's neck is broken, external skull traction is used to immobilize the head and neck for up to 3 months. With this type of traction, called a *halo device,* the head is kept from moving by tongs, ropes, weights, or other devices.

If the person is unconscious, don't move him or her. Place folded blankets, towels, or clothing at the person's sides, head, and neck. Keep the person's body aligned at all times.

Supporting the person's head and neck

Let's say you've witnessed someone suffer a serious blow to the back. After you call for emergency medical assistance, you'll need to stabilize the person to prevent further injury. Here's how.

Support and immobilize the head

To keep the person from moving, grasp the collarbone and shoulder on both sides of the neck, cradling the head between the insides of your forearms. Hold the head and neck still until the emergency rescue team arrives. Remind the person not to move.

Form a barrier

If you tire from holding the person's head, place objects on both sides of the head to keep it from rolling from side to side.

How to provide support in the water

If the injured person is in shallow water, provide support in the water. *Don't move the victim out of the water until a backboard is available.* To prevent further spinal damage, wait for emergency help

Surgery

The person may need surgery if diagnostic tests show pressure on the spinal cord or a broken vertebrae that can't be corrected any other way. During the operation, part of the damaged bone is removed and fused to a neighboring vertebra.

After surgery, the person may have to wear a body cast and be placed in a special bed to prevent bedsores and other complications of long-term immobility.

What else should you know?

If the spinal injury causes permanent paralysis, the person will need long-term care and special equipment. Examples include:

- a mechanical ventilator
- a wheelchair
- special utensils for eating
- adapted clothing to aid dressing.

Adaptive assistance: An aid to rehabilitation

To help a paralyzed person adapt, rehabilitation also includes:

- helping the person to grieve
- assisting the person to adapt to dependence and the change in body image
- teaching special techniques for emptying the bowel and bladder
- helping the person achieve reasonable goals.

SPLINTERS

A splinter is a sharp fragment of glass, wood, or other material that has become embedded under the surface of the skin. Most often, people get splinters (also called *slivers*) in their hands or feet from walking on or handling a surface that has shards of glass or rough wood. (See *Gaining the upper hand on splinters,* page 482.)

What are the symptoms?

Splinters typically cause redness with local pain or irritation. The person usually notices the splinter right away. However, occasionally, a splinter goes unnoticed until it becomes painful, infected, or swollen.

Symptoms of infection

Left untreated or treated with unsterile equipment, a splinter can become severely infected. Then it might cause such symptoms as:
- throbbing
- pus
- swelling or warmth of the skin overlying the splinter
- red streaks on the skin running from the wound toward the center of the body.

What should you do?

You can handle most splinters at home by following the simple steps below. If the victim is a young child, try to get assistance from another adult or an older child.
- Wash your hands and the area around the splinter with soap and warm water.
- Pass a sewing needle and tweezers over an open flame twice to sterilize them. If they turn black, clean them off and hold them over a flame again. Or boil the needle and tweezers in a pot of boiling water for 5 minutes to sterilize them.
- Then follow the steps below.

How to remove a splinter near the skin surface

- If the splinter isn't deeply embedded under the skin, use the sterilized tweezers to get it out. Try to pull the splinter out at the same angle that it entered the skin.
- If the splinter is small, you may be able to remove it by simply passing the edge of a credit card over it — again in the same direction that the splinter entered.

> ❌ Don't treat the splinter until you've washed your hands. Otherwise, dirt under your fingernails could cause an infection.
>
> ❌ Never use an unsterilized needle or tweezers.
>
> ❌ Be sure not to try to retrieve the splinter using your bare hands. You could break it, making the part that's still in the skin harder to remove.

Usually, the person notices the splinter right away. But some splinters go unnoticed until they become painful, infected, or swollen.

Gaining the upper hand on splinters

As any parent knows, splinters are a normal part of growing up. No family is immune to this annoying, though usually minor, injury. But you can reduce the number of splinters that you and your kids get by taking these steps.

Keep your home clean and well-maintained

■ Promptly and thoroughly clean up broken glass to help protect your family from glass slivers.
■ Keep your wooden deck and playground equipment in good shape.

Other precautions

■ Don't let your children play on rough, unsanded wood.
■ Wear gloves and have your children wear them when performing tasks that are likely to cause splinters — for example, bringing in firewood.

Be prepared

Keep a first-aid kit at home and in your vehicle. Besides first-aid basics, the kit should contain supplies for removing splinters: tweezers, a sewing needle, matches (for sterilizing), and an assortment of adhesive bandages.

How to remove an embedded splinter

■ If the embedded splinter is clearly visible, use the sterilized needle to gently loosen the skin so you can reach it. Then remove the splinter carefully using the tweezers. Move the tweezers backwards at the same angle that the splinter entered the skin.
■ If the splinter is deeply embedded or breaks when you try to remove it, get medical attention for the person.
■ If the splinter is small and you have trouble removing it, try soaking it in warm, soapy water for 15 minutes three times a day for 2 days. If this doesn't help the splinter work its way to the surface, call the doctor.

What to do after you've removed the splinter

■ Wash the wound under running water to flush out germs. Then wash the area with soap and warm water again.
■ Apply an antibiotic ointment, such as Neosporin. Then cover the wound with an adhesive bandage.
■ Watch the person for symptoms of infection, such as pus, redness, or red streaks that seem to extend from the wound toward the center of the body. Get immediate medical attention for the person if you see red streaks.

How are splinters treated?

The doctor may remove a deeply embedded splinter in the office. If the splinter is totally covered by skin, the doctor may use surgical tools to make a tiny incision. To help prevent infection, the person should get a tetanus booster if he or she hasn't had one in the past 5 to 10 years.

What else should you know?

If your infant has a deep puncture wound from a splinter and you're not sure whether his or her tetanus shot is up-to-date, call your pediatrician's office to ask whether a booster is required.

SPRAINS AND STRAINS

A *sprain* is a tear in a ligament — a fibrous band that attaches one bone to another. This injury typically occurs when a joint is overextended or twisted beyond its normal range of motion. If you twist your ankle, for instance, you will probably sprain it.

A *strain* is a tear in a muscle or a tendon — a fibrous band that attaches muscle to bone. A strain typically comes from sudden movement or overexertion. For example, you may strain your back muscles if you lift a heavy box without bending your knees.

What are the symptoms?

Symptoms of a sprain and strain are similar, although certain symptoms may suggest one injury rather than the other. For instance, if a joint is forced into an awkward position and immediately begins to hurt, the injury is probably a sprain; it could even be a fracture. On the other hand, if your muscles feel sore the day after you start a new exercise routine, chances are you've suffered a strain.

A sprain occurs when a joint is twisted or extended too much. A strain comes from sudden movement or overexertion.

Symptoms of a sprain
The person with a sprain usually has:
- pain, especially when moving the injured joint (some sprains hurt more than fractures)
- swelling of the injured joint
- tenderness when the injured area is touched
- discoloration or bruising.

Symptoms of a strain
Symptoms may arise immediately or not until the next day. The person may have:
- intense pain
- moderate swelling
- painful and difficult movement
- discoloration (but less than with a sprain).

What should you do?

Your actions depend on the person's symptoms.

What to do for a sprain

■ If the joint looks deformed, the sprain may be severe or a bone may be broken. Support the joint by splinting it. If you don't have a splint available, improvise one as you would for a fracture. (See "Fractures [broken bones]," page 251.) Get medical attention for the person as soon as possible.

■ For a less severe sprain, apply ice or a chemical cold pack to the injured area for 15 minutes every hour for the first 24 hours. Be sure to wrap the bag of ice in a wet cloth. If you don't have a cold pack or ice, apply a bag of frozen vegetables (such as peas or loose corn) on the injury until you can obtain a cold pack or make some ice.

■ Call the doctor. He or she may want to take an X-ray to rule out a broken bone.

■ After thoroughly icing the injury, wrap it in an elastic bandage. This will reduce swelling and promote comfort. (Keep using the bandage for several days.)

■ Elevate the injured joint above the level of the person's heart to decrease blood flow to the injured area. (See *Do the RICE thing.*)

■ Give aspirin or ibuprofen (such as Advil or Motrin) to reduce pain.

■ Have the person rest the injured part.

■ If pain and swelling don't go away, make sure the person gets medical attention if he or she hasn't already done so.

> ❌ Never apply ice directly to the skin.
>
> ❌ Don't let the person use the injured joint.
>
> ❌ Don't apply heat, hot soaks, or a heating pad for the first 72 hours. You could aggravate the injury.

What to do for a strain

■ For the first 24 hours, apply ice to the injured area for 15 minutes every hour.

■ Have the person rest and elevate the injured area.

■ For the next 2 days, ice the injured area several times a day for 15 minutes.

■ Wrap the injured part in an elastic bandage. (Keep using the bandage for several days.)

■ Give aspirin or ibuprofen (such as Advil or Motrin) to relieve pain.

■ Have the person get medical attention if he or she hasn't already done so.

If the joint looks deformed, the sprain may be severe or a bone may be broken. Splint the injury, and get medical attention for the person as soon as possible.

Do the RICE thing

After the doctor has ruled out a more serious injury, you can treat a sprain or strain at home. How? By using the RICE formula. This acronym stands for:

- *R*est
- *I*ce
- *C*ompression
- *E*levation.

Rest the injured part

Try to use the injured part as little as possible for the next few days. If necessary, use a sling or crutches to get around.

Once the initial pain subsides, *gradually* start using the injured part. Too much rest can cause loss of strength and flexibility.

Apply ice

Ice reduces swelling by constricting blood vessels in the injured area. This, in turn, dulls pain and relieves muscle spasms.

Start using ice as soon as possible after the injury, before swelling begins. Even a minute's delay can slow healing.

Use ice every hour

Keep ice on the injured part for 15 to 20 minutes at a time every hour (or at least three or four times daily) for the first 24 hours. Then follow your doctor's instructions. He or she may want you to switch to heat application at this time. However, for a severe injury, you may be instructed to keep applying ice for 72 hours.

Protect your skin

Placing ice directly on the skin can cause frostbite. Be sure to place ice cubes in a double plastic bag or wrap them in a cloth. Or use a chemical or fabric cold pack instead of ice cubes, and follow instructions on how to insulate the pack. Don't apply ice for more than 20 minutes at a time.

Compress the area

Compressing (squeezing) the injured part limits swelling and internal bleeding by squeezing fluid and other matter out of the area. An elastic bandage is unbeatable for compression.

Wrap in a spiral

Start wrapping the bandage a few inches below the injury site. Continue wrapping upward in an overlapping spiral. Start with moderately tight pressure and gradually wrap more loosely above the injury.

Wear the bandage continuously for 18 to 24 hours. At night, loosen it — but don't remove it.

Take precautions

Don't wrap the bandage too tightly. You could impede blood flow to the injured area. Leave the fingers or toes exposed so you can watch for color changes, which can tell you if the bandage is too tight.

If the exposed skin turns pale or gets numb or tingly, remove the bandage and leave it off until the normal color and sensations return. Then rewrap it, but less tightly.

Elevate the injured area

Like ice and compression, elevation limits circulation to the injured area. This reduces swelling and internal bleeding. Try to elevate the injured part above the level of the heart for the first 24 to 48 hours after the injury.

❌ Be sure not to delay seeking medical treatment. Misdiagnosis and incorrect treatment can slow the person's recovery.

❌ Take care not to let the person use the injured part too much (although light weight-bearing is permitted).

❌ Don't apply heat, hot soaks, or a heating pad for the first 72 hours. You could aggravate the injury.

How are sprains and strains treated?

Sprains and strains call for similar treatment.

Treating a sprain

For a severe sprain or one that accompanies other injuries, the person may be treated in the hospital and receive codeine for pain. The doctor may splint the injury, possibly with an air cast, to reduce swelling. If the ligaments are completely torn, surgical repair may be required. Physical therapy can help restore full range of motion to the joint.

For a mild or moderate sprain, the doctor prescribes the same treatment a person would use at home — rest, ice followed by heat, elevation, and pain relievers. The doctor may apply an elastic bandage and instruct the person to avoid all but minimal weight-bearing on the injured part for 3 days, or until pain and swelling subside. The person may need crutches.

Treating a strain

The doctor may prescribe aspirin or ibuprofen for pain, apply an elastic bandage, and instruct the person to elevate the injured limb and apply ice for 48 hours (depending on the severity of the strain).

The amount of weight-bearing permitted varies with the severity of the injury:
- With a mild strain, weight-bearing is permitted.
- With a moderate strain, only light weight-bearing is permitted.
- With a severe strain, no weight-bearing is permitted.

For a back strain, the doctor usually recommends ice, rest, pain relievers, and then moist heat.

What else should you know?

The doctor may refer a person with a sprain to a physical therapist for range-of-motion exercises. These exercises can help prevent weakening of the injured joint; such weakening could lead to loss of joint mobility.

To treat a strain, the doctor may prescribe aspirin or ibuprofen for pain, apply an elastic bandage, and instruct the person to elevate the injured limb and apply ice for 48 hours.

STABBING

A stab wound occurs when a sharp object, such as a knife blade or an ice pick, penetrates the body. In the United States, stab wounds send many people to hospital emergency departments every day. Some stab wounds are fatal.

Dangerous damage

Stab wounds vary enormously in size and severity. The wound may damage:
- bones
- soft tissue
- blood vessels
- nerves
- vital organs.

A stab wound to the *abdomen,* for instance, may threaten the victim's life by damaging major blood vessels and internal organs.

A stab wound to the *chest* may tear major blood vessels and cause shock from massive bleeding. This injury can be fatal if it allows blood or air to enter the chest cavity. When blood enters, the condition is called *hemothorax;* when air enters, it's called *pneumothorax.* Both conditions prevent lung expansion and may cause the person's heart to beat irregularly or to stop beating entirely. (See *What happens in a stab wound,* page 489.)

What are the symptoms?

A stab wound to the abdomen or chest causes profuse bleeding. The bleeding may be visible on the outside of the person's body. If the person is awake and alert, he or she may be in severe pain.

Other symptoms to watch for

A stab wound may also cause:
- anxiety
- pale or bluish skin
- rapid breathing or shortness of breath
- a visible wound, which may make a sucking sound if air enters the chest cavity through the wound
- changes in the person's level of awareness, from confusion to unconsciousness
- a rapid or weak pulse.

A stab wound to the abdomen may threaten the victim's life by damaging major blood vessels and internal organs. A stab wound to the chest may tear blood vessels and cause massive bleeding.

What should you do?

 WHEN SECONDS COUNT

If you hear a sucking sound at the chest as the person breathes, you must seal the wound right away — even before emergency rescuers arrive. Be sure to immediately send someone to call 911 or your local emergency medical services.

Next, tell the person to take a breath and exhale. After he or she exhales completely, press on the chest. Then quickly seal the wound with plastic wrap, a plastic bag, or any other available material that will stop air from entering the chest. Tape the sealing material in place. If the victim has trouble breathing or seems to get worse, remove the plastic wrap, let the air escape from the chest, and cover the wound again.

While waiting for help to arrive, keep checking to see if the person has a clear airway and a pulse and is breathing. If the person is conscious, keep him or her sitting up or elevate the head and shoulders. If the person can't sit up, have him or her lie with the injured side down. This prevents blood from filling the uninjured side of the chest and allows the good lung to keep functioning.

> Don't give the person anything to eat or drink. If you're hours from the nearest medical facility, offer a clean cloth soaked in water to relieve a dry mouth.

What to do if the object is still impaled

If the knife or other penetrating object is still impaled in the person's body, *don't remove it.* Instead, stabilize it by placing bulky dressings or taping pieces of cloth around it to keep it from moving. Get immediate medical attention for the person.

> Never remove a penetrating object that is impaled in a person's body — you'll only increase bleeding by making a hole where the knife was.

What to do if an organ is protruding from the body

If you see part of an organ exposed or protruding from the person's abdomen, cover it with a sterile bandage or a clean cloth. To prevent the organ from drying out, pour clean drinking water on the dressing.

If the person is conscious, keep him or her sitting up or elevate the head and shoulders while waiting for help to arrive.

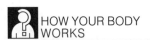

HOW YOUR BODY
WORKS

What happens in a stab wound

A penetrating object like a knife may damage many organs at once as it enters a person's chest or abdomen. For instance, it may penetrate the person's:

- stomach
- large intestine
- pancreas
- aorta — a very large artery
- inferior vena cava — the main vein that returns blood to the heart from the pelvis, abdomen, and legs.

When the heart is stabbed

A stab wound to the heart can cause an injury called *cardiac tamponade.* The penetrating object injures a blood vessel, which bleeds into the sac around the heart (pericardium), as shown below. Or it may injure the heart itself.

Overfilled sac

Blood then builds up in the sac, squeezing the heart and impairing its function. To save the person's life, blood must be removed from the sac; the person may need surgery to repair the injury.

STABBING OF HEART

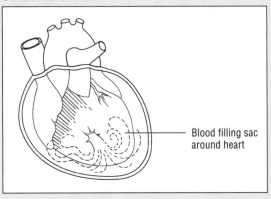

Blood filling sac around heart

When the lung is punctured

A stab wound to the chest can puncture a lung. The wound creates a valvelike opening in the chest wall, causing a condition called *tension pneumothorax.* In this injury, air gets trapped in the lung and pressure outside the lung rises.

Trapped air, endangered heart

The increased pressure may squeeze the heart, impeding its function. To remove the trapped air, the doctor inserts a tube in the person's chest.

STABBING OF LUNG

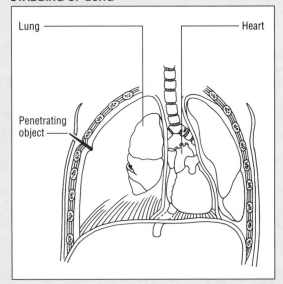

Lung

Heart

Penetrating object

Never try to push a protruding organ back into the body.

 Be sure not to touch an organ that is protruding from a wound.

 Don't cover a protruding organ tightly or with a material that may disintegrate or stick to the organ — say, a tissue or paper towel.

How is a stabbing treated?

The medical team first makes sure the person is breathing adequately. They may need to insert a tube in the chest to keep the lung inflated, ensure proper pressure within the chest, and permit blood to drain from a hemothorax. The person may need oxygen or a mechanical ventilator to keep breathing.

Stopping further blood loss

The team's next priority is to stop the bleeding. The person may need surgery to repair the wound. With less serious bleeding, the medical team bandages the wound with sterile dressings. If the person has a sucking wound, they may apply a gauze dressing coated with petroleum jelly.

Depending on how much blood the person has lost, he or she may receive blood transfusions and intravenous fluids to prevent shock. The doctor may prescribe pain relievers to reduce pain and antibiotics and a tetanus booster to help prevent infection.

What else should you know?

The severity of a stab wound depends on:
- the type and size of the penetrating weapon
- the location and angle of the weapon's entry
- which organs or structures are injured.

The small intestine is the organ most often injured by stabbing. Unfortunately, injury to the small intestine is likely to cause widespread infection, especially if the intestine is full of feces at the time of injury. Here's why: A full intestine readily empties into the abdominal cavity. The contents then may contaminate other organs in the cavity, leading to a life-threatening infection.

The severity of a stab wound depends on the type and size of the weapon, the location and angle of the weapon's entry, and which organs or structures are injured.

STINGS BY MARINE LIFE

A person who has been stung by marine life can have a reaction ranging from itchy skin or mild pain to severe, life-threatening shock. Fortunately, most victims recover without medical intervention.

The severity of the reaction depends on:

- the person's age
- whether the person is allergic to these stings
- the toxicity of the injected venom.

Usually, people who are very young, very small, or very old are more severely affected by these stings because of their small size or greater sensitivity.

Marine animals with tentacles

The most common stinging animals from the sea include the many varieties of *jellyfish* and the *Portuguese man-of-war.* These animals have stinging cells on their tentacles. A tentacle can sting even after it has been detached.

Sea coral may resemble rocks more than animals, but they're actually sea creatures. Gracefully floating in the water, *anemones* may be mistaken for plants, but beware — these brightly colored creatures can cause a painful sting.

Another stinging animal, the *hydra,* has a hollow, tube-shaped body that is closed at one end. At the other end is a central mouth surrounded by tentacles armed with stingers.

Poisonous fish and stingrays

Poisonous fish are equipped with venom, but the poison is located in their rear spines. *Stingrays* burrow in the sand, where they're often stepped on by unwitting beachgoers.

While fishing, a person may be injured by handling stinging fish. Some examples of stinging fish are:

- catfish
- weever fish
- scorpion fish (including zebra fish)
- toadfish and surgeonfish.

Spiny sea creatures

Sea cucumbers, starfish, and *sea urchins* are spiny sea creatures that sting only in defense. With their sharp spines, they puncture the skin of their victims. Typically, a person is stung when accidentally

> *The most common stinging animals from the sea include the many varieties of jellyfish and the Portuguese man-of-war.*

stepping on one of these animals or when picking one up and mishandling it.

What are the symptoms?

A person who's been stung by marine life may have some or all of the following symptoms:

- intense burning pain
- reddened skin
- muscle cramps.

Other symptoms vary with the type of marine life.

Symptoms of Portuguese man-of-war stings

This sting produces welts — either scattered or appearing in a row. These reddened patches usually disappear within 24 hours.

Symptoms of jellyfish, anemone, and coral stings

These stings usually cause multiple thin lines of welts in a zigzag pattern. The welts often disappear within an hour. Burning pain may spread from the sting site into the groin and abdomen; the pain typically lasts 10 to 30 minutes. Blisters may occur, too.

Symptoms of sea cucumber, starfish, and sea urchin stings

These stings cause puncture wounds, which may be extremely painful. A person who has multiple punctures may suffer a dangerous body-wide reaction.

Other symptoms to watch for

Sometimes, a person has a severe allergic reaction and goes into shock. When this happens, you might see these symptoms:

- anxiety
- swelling
- fainting
- nausea and vomiting
- wheezing or difficulty breathing.

If the person experiences difficulty breathing, get emergency medical help. If a bee sting kit is available, help the person administer Adrenalin.

What should you do?

WHEN SECONDS COUNT

- If the person develops symptoms of shock (difficulty breathing, wheezing, fainting, and anxiety), get emergency medical help. If an anaphylaxis (bee sting) kit is available, help the person administer a shot of Adrenalin.

■ If the person seems to have stopped breathing, check for a clear airway. Then look, listen, and feel for breathing, and check for a pulse. If breathing and pulse are absent, begin CPR if you know how. (See *Performing CPR on an adult,* page 579, *Performing CPR on a child,* page 585, or *Performing CPR on an infant,* page 590.) If you're at a beach with a lifeguard, the lifeguard should be able to perform basic first aid and even CPR and may be able to use a radio to get help.

What to do for jellyfish and Portuguese man-of-war stings
■ If needed, perform CPR.
■ Wash the sting site with vinegar. If vinegar isn't available, use 40% to 70% rubbing alcohol.
■ Cover your hands with a towel or a piece of cloth, and then scrape the tentacles away from the skin with a credit card.
■ Usually, removing the tentacles brings relief from pain. You may also give the person a mild pain reliever. If the person continues to have severe pain, consult a doctor.

 Avoid pouring fresh water on the wound.

 Be sure not to give aspirin to a child under age 16 without a doctor's approval. Give Tylenol (or another form of acetaminophen) instead, or follow the doctor's instructions.

What to do for stings from spiny sea creatures, poison fish, and stingrays
To inactivate the poison of a sea cucumber, starfish, or sea urchin, have the person place both feet in a bucket of very hot water (113° F [45°C]) for 30 to 90 minutes. Although both feet are seldom stung, the person should immerse them both; the uninjured foot serves as a thermometer for the injured foot, which may be numb and oblivious to water temperature.

 Don't scrub the injured area.

How are stings by marine life treated?
The doctor orders treatments that will:
■ stabilize the person's overall condition
■ counteract the effects of the poison
■ relieve pain.
    If the spines or tentacles haven't already been removed, the doc-

To inactivate the poison of a sea cucumber, starfish, or sea urchin, have the person place both feet in a bucket of hot water for 30 to 90 minutes.

tor or nurse removes them. Some people may need a tetanus shot to prevent infection. A few people who have been stung by marine life even need surgery to repair the wound.

Treating a severe allergic reaction

A person who's having a severe allergic reaction needs emergency treatment to keep the airway open and restore and maintain breathing and circulation. For instance, a breathing tube may be inserted and oxygen may be administered. Fluids may be given intravenously to treat low blood pressure, and drugs are prescribed to relieve pain.

What else should you know?

Divers are especially vulnerable to injuries from marine life. Some stings may be deadly because the diver is too far from shore to swim to safety and drowns from excruciating pain or a severe allergic reaction.

STROKE

Strokes affect about 500,000 Americans each year. They occur in people of all ages.

A stroke comes from a dramatic decrease in blood flow to a part of the brain. Without adequate blood, the brain doesn't get enough oxygen, and brain cells may quickly be damaged or destroyed.

Strokes affect about 500,000 Americans each year. Although they mainly affect older adults, they occur in people of all ages. Strokes are more common in men than women and more common in blacks than whites.

Disastrous effects

About half of the people who suffer strokes die. Of those who survive, roughly half remain permanently disabled and experience a recurrence within weeks, months, or years. (See *How to avoid another stroke.*)

Here are some of the problems a stroke can cause:
- paralysis on one side of the body (the side opposite the affected side of the brain)
- weakness
- numbness
- reduced ability to feel sensations

PREVENTION TIPS

How to avoid another stroke

You can help reduce the risk of having another stroke by controlling any underlying diseases, such as diabetes or high blood pressure. For instance, be sure to take prescribed medication for these diseases. Read on for more advice.

Watch what you eat
If you have high blood pressure, you can help reduce it by eating a low-cholesterol, low-salt diet. If you're diabetic, follow your doctor's advice about meal planning and exercise.

Watch your weight
If you're overweight — a risk factor for stroke — try to lose weight. For instance, reduce your calorie intake and increase your activity level.

Get regular exercise
You'll feel best if you can schedule regular activities, such as walking or dancing. In urban and suburban areas, many senior citizens' organizations offer exercise or dance programs tailored for the lifestyle of the older person.

Other instructions
- If you're a smoker, try to quit.
- Find ways to reduce stress in your life.
- Avoid prolonged bed rest if possible. Bed rest may increase the risk of a stroke.

- partial blindness
- eyelid drooping
- speech defects
- problems understanding language
- memory loss.

However, many stroke victims can regain some skills through rehabilitation. The prognosis depends not just on the extent of damage from the stroke, but also on the person's attitude toward rehabilitation.

Three paths to a stroke
Strokes involve disruption of blood flow to the brain. The disruption is caused by one of these three problems:
- a blood clot
- an obstructed blood vessel
- bleeding within the brain.

Blood clot: Most common cause of stroke
A stroke-causing blood clot is usually brought on by plaque buildup (atherosclerosis) in an artery that supplies the brain. The blood clot

blocks the blood vessel, cutting off blood flow to the brain tissue supplied by the vessel. The clot also causes congestion and swelling.

The risk of blood clot formation rises with age because of the higher incidence of such diseases as atherosclerosis, diabetes, and high blood pressure in older people. Obesity, smoking, and use of birth control pills can also predispose a person to a stroke from a blood clot. Some younger people have suffered cocaine-induced strokes.

How an obstructed blood vessel can cause a stroke

If an embolus — a piece of a blood clot, a bit of tissue or tumor, some air or gas, or a foreign object — becomes lodged in a blood vessel in the brain, it can block the vessel. This brings on a stroke by reducing blood flow to the brain.

Strokes from an obstructed blood vessel can occur at any age, especially among people who have undergone open-heart surgery or who have a history of:
- rheumatic heart disease
- inflammation of the heart's inner lining
- heart valve disease
- irregular heartbeats.

This type of stroke usually develops rapidly — in 10 to 20 seconds — and without warning. It is generally more severe and life-threatening than a stroke caused by a blood clot.

Bleeding within the brain: A threat at any age

Chronic high blood pressure or a ballooned-out portion of an artery (called an *aneurysm*) can cause a brain artery to burst suddenly. The area of the brain served by the burst artery no longer receives the oxygen it needs to survive. What's more, blood builds up deep within the brain. This further squeezes brain tissue and causes even greater destruction of brain cells.

A stroke from bleeding within the brain can occur suddenly at any age.

Little strokes

Many people have little strokes — temporary interruptions of blood flow to the brain. These episodes, which doctors call *transient ischemic attacks,* are warnings that a stroke is imminent. They may occur days, weeks, or even months before a stroke. With prompt medical attention, the person may be able to prevent a major stroke or at least decrease the damage. (See *Dinner with Uncle Mike,* page 499.)

Little strokes are temporary interruptions of blood flow to the brain. These warnings may occur days, weeks, or even months before a stroke.

What are the symptoms?

Symptoms depend on the severity of the stroke and the part of the brain that is affected.

Symptoms of a major stroke

A major stroke usually causes progressive symptoms. They may include:

- sudden headache
- weakness, numbness, or paralysis on one side of the body
- drooping of the corner of the mouth
- difficulty speaking; this may range from slurring of words to loss of speech
- difficulty understanding speech
- blurred, double, or impaired vision in one or both eyes
- difficulty breathing or swallowing
- loss of balance
- loss of bladder and bowel control
- pupils of different sizes
- seizures
- confusion
- possible collapse and loss of consciousness.

Symptoms of a minor stroke

A minor stroke may cause symptoms that last for only a few minutes or a few hours, but they shouldn't be ignored. They include:

- slight dizziness
- headache
- sudden memory loss
- weakness in an arm or a leg
- minor speech difficulty, such as slurring
- slight confusion.

Symptoms of a transient ischemic attack

Suspect a transient ischemic attack if the person has:

- minor speech difficulty
- slight confusion
- slight dizziness
- muscle weakness.

> *A major stroke can cause a sudden headache, weakness or paralysis on one side of the body, and difficulty speaking.*

What should you do?

 WHEN SECONDS COUNT

■ If you suspect a person has had a *major stroke,* call for immediate medical help.
■ Make sure the person's airway is clear. Check for a pulse, and look, listen, and feel for breathing. If a pulse and breathing are absent, start CPR if you know how. (See *Performing CPR on an adult,* page 579, *Performing CPR on a child,* page 585, or *Performing CPR on an infant,* page 590.)
■ Loosen tight clothing around the person's neck, chest, or waist.

> Don't give the person anything to eat or drink. He or she may not be able to swallow.

Position the person properly
■ Keep the person quiet and at rest.
■ Unless the head, neck, or spine has been injured, help the person roll over onto the weak side, with the upper arm bent and the head resting on one hand for support. Bend the person's upper leg at the knee for stability.
■ Next, slightly elevate the person's head and chest on rolled-up blankets or firm pillows. Keep him or her warm and comfortable.

> Don't move a person who has fallen unless you're certain he or she hasn't suffered an injury to the head, neck, or spine.

What to do for a minor stroke or transient ischemic attack
Protect the person from falling. Seek medical help immediately so the person can be evaluated. Watch for further symptoms. Reassure and calm the person.

> Never ignore symptoms of a minor stroke or a transient ischemic attack. Get medical help for the person as soon as possible.

How is a stroke treated?
Emergency rescuers make sure the person has a clear airway and a pulse and is breathing. In the hospital, once the person is medically stable, the doctor tries to pinpoint the origin of the stroke based on symptoms. For instance, a stroke affecting the left side of the brain

Never ignore symptoms of a minor stroke or a transient ischemic attack. Get medical help for the person as soon as possible.

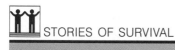

STORIES OF SURVIVAL

Dinner with Uncle Mike

My wife and I always enjoyed having Uncle Mike over for dinner. I had grown up with Uncle Mike, going with him to baseball games, heading down to the corner store for an ice-cream cone, and especially lacing up our shoes together for a game of bowling. He loved to bowl. He was so active then, so alive.

Age takes its toll

Age had taken a toll on him, though. Stricken with arthritis, cataracts, a thyroid condition, and a bad heart, my 85-year-old uncle had slowed and become, almost before my eyes, a very old man.

I thought we had lost him

Then one night at dinner, I thought we had lost him. We were eating liver and onions — his favorite dish — when he started to sweat. "I feel dizzy," he told us. Then he slumped in his chair.

We tried to lay him on the floor, but at 6 feet, 200 pounds, we were afraid we might drop him, so we left him in the chair. He was drenched in sweat and couldn't answer our questions. He could only mumble.

I took off his sweater and scarf, which he had insisted on wearing throughout dinner, and wiped his face with a cold washcloth in an attempt to arouse him. Nothing helped.

No response

Then he stopped responding at all.

We felt his pulse — it was present, thank goodness — and we could see his chest rise and fall, so we knew he was still breathing. But we were so scared....

Mary called 911 while I put Uncle Mike's feet on a pillow. Then we waited for the ambulance, the longest few minutes I've ever spent in my life.

Help arrives

When the EMTs arrived, they gave Uncle Mike oxygen, put him on a heart monitor, and rushed him to the hospital. The doctor in the emergency department said Uncle Mike had an irregular heartbeat and had suffered what he called a TIA or a "little stroke."

Then, while we were sitting with him in the emergency department, Uncle Mike woke up, asked, "What's for dinner?" and winked at me.

I nearly cried. Uncle Mike spent 3 days in the hospital, then went home. He's doing great now. He has lost some weight and actually looks like his old self. In fact, the last time I saw him, he was bowling — and winning.

AfterWords

Mike's nephew and wife did most things right while trying to help their uncle. First and most important, they called 911 when they realized something serious was wrong. They also assessed the situation properly, checking Mike's pulse and watching for chest movement to see if he was breathing.

However, they shouldn't have taken the time to remove Mike's sweater and scarf — at least not before calling for help. Any time someone stops responding or becomes unconscious, you've got a medical emergency on hand. Removing clothing, if it's necessary at all, should come *after* the call to 911 or to your local emergency medical service.

typically produces symptoms on the right side of the body, and vice versa.

To help diagnose the stroke, the doctor evaluates the person's symptoms, performs a physical exam, checks the medical history

The person may undergo surgery to improve blood flow to the brain. The doctor may prescribe various medicines.

for risk factors, and orders various diagnostic tests. These may include:

■ computed tomography scan (commonly called a CAT scan)
■ magnetic resonance imaging (commonly called MRI) or a brain scan
■ spinal tap (also called lumbar puncture)
■ a special X-ray of the inside of the brain's blood vessels (called an *angiogram*)
■ an eye exam to detect symptoms of high blood pressure and hardening in the arteries of the eye's retina.

What happens next

If the stroke was caused by a blood clot or an obstructed blood vessel, the person may undergo surgery to improve blood flow to the brain. In an operation called an *endarterectomy,* the surgeon removes any plaque blocking the artery's inner walls. In a procedure called a *microvascular bypass,* the surgeon joins a blood vessel outside the skull to one inside the skull.

Drug therapy

The doctor may prescribe various medicines. Drugs useful for treating a person who has had a stroke include:

■ Ticlid, which may be more effective than aspirin in preventing stroke and reducing the risk of recurrence
■ tissue plasminogen activator (also called t-PA or Activase) to help dissolve blood clots
■ antiseizure drugs, such as Dilantin, to treat or prevent seizures
■ stool softeners to prevent straining at stool (which increases pressure within the skull)
■ steroids, such as Decadron, to minimize brain swelling
■ pain relievers, such as codeine, to ease the headache that typically follows some strokes.

Treating a transient ischemic attack

After a transient ischemic attack, the person may receive treatments to prevent a full-fledged stroke. For instance, aspirin or blood thinners can minimize the risk of blood clots. Or the person may undergo surgery to try to reduce the risk of future strokes.

What else should you know?

After a stroke, everyday activities can be difficult. However, physical

How to make eating easier after a stroke

If you find it difficult to eat after a stroke, your doctor, nurse, or physical therapist can advise you on where to get special glasses, cups, plates, and utensils designed especially for people like you. Here are some suggestions for using these assistive devices.

Use plastic tumblers

If you have trouble holding onto a glass, use a plastic tumbler instead. Because plastic is lighter and less slippery than glass, it's easier to hold onto. If you prefer, use terrycloth sleeves over glasses to make them easier to grasp.

Drink from special cups

You can choose from many specially designed cups. A cup with two handles is easier to keep steady than a cup with one handle. A pedestal cup or a T-handled cup are both easy to grasp. You can also try a cup with a weighted base that helps prevent spills.

If your neck is stiff, use a cup with a V-shaped opening on its rim. You can easily tip this cup to empty it without bending your neck backward.

A cup for unsteady hands

If your hands are unsteady, you may find it easier to hold a cup with a large handle. Or drink from a lidded cup with a lip to help decrease spills. If you have decreased sensation or feeling in your hands, use an insulated cup or mug to avoid burning yourself.

Use drinking straws

Flexible or rigid straws come in several sizes. You can find disposable or reusable straws — some are even wide enough to use for drinking soups and thick liquids. To hold the straw in place, use a snap-on plastic lid with a slot for the straw.

Eat from unbreakable dishes

Try to use only unbreakable dishes. To keep a plate from sliding, place a damp sponge, washcloth, paper towel, or rubber disk under it.

Consider using a plate with a nonskid base or placemats made of dimpled rubber or foam underneath the plate. Suction cups attached to the bottom of a plate or bowl also help prevent slipping.

Try out plate guards and scooper plates

You may want to consider using a plate guard. This device prevents food from falling off the plate so that it can be picked up easily with a fork or spoon. Attach the guard to the side of the plate opposite the hand you use to feed yourself.

A scooper plate has high sides that provide a built-in surface for pushing food onto the utensil. Eating from a sectioned plate or tray may also be convenient.

Use easy-grasp flatware

If your hand is weak or your grip is shaky, you may want to try ordinary flatware with ridged wood, plastic, or cork handles — all easier to grasp than smooth metal handles. Or try building up the handles with a bicycle handgrip, a foam curler pad, or tape.

This technique also works for making pens and pencils, toothbrushes, or razors easier to hold. You can also try strapping the utensil to your hand.

therapy and speech therapy can help restore much lost function. To make eating easier, for instance, the person may need to use adapted utensils and dishes. (See *How to make eating easier after a stroke.*)

Show support

Keep in mind that the person who has had a stroke needs a great deal of emotional support. In frustration, he or she may lash out at friends and family members.

Despite any outbursts, try to be supportive. Family members may need to take time out and return when both they and the person who has suffered the stroke are calmer.

Also, be sure not to shout, talk down, or act as though the person is less intelligent after a stroke. The brain's speech and motor centers may be impaired but the brain is still functioning.

SUICIDE POTENTIAL

A depressed person who often thinks about ending his or her life has suicide potential. Actually, many people think or fantasize about killing themselves — say, in reaction to upsetting events. Feeling sad or dejected every now and then is a normal part of life. Usually, these emotions pass in a few hours or days.

But a person who has intense feelings of sadness or dejection lasting longer than usual may be suffering from depression. This puts the person at significant risk for suicide.

Who's at risk?

People of all ages consider — and attempt — suicide. However, suicide is more prevalent in some age-groups. (See *Identifying suicide risk factors*.)

Sometimes, a person shows unmistakable suicide potential — for instance, stepping out onto a window ledge. Some very depressed people threaten to commit suicide. Still others don't talk about their suicidal feelings but act in ways that suggest they're thinking of suicide.

What are the symptoms?

Suspect suicide potential in someone who:
- expresses feelings of guilt, shame, or low self-esteem
- takes responsibility for everything that goes wrong
- feels profoundly hopeless

Sometimes, a person shows unmistakable suicide potential — for instance, stepping out onto a window ledge. Other depressed people don't talk about their suicidal feelings but act in ways that suggest they're thinking of suicide.

- says that he or she feels like a burden to others
- is sad and dejected or inappropriately elated
- takes no pleasure in anything
- has trouble eating and sleeping
- lacks a sense of humor
- has lost interest in sex
- cries without tears
- wrings the hands
- laughs inappropriately
- has scratches on the skin from compulsive picking.

Stay alert for suspicious behavior
Some suicidal people seem apathetic, lethargic, or withdrawn. Others are agitated and restless. Drinking heavily, making out a will, and failing to renew a rental lease may also warn of suicide potential.

Be especially concerned if the person causes self-injury, takes an "accidental" drug overdose, starts giving away personal property, says goodbye in a way that implies you'll never see him or her again, or reveals a suicide plan that's likely to succeed.

On the other hand, don't make the mistake of assuming that everyone who feels suicidal is severely depressed. A person may attempt suicide weeks or months after beginning to recover from severe depression. (See *Separating suicide facts from fiction,* page 504.)

What should you do?
Take all hints and threats of suicide seriously. Often, the threat or attempt is a cry for help. Most people thinking of suicide want help and may change their minds if given the chance.

If you believe someone is at serious risk for suicide, urge that person to see a mental health professional, such as a psychiatrist, or to ask the family physician for an appropriate referral. Or call the suicide hotline; you can find the number in the telephone book.

If a child threatens suicide, take the threat very seriously. Don't leave the child alone until a thorough psychiatric evaluation is done.

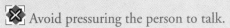 Don't be afraid to ask directly if the person is considering suicide. Asking won't put the idea into his or her head. But it may help the person to discuss feelings, which can show how serious the suicide risk is.

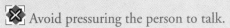 Avoid pressuring the person to talk.

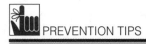 PREVENTION TIPS

Identifying suicide risk factors

Although a person of any age, sex, or economic class can be suicidal, certain risk factors make suicide more likely. Learning about these risk factors can help you become more alert to suicide potential in family members and friends.

Age, sex, and marital status
Women try suicide more often, but men are three times more likely to succeed. People under age 19 and over age 45 are at higher risk for suicide. So are people who are single, separated, divorced, or widowed.

Physical and mental health
People with serious or chronic physical illnesses, alcoholics, depressed people, and those with mental illness have a higher suicide risk.

Past suicide attempts
People who have tried suicide before are more likely to try it again.

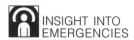
INSIGHT INTO
EMERGENCIES

Separating suicide facts from fiction

The myths that surround suicide could prevent you from recognizing suicidal impulses in family members or friends. Or they could stop you from showing the concern and empathy that could prevent a tragedy. Compare the myths about suicide, shown in the left column below, with the facts, shown in the right column.

Fiction: Suicide typically strikes the very rich or the very poor.	**Fact:** People from all levels of society kill themselves.
Fiction: Suicidal tendencies run in certain families.	**Fact:** Suicidal tendencies occur in individuals, not families.
Fiction: All suicidal people are mentally ill.	**Fact:** Suicidal people are very unhappy, but not necessarily mentally ill.
Fiction: People who talk about committing suicide don't kill themselves.	**Fact:** About 80% of the people who commit suicide have given clear warnings of their intentions.
Fiction: You can't stop a person who's suicidal from carrying out the act.	**Fact:** Most suicidal people can't decide whether they want to live or die. Timely intervention can save them.
Fiction: Once a person starts to recover from severe depression, little risk of suicide remains.	**Fact:** Typically, people commit suicide during the first 3 months of their recovery from depression. As they improve, they gain the energy to carry out their suicidal intentions.

WHEN SECONDS COUNT

If a suicide attempt seems imminent — say, the person is holding a gun or knife — get the situation under control at once. Stay calm, and call 911 or your community's local emergency number; a dispatcher will send the police. Speak softly and don't make sudden movements. Don't argue with or show anger toward the person. Urge the person to talk, and listen attentively. Show concern for what he or she is saying.

Once the immediate crisis is under control, get professional help for the person. If possible, accompany him or her to a hospital or psychiatric facility.

How is suicide potential treated?
Safety takes highest priority. The medical team removes from the

person's reach any object that he or she could use as a weapon or put in the mouth. This may involve removing the person's clothes. For increased safety, one staff member may be assigned to stay within arm's reach of the person at all times. Restraints may be applied if the person's behavior gets out of control.

Ruling out drug use and diseases

A blood or urine specimen may be taken to check for drug use. The doctor may administer an anti-anxiety medication like Ativan to calm the person and perform a medical exam to rule out an underlying medical condition that could be causing suicidal feelings.

If the exam fails to turn up such a condition, a psychiatrist evaluates the person to gauge the extent of the suicidal urges. A person whom the psychiatrist believes is strongly suicidal may be admitted to the hospital.

What else should you know?

Many depressed people get relief from drugs. Medications used to treat depression include:
- Prozac and similar drugs, called selective serotonin uptake inhibitors
- tricyclic antidepressants, such as Tofranil
- antidepressants called monoamine oxidase (MAO) inhibitors, such as Marplan
- Lithobid, used to treat manic-depression (bipolar disorder).

Some people also receive electroconvulsive therapy (sometimes called shock treatments). For more information on treatment of depression, see "Depression," page 176.

The medical team removes from the person's reach any object that he or she could use as a weapon or put in the mouth.

SUNBURN OR SUN POISONING

Many people think of sunburn as a tolerable nuisance on the road to a great suntan. However, overexposure to the sun can cause a real burn — ranging from mild (first-degree) to serious (second-degree).

Sun exposure can also lead to these long-range problems:
- an increased risk for skin cancer, including the potentially fatal malignant melanoma
- wrinkling, freckling, and roughening of the skin.

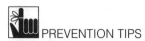
PREVENTION TIPS

How to reduce your risk for sunburn

The easiest way to prevent sunburn and skin cancer is to reduce your exposure to the sun. Most skin cancers occur after age 50, but the sun's damaging effects begin in childhood. Blistering burns in childhood may be the most damaging of all.

You can begin protecting yourself from skin cancer no matter what your age. Here's how.

Wear sunscreen

Protect your skin with a lotion or cream containing para-aminobenzoic acid (PABA). For infants or those allergic to PABA-based sunscreen, look for sunscreens labeled "PABA-free."

Sunscreens are rated in strength according to the familiar skin protection factor (SPF). Ranging from a low of 2 to a high of 30 or more, the SPF rates products by the length of protection they give. If you would normally burn within an hour and you used a product with a rating of 15, it would take 15 hours of sun exposure to burn using that product. If you're fair and burn easily, choose a sunscreen with an SPF of 15 or higher.

When to apply sunscreen

Apply sunscreen 30 minutes before you go outside. Then reapply every 2 to 3 hours. Apply sunscreen more frequently if you perspire heavily. Always reapply after swimming or exercising.

Should you use a water-resistant product?

Consider using a water-resistant sunscreen if you plan to swim. But keep in mind that you'll still need to reapply such a product — it's merely water-resistant, not waterproof.

Sunscreen isn't just for summer

Apply sunscreen routinely before you go outside, even in the winter, because the sun's rays can damage your skin whether you're on the way to work or school or lounging at the pool. With the new holes in the protective ozone layer, more damaging ultraviolet rays are reaching the earth than ever before.

Consider storing your sunscreen in a safe place near your front or back door, and encourage the whole family to wear it. Keep an extra container in the trunk of your car. (Don't leave it on the seat or it may get too hot.)

Cover up in the sun

Wear protective clothing, such as a wide-brimmed hat, long sleeves, and sunglasses. If your skin is extremely sensitive, remember that flimsy, lightweight clothes may not protect you against sunburn. Why? Because the sun's rays can penetrate them.

Also, don't rely entirely on a shady tree or an umbrella to prevent sunburn. Although these objects can screen out some rays, they can't offer you complete protection.

Heed advisories

Weather reports in some areas now include advisories about the risk of ultraviolet exposure during the summer months. Heed these warnings and cover up well on the brightest, most dangerous days.

Choose your time in the sun

To further reduce your exposure, avoid outdoor activities when the sun's rays are strongest — between 10 a.m. and 3 p.m. (11 a.m. and 4 p.m. daylight saving time). If you can, schedule outdoor activities such as swimming, tennis, and yard work for early in the morning or late in the afternoon.

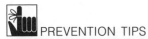

PREVENTION TIPS

How to reduce your risk for sunburn *(continued)*

Other points to remember

■ Keep in mind that no matter how attractive a suntan may be, it means your skin has been damaged. There's no such thing as a "healthy" tan. Spread the word that pale can be beautiful or handsome. Remind sun worshipers that the skin stays unlined and youthful longer if you don't damage it by tanning.

■ Don't use oils or a reflector device to promote a suntan.

■ Check with your doctor or pharmacist to find out whether any prescription or over-the-counter medicines you're taking may make you more sensitive to sunlight.

■ Avoid artificial ultraviolet light, including sunlamps.

■ Steer clear of tanning parlors or booths.

How sunburn occurs

When a person is exposed to the sun, the skin tries to protect itself from the sun's ultraviolet rays by producing more melanin, a brown pigment. If melanin production lags behind ultraviolet exposure, the skin gets burned. (See *How to reduce your risk for sunburn.*)

The sun's aging effects

The sun ages the skin by damaging blood vessels near the skin surface. It also destroys connective tissue in the skin's inner layer and breaks down the skin's elastic fibers.

What are the symptoms?

The severity of the person's symptoms depends on how much skin was burned and the degree of the burn. Any or all of these skin symptoms may occur:

■ redness

■ pain

■ mild to severe swelling

■ blisters (with a second-degree burn).

Sunburn can also cause a fever, chills, nausea, and fatigue.

What should you do?

Your actions depend on the severity of the burn.

What to do for a severe sunburn

Get prompt medical attention for a person with a severe burn, especially a young child.

What to do for a blistering sunburn

Make sure the person sees a doctor. After medical treatment, here are some home treatments to use.

■ Immerse the burned area in cool water. Soak burned hands or feet directly in cool water. Apply towels soaked in cool water to burns of the face, back, chest, or abdomen. Cover the wet towels with sheets to prevent chilling.

■ Elevate the person's arms and legs if they're badly sunburned.

■ Give aspirin or ibuprofen (such as Motrin or Advil) to relieve pain and inflammation.

■ After the sunburn cools, put dry sterile bandages on any open blisters, if possible.

■ Have the person drink plenty of water to prevent dehydration and heat exhaustion.

■ Make sure the person avoids further exposure to the sun until the skin has healed.

Immerse the burned area in cool water. Raise the person's arms and legs if they're badly sunburned.

 Don't apply oil or lotion to sunburned skin.

 Never put butter or margarine on a sunburn.

 Avoid breaking blisters or peeling sunburned skin.

 Don't rub the sunburned skin. Treat it gently.

What to do for mild sunburn

■ Apply wet compresses to the sunburned area to relieve pain. Remoisten the compresses as they warm up.

■ Give the person aspirin or ibuprofen (such as Advil or Motrin).

■ Have the person take a cool bath with baking soda (a half cup to one cup of baking soda per bath) or Aveeno powder (available at the drug store).

■ Apply aloe vera gel to the sunburned skin.

 Don't give Tylenol or other forms of acetaminophen because it doesn't reduce inflammation. An exception: You may give Tylenol if the person can't take aspirin or ibuprofen.

What is basal cell cancer?

Basal cell cancer is a slow-growing skin tumor that most often occurs in people over age 40. The most common cancerous tumor in whites, it's most prevalent in blond, fair-skinned men.

Learning about the causes

Most of the time, basal cell cancer comes from prolonged sun exposure. Less common causes are:

- radiation exposure
- burns
- suppression of the immune system, as in certain diseases
- arsenic poisoning
- vaccinations.

Options for treatment

Treatment depends on the size, location, and depth of the tumor as well as the person's age and health. The doctor may recommend one or more of the following treatments:

- cutting away the tumor and then vaporizing it with a laser if it is small
- chemotherapy if the cancer is restricted to the surface of the skin
- surgery to carefully remove layers of skin until a tumor-free layer is reached
- radiation therapy if the tumor would be hard to reach during surgery, or if the person is older or unable to endure surgery
- special cold treatments that freeze and kill cancerous cells
- destruction of the tissue using a chemical if the tumor persists or comes back.

Self-care

If you have basal cell cancer, taking the following steps can ease symptoms and help prevent a recurrence.

- If the tumor is on your face, wash your face gently when ulcers and crusting occur. Scrubbing too vigorously may cause bleeding.
- To relieve skin inflammation from chemotherapy, apply cool compresses or a steroid ointment prescribed by your doctor.
- If the cancer has invaded your mouth and is making eating difficult, eat egg nog, pureed foods, or liquid protein supplements instead of solid foods.
- Avoid excessive sun exposure to help prevent another bout of skin cancer.

How is sunburn or sun poisoning treated?

Unless the sunburn is severe and covers most of the body, the person doesn't need hospital treatment. The doctor or nurse cools the burned skin by applying cold compresses or immersing the burned parts in cool water. The doctor prescribes anti-inflammatory drugs to relieve pain and reduce inflammation and swelling. If the person has open blisters, the doctor may prescribe a topical antibiotic.

For severe sunburn, the person may need to be hospitalized to receive intravenous fluids and other treatments that help prevent shock.

What else should you know?

Certain ethnic groups are at higher risk for developing skin cancer from overexposure to the sun. For instance, you are more likely than other people to burn — and thus have an increased risk for skin cancer — if you:

- are of Scottish, Irish, English, or German ancestry
- have blond hair and pale skin.

Be aware that even people in the same family can vary tremendously in their ability to withstand the sun's harsh rays. Your brother or sister may be able to tan quickly without burning, but that doesn't necessarily mean you can. (See *What is basal cell cancer?* page 509.)

SWALLOWING DIFFICULTY

A person may have difficulty during any part of the swallowing process:

- when chewing
- when beginning to swallow
- after swallowing, when the food moves through the food tube (esophagus) into the stomach.

What happens when you swallow

Normally, when you swallow food, the back of the tongue pushes the food into the esophagus — the muscular tube that runs from the back of your throat to your stomach.

As food enters the esophagus, the top of the windpipe (called the *trachea*) temporarily closes to prevent food from entering your lungs. Rhythmic contractions of the esophageal muscles then sweep food down the esophagus to the stomach.

Understanding the causes

Swallowing can become difficult for many reasons. Common causes include:

- spasms of the muscles of the esophagus
- inflammation of the esophagus (called *esophagitis*)

A person may have difficulty when chewing food, when beginning to swallow, or after swallowing when the food moves through the food tube into the stomach.

■ hiatal hernia, in which part of the stomach slips through an opening in the diaphragm and juts into the chest cavity

■ stroke

■ persistent sore throat.

Less common causes of swallowing difficulty are:

■ nervous system or neuromuscular disorders (such as myasthenia gravis) that affect the muscles, especially those in the head and neck

■ botulism, a type of food poisoning

■ a blocked food tube caused by something *inside* it (like a tumor or foreign body) or something *outside* it (like a growth on the voice box). (See *When your child has trouble swallowing,* page 512.)

A person who has had a tube in the throat during hospitalization may also have difficulty swallowing if the tube irritates the throat. Radiation therapy directed against cancer of the mouth may cause temporary swallowing difficulty.

What are the symptoms?

The person may have trouble swallowing either liquids or solid foods. For some people, swallowing liquids is harder than swallowing solids. Sometimes, the symptoms disappear if the person changes position or swallows repeatedly.

Swallowing difficulty can make the person choke on food or inhale a foreign object into the lungs. In this case, the person may put a hand to the throat and start to turn blue. If the windpipe is completely blocked, the person won't be able to cough, speak, or breathe.

If swallowing difficulty lasts a long time, the person may become malnourished and dehydrated.

A person who experiences difficulty swallowing should consult a doctor promptly. This is especially important if the person has lost a lot of weight recently.

What should you do?

A person who experiences difficulty swallowing should consult a doctor promptly to find out the cause. This is especially important if the person has lost a lot of weight recently; the cause could be cancer of the esophagus.

WHEN SECONDS COUNT

If a person suddenly complains of difficulty swallowing and starts to have trouble breathing, suspect that something is blocking the airway. If the person can't talk and points to the throat, assume he or she is choking and quickly perform the Heimlich maneuver. (For instructions, see *Clearing a blocked airway,* page 593.)

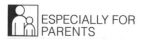
ESPECIALLY FOR
PARENTS

When your child has trouble swallowing

Swallowing difficulty in a young child is most likely to result from a foreign object blocking the esophagus (food tube) or from swallowing a poison.

Observe your infant

How can you tell if your infant is having trouble swallowing? Observe the way he or she sucks and swallows during feedings. Then ask yourself these questions:

- Does my child cough during feedings?
- Does my child seem to choke during feedings?
- Does my child regularly regurgitate after feedings?

How much regurgitation is normal?

Most infants spit up some formula or breast milk from time to time. But if regurgitation seems unusual or excessive, call your pediatrician.

Get immediate help

If your child seems to be choking or if you suspect he or she has swallowed a poison, call for emergency medical help immediately. Be prepared to perform CPR if necessary.

How is swallowing difficulty treated?

The person undergoes a complete diagnostic evaluation to pinpoint the cause of the swallowing difficulty. Diagnostic tests may include:

- endoscopy — passage of a tube through the mouth to inspect the esophagus and other respiratory or digestive organs
- esophageal manometry — passage of a tube through the nose and into the stomach to allow inspection and measure important pressures within the esophagus.

Specific treatments depend on what disorder the diagnostic tests uncover.

What else should you know?

Once the person's condition has been diagnosed, the following self-care measures may help relieve symptoms.

- Avoid foods with a sticky texture, like peanut butter and bananas.
- At mealtimes, sit upright, with your neck bent forward slightly and your face forward. This position uses gravity to ease swallowing.
- During meals, separate solid foods from liquids, which are harder to swallow. If your mouth feels dry, moisten the food with a little liquid.

SWEATING

We sweat to reduce our body temperature: When heat or exercise increases the body temperature, sweating cools it.

But some people sweat *excessively* for reasons other than physical activity or hot weather. Whatever the cause, someone who sweats profusely can lose up to 1 quart of sweat an hour.

Understanding the causes
Excessive sweating can come from these causes.
- *Fever.* Sweating usually occurs with a fever.
- *Acute pain.* This may bring on an isolated episode of profuse sweating.
- *Heart attack.* Excessive sweating may occur early in this emergency.
- *Stress.* A stressed-out person may sweat from any part of the body or just from the palms, soles, and forehead.
- *Obesity.* Even minimal activity can make an overweight, out-of-shape person sweat a lot.
- *Hormonal changes.* Menstruation, menopause, or the hormonal changes of adolescence can cause excessive sweating.
- *Some drugs.* For instance, aspirin can cause sweating when taken in large doses.
- *Alcohol.* Drinking alcohol widens the blood vessels, producing a brief warming flush.

Excessive sweating can result from such conditions as a fever, acute pain, heart attack, stress, hormonal changes, alcohol, and some drugs.

What are the symptoms?
Usually, profuse sweating begins abruptly. When sweating comes from a fever or a high environmental temperature, the person usually sweats from all parts of the body.

Other symptoms to watch for
Symptoms that may go along with sweating include:
- anxiety
- extreme thirst
- ashen or gray skin
- fever
- rapid pulse
- headache and dizziness (from high blood pressure).

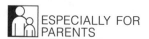

Is your child dressed to sweat?

When a child sweats a lot, it is usually because he or she is overdressed for the weather or the room temperature. Here are some ways you can prevent your child from getting hot and bothered.

Don't overdress your child

■ Dress your child as you would dress yourself rather than bundling the child up. Children are more physically active than adults, so they're often more comfortable with fewer layers than are sedentary adults.

■ When your child complains about being too hot to wear that extra sweater, don't force the sweater on him or her. Usually, you have no reason to doubt your child.

When to consult a doctor

Sometimes excessive sweating in a child signals an underlying illness. If your child starts sweating a lot for no apparent reason, call the doctor.

Medical conditions that can make a child sweat include:

■ congestive heart failure

■ a severely overactive thyroid gland

■ use of drugs such as antihistamines (commonly given for coughs and colds).

Night sweats: Possible warning sign

Some diseases may cause a person to sweat at night. For instance, night sweats are an early symptom of AIDS and Hodgkin's disease. Tuberculosis, lung abscess, and infection of the heart's inner lining (a condition called *endocarditis*) can also cause night sweats.

What should you do?

Anyone who sweats should replace lost fluids and body salts by drinking fluids. If the person has been sweating from a fever, taking tepid baths and using a drug containing ibuprofen or acetaminophen may bring the body temperature down.

Someone with *unexplained* excessive sweating should contact a doctor.

WHEN SECONDS COUNT

Excessive sweating is an early sign of certain life-threatening emergencies. Get immediate medical help if the person who is sweating also has these symptoms:

■ blurred vision, dizziness, irritability, and hunger (these are symptoms of a low blood sugar crisis)

■ weakness, fatigue, confusion, anxiety, a thready pulse, dizziness, and cold, clammy skin after being exposed to high temperatures (heatstroke could be the culprit)

■ chest pain, shortness of breath, nausea and vomiting, and pale, clammy skin (these symptoms could mean a heart attack).

> ✖ Don't ignore excessive sweating that accompanies weakness or nausea.

How is excessive sweating treated?

If the person needs to be hospitalized for a serious underlying disorder, he or she receives intravenous fluids to replace the lost fluids. The person is encouraged to drink extra fluids, if possible.

To find the cause of sweating, the doctor may order diagnostic tests, such as:

■ blood tests

■ specimens of certain body fluids to look for dangerous organisms

■ chest X-rays

■ immunologic studies

■ biopsy

■ computed tomography scans (commonly called CAT scans).

Other treatments depend on the specific cause of the excessive sweating.

What else should you know?

Infants and elderly people may not sweat profusely. In infants, the reason is immature sweat glands; in older people, it's less active sweat glands.

However, older children lose fluids quickly and may become ill more rapidly than adults. If your child is sweating excessively, encourage him or her to drink plenty of fluids to replace the lost fluid. Try to avoid soft drinks; water is the best drink for thirsty children. (See *Is your child dressed to sweat?*)

Children lose fluids quickly and may become ill rapidly. Give plenty of water to a child who is sweating.

SWELLING

Swelling occurs when too much fluid collects in a part of a person's body (local swelling) or when excess fluid builds up all over the body (generalized swelling).

Understanding the causes

There are many reasons why fluid may collect in the body, some relatively minor and some life-threatening. Something as simple as eating too much salt can lead to generalized swelling. Other causes of swelling include:

- heart, kidney, liver, and hormone disorders
- severe burns
- malnutrition
- the effects of certain drugs or treatments. Drugs that make you retain salt can cause, or worsen, generalized swelling. These include some blood pressure medications, steroids, hormones (such as estrogen), and nonsteroidal anti-inflammatory drugs (such as the pain relievers Advil and Anaprox).

Swelling of the *face* can come from a sinus infection or an eye disorder, such as pinkeye or a stye. Sometimes it signals a life-threatening allergic reaction.

Swelling of an *arm* or a *leg* usually stems from an injury, an infection, or poor drainage of blood or lymph (the fluid that circulates through the lymphatic system). Poor drainage can result from a kidney problem or another serious condition.

Swelling in children

Children may experience swelling for different reasons than adults. Kids with heart or kidney problems tend to swell up around their eyes rather than in the arms or legs, as adults do. And mumps causes facial swelling in children much more often than in adults. A child's calf muscles can become swollen and firm from one form of muscular dystrophy, a disease that causes muscles to lose protein and enlarge with fat and connective tissue.

What are the symptoms?

Swelling makes the affected area grow puffy and large. The skin over the swollen place may become shiny, taut, and cool. In severe swelling, the area may become rock-hard. If swelling results from an injury or a broken bone, the person may also have:

- redness
- pain
- bruising.

Infection can also cause redness and pain. If nerves are involved, the person may experience numbness and tingling.

Swelling can come from something as simple as eating too much salt or from something as serious as a heart or kidney disorder.

What should you do?

WHEN SECONDS COUNT

Rapid swelling of the face, especially with difficulty breathing, may signal a severe allergic reaction. If the person's throat swells, he or she may be unable to breathe. Your rapid response to this emergency could save the person's life. (See *Recognizing allergic swelling,* page 518.)

Also suspect an emergency if the swelling:
- comes on rapidly
- follows a serious injury
- is coupled with shortness of breath
- results from a snake or insect bite
- involves the head and neck.

If the person's entire body is swollen, check to be sure he or she is alert, breathing, and not turning blue. Depending on the circumstances, you may need to call an ambulance or get immediate medical attention for the person.

What to do if a limb is swollen

If just one limb is swollen, compare it to the one on the other side to judge how swollen it is. Look at the skin color, and feel whether the area is overly warm or cool. Check for a pulse on the swollen limb. Then ask the person if the limb is painful. Finally, see if the swelling is affected by the person's body position.

If the limb (or any other part of the body) is *severely* swollen, call the doctor promptly. If you think the swollen limb is broken, splint it as described in "Fractures (broken bones)," page 251. Then get medical care for the person right away. Unless the swelling is from a venomous bite, you should position the swollen limb above the level of the person's heart. This will help the swollen area to drain.

What to do if the ankles are swollen

If the ankles and lower legs are swollen from poor circulation, instruct the person to:
- keep the legs elevated as much as possible
- avoid crossing the legs when sitting down
- avoid sitting or standing for long periods
- wear support socks or stockings (they must be put on *before* the person gets out of bed in the morning).

Assume the swelling is an emergency if it comes on rapidly, follows a serious injury, or is coupled with shortness of breath.

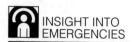

INSIGHT INTO
EMERGENCIES

Recognizing allergic swelling

A person whose face swells rapidly could be having a serious allergic reaction. Because facial swelling can affect the airways and impede breathing, the situation could be life-threatening.

Take quick action
If the person is hoarse or having trouble breathing, find out if he or she has an anaphylaxis (bee sting) kit. (Many people at risk for serious allergy carry them.) If so, get the Adrenalin injector out of the kit and prepare to use it, if necessary. Adrenalin is the only antidote to this kind of life-threatening allergic reaction.

Immediately after you give the Adrenalin, call for emergency medical assistance.

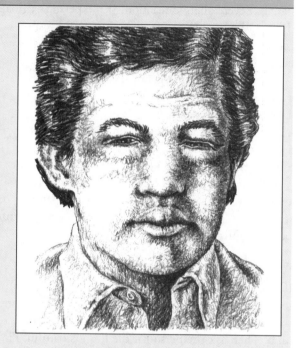

How is swelling treated?
For sudden, severe, generalized swelling, the medical team makes sure that the person can breathe and that the heart is functioning as it should. Then they take these steps:
- place the person in the position that best promotes breathing
- give oxygen, if necessary
- administer intravenous drugs to help the person get rid of excess fluids.

Treating swelling from a circulation problem
The doctor may prescribe:
- medications
- changes in the person's diet and exercise
- elastic support stockings.

Treating swelling from an injury
For swelling caused by an injury, treatment may include:
- X-rays
- stitches
- cosmetic or other surgery
- a cast
- crutches
- other implements.

Home treatment may include applying heat and cold to help limit the injury and reduce swelling.

Investigating the underlying condition
Once the person is stable, the doctor finds out these important details about the swelling:
- when the swelling started
- what seemed to bring it on
- if the swelling changes with the person's position
- if the person has been urinating more or less frequently than usual.

The doctor also asks about previous burns and finds out whether the person has a heart, kidney, liver, hormone, or digestive problem. Asking about the person's usual diet and any medications he or she takes can also help the doctor diagnose the condition.

What else should you know?
If you have injured yourself, you can help reduce pain and swelling by applying heat and cold to the hurt area. The latest research from sports medicine shows it's best to apply ice for the first 48 hours after the injury, then switch to heat. (However, your doctor may give you other instructions.)

You have many different options for applying both heat and cold. You can probably find the required supplies in your kitchen, linen closet, or your local drug store.

Heat treatments
To apply heat, you can use:
- a hot water bottle
- a heating pad
- washcloths soaked in hot water
- gel packs that you heat in a microwave oven.

Cold treatments

To apply cold, your options are to:

- place crushed ice in a sealable plastic bag and then place the bag in a pillowcase or towel
- use a gel pack designed to stay cold and pliable in the freezer.

Points to remember

- Whichever method you use, be sure to apply the heat or cold for no longer than 20 minutes at a time.
- Never put a hot or cold object directly on your skin. First pad and insulate it with a towel or similar covering.
- If the swelling comes from an injury, such as a sprain, seek medical attention to check for possible broken bones.

T

TEARING

Tears bathe the eyes, keeping them moist and washing away debris. Usually, we produce about 0.002 ounces of tears each day in a process called *lacrimation*. (See *Where tears come from*, page 522.)

Too many tears
Sometimes the eye produces an excessive amount of tears. Increased tearing can result from:
- sadness
- frustration
- anger
- some other emotions.

In *reflex lacrimation,* the person tears up when yawning, vomiting, or laughing.

But increased tearing is also the body's natural response to certain emergencies, such as an eye injury. Or it may come from exposure to environmental stresses, such as:
- a strong or hot wind
- bright light
- an allergy-causing substance like pollen in the air.

What are the symptoms?
Symptoms depend largely on the cause of the increased tearing. Any injury or infection involving the eye's cornea can produce severe pain. For example, getting a chemical or some other irritating substance in the eye can produce copious tearing and considerable pain.

Symptoms of penetrating eye wounds
An object that penetrates to the inside of the eyeball is likely to cause bleeding and severe pain along with increased tearing. The person may not even be able to open the eye for you to look. But if you see a cut on the eyelid, assume the person could have a penetrating

Increased tearing is the body's natural response to certain emergencies, such as an eye injury. Or it may come from exposure to bright light or a strong or hot wind.

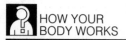

HOW YOUR BODY WORKS

Where tears come from

Tears are produced by the *lacrimal (tear) gland*, located just above and to the outside of each eye. Tears travel across the eye, keeping the eye moist and sweeping tiny bits of debris away from the cornea.

Tracks of our tears

When tears and debris get to the inside corner of the eye, called the inner canthus, they are "vacuumed" up into the lacrimal canals.

From sac to nose

The lacrimal canals dump excess tears into the lacrimal sac, which in turn deposits them inside the nose. That's why your nose runs when you cry or when your eyes water.

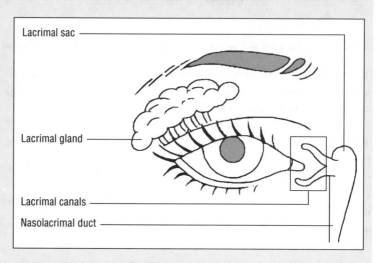

Lacrimal sac

Lacrimal gland

Lacrimal canals

Nasolacrimal duct

wound. A foreign body embedded in the cornea may cause rapid blinking, blurred vision, and pain.

Symptoms of infection

A corneal infection can produce increased tearing with severe pain. The infection may cause the white part of the eye, called the *sclera*, to turn red. If the person has an infection of the lacrimal sac — the part of the tear duct where tears are stored — you may see a pronounced bump between the nose and the inner corner of the eye.

What should you do?

If you suspect a penetrating eye injury, seek emergency medical attention for the person. Also seek prompt attention if the person has a foreign body lodged in the cornea or an infection of the cornea or lacrimal sac.

If the person got a chemical or other irritating substance in the eye, you may be able to wash it out. This will ease the person's symp-

When the well runs dry

As we age, we produce fewer tears. But some other conditions can make the eyes dry up and cause discomfort.

Naming the causes
Here's a partial list of the conditions that can cause dry eyes.

Eye conditions
- Absence of the tear glands from birth
- Dry-eye syndrome, which causes the tear glands to shrink
- Scar tissue that forms after an eye injury

Body-wide illnesses
- Sarcoidosis, a disease that affects many body systems and inflames the tear glands
- Stevens-Johnson syndrome, a severe reaction to drugs and some other conditions, in which the person has decreased tearing along with pinkeye and severe eye pain
- Vitamin A deficiency, which leads to decreased tearing and poor night vision

Drugs
- Medicines used to widen the pupils, such as atropine, Transderm-Scōp, Cyclogyl, and Tropicacyl

An artificial boost
Unless decreased tearing comes from an eye injury, the doctor usually prescribes a preparation of artificial tears in drops or an ointment.

toms and relieve the injury until he or she can get medical help. (See *How to flush the eye*, page 106.)

Flushing the eye is especially important if the chemicals involved are alkaline substances, such as plaster, drain cleaners, cleaning agents, ammonia, and cement.

How is excessive tearing treated?
Treatment depends on the cause of the increased tearing. An eye infection or injury may require medications, stitches, and patching. To remove a foreign object, the doctor may need to numb the eye and use a tiny instrument.

What else should you know?
Sometimes a person's tears decrease rather than increase. This condition makes the eyes feel uncomfortably dry. (See *When the well runs dry*.)

TESTICLE PAIN

In this uncommon problem, a boy or man gets severe pain in the testicle, either suddenly or over a few hours or days. Depending on the cause, testicle pain may call for emergency treatment.

Understanding the causes

The most dangerous cause of testicle pain is *testicular torsion*. In this emergency, a testicle gets twisted up inside the scrotum, cutting off its own blood supply. (See *Learning about testicular torsion*.)

Testicular torsion occurs mainly in infants and boys nearing or going through puberty. Sometimes strenuous physical activity seems to bring on the pain. Nine times out of 10, the pain affects just one side of the scrotum — the left side more often than the right.

Another cause of testicle pain is *epididymitis.* In this condition, the epididymis — the tube that carries sperm to another tube called the vas deferens — becomes inflamed. Epididymitis usually stems from a bacterial infection.

Finally, a problem called *orchitis* can cause testicle pain. In this condition, one or both testicles become inflamed. Orchitis usually results from:

■ mumps
■ an infection of the prostate gland or epididymis
■ tuberculosis
■ syphilis.

Orchitis can permanently damage one or both testicles, leading to infertility.

What are the symptoms?

In *testicular torsion,* the person feels sudden, excruciating pain in or around the testicle. The pain may spread to the lower abdomen. The scrotum swells up, with the affected side growing red and tender. The testicle may seem to be raised inside the scrotum. The pain gets worse when the person stands. The person may also have:

■ nausea
■ vomiting
■ fever
■ fainting or light-headedness.

In *epididymitis,* severe pain develops gradually over several hours or days. Heat and swelling may spread across part of the scrotum.

The most dangerous cause of testicle pain is testicular torsion. In this emergency, a testicle gets twisted up inside the scrotum, cutting off its own blood supply.

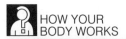

HOW YOUR
BODY WORKS

Learning about testicular torsion

The testicles produce sperm and male hormones such as testosterone. A spermatic cord suspends each testicle in the scrotum as shown in the large illustration. Blood vessels in this cord supply the testicle with oxygen and other nutrients.

A dangerous twist

In torsion, the testicle twists on its spermatic cord, as you can see in the close-up below. Such twisting cuts off the testicle's blood supply. Without treatment, the testicle could suffer damage or turn gangrenous within hours.

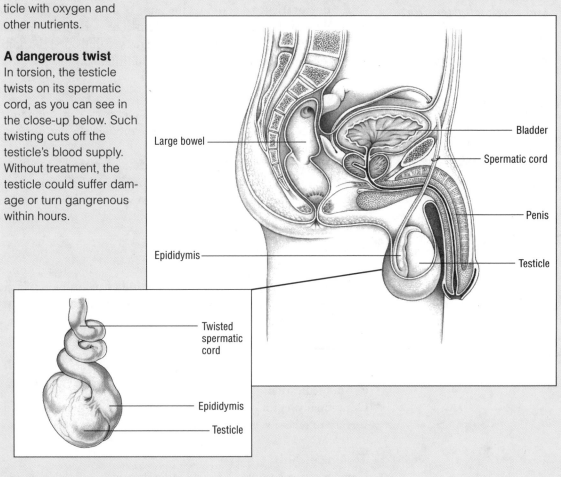

Usually, the pain occurs only on one side and may decrease a bit if the person lifts the painful testicle while standing. The person may have a fever.

In *orchitis,* the person usually develops a painful, swollen scrotum on one side. His scrotum may feel unusually heavy.

What should you do?

Get medical attention immediately if testicle pain occurs without a known cause. This is especially important with an infant or a boy at the age of puberty. If testicular torsion is causing the pain, the testicle could suffer damage or turn gangrenous within just a few hours.

How is testicle pain treated?

As the doctor tries to determines the cause of the problem, ice packs are applied to the scrotum to reduce pain. The person may receive pain medication and undergo ultrasound tests to find out if the problem is testicular torsion or some other condition.

Treating testicular torsion

The doctor may try to gently untwist the spermatic cord and return the testicle to its normal position. Usually, though, the person needs immediate surgery to unkink the cord.

If treatment is delayed and the testicle is damaged, the doctor may have to remove the testicle during surgery. After surgery, treatments include ice packs, pain medications, a scrotal support, and bed rest.

Treating epididymitis

Epididymitis usually is treated with medication. Because it comes from a bacterial infection, the doctor prescribes an antibiotic. If the person is sexually active, his sexual partner will probably need treatment for the infection, too.

Other treatments for epididymitis include:
- ice packs
- supporting the scrotum
- pain medication.

Occasionally, epididymitis becomes chronic and the person needs surgery to relieve symptoms.

Treating orchitis

If orchitis stems from the mumps, the doctor can do little to treat this viral infection. The person receives supportive treatments, such as rest and pain medications.

If the cause of orchitis is a bacterial infection, the doctor prescribes antibiotics.

Get medical attention immediately if testicle pain occurs without a known cause. If torsion is causing the pain, the testicle could suffer damage or turn gangrenous within a few hours.

What else should you know?
If the testicle must be removed, the person may be a candidate for an artificial (prosthetic) testicle.

TOOTHACHE

A toothache usually results from tooth decay or an abscess (a sac of pus) in or near a tooth. *Decay* occurs when bacteria eat through the tooth's hard surface to the inner layers. An *abscess* develops when bacteria infect the tooth's innermost pulp layer, possibly down to the underlying bone. (See *An inside look at a tooth,* pages 528 and 529.)

What are the symptoms?
At first, tooth decay doesn't cause symptoms. But as bacteria invade the tooth's inner layers, the person starts to feel pain.

Often, the first sign of decay is tooth pain when eating something sweet, very hot, or very cold. *Sharp* pain when eating these things may indicate a more serious cavity.

Warning signs of abscess
A tooth abscess can cause:
■ aching or throbbing tooth pain
■ unusual tooth sensitivity to hot and cold
■ pain when chewing
■ swollen glands in the neck
■ fever
■ a general ill feeling.
The abscess may form a swollen area on the gum that could burst into the mouth. If that happens, the pain may go away. But the abscess releases thick, pus-filled liquid that tastes and smells foul.

What should you do?
First, have the person rinse the mouth with warm water to clean out debris. Then instruct him or her to use dental floss to remove any food trapped between the teeth.

A toothache usually results from tooth decay or an abscess in or near a tooth. Often, the first sign of decay is tooth pain when eating something sweet, very hot, or very cold.

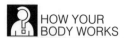

An inside look at a tooth

A tooth is a living part of your body. Supplied by nerves and blood vessels, it is vulnerable to bacteria and poor care. The picture below shows the many parts of a tooth.

NORMAL TOOTH

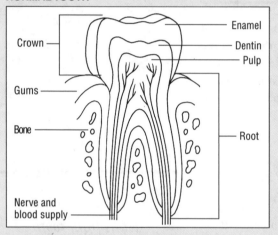

How decay sets in

Usually, teeth get decayed from the interaction of bacteria, sugar in the foods you eat, and poor tooth care. Bacteria in the mouth convert sugars to acids. Together with food particles and mucus, the bacteria and acids form a sticky coating on the teeth. This coating is called *plaque.*

Tiny holes for bacteria

The acid in plaque eats at the hard enamel coating on your teeth, eventually creating tiny openings. Bacteria that pass through these openings start to spread through the next tooth layer (dentin), as you see in the picture below.

DECAYED TOOTH

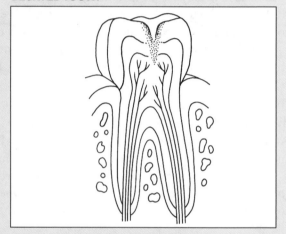

What makes a tooth hurt

Eventually, bacteria can work their way to the pulp, the tooth's innermost layer. It's here that the potential for toothache reaches its peak. That's because the pulp is filled with blood vessels and nerves that can swell when infected. Those vessels are surrounded by a hard tooth shell, so you feel pain when they swell inside it.

If the tooth still hurts, suspect a cavity or an abscess. To ease the pain, take these steps:
- Give the person aspirin, acetaminophen (such as Tylenol), or ibuprofen (such as Advil).
- Apply hot or cold compresses to the person's face (some people prefer hot compresses; others prefer cold).

HOW YOUR BODY WORKS

An inside look at a tooth *(continued)*

How an abscess forms

Once bacteria reach the pulp layer, they can spread all the way to the jaw bone. As they try to spread, your body begins to combat the infection by sending more white blood cells to the site. When a pocket of these cells forms, it's called a tooth abscess, as shown in the picture at right.

Get rid of an abscess for good

A tooth abscess can cause considerable pain. It can also kill the tooth's nerves and blood vessels. When this happens, the toothache may disappear, but then come back any time — even years later. The only way to get rid of a tooth abscess for good is through complete dental care.

ABSCESSED TOOTH

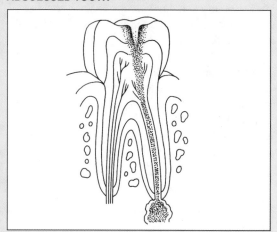

Never put aspirin directly on the tooth or the gum because it could cause an acid burn.

Don't put a cotton ball on the tooth if you see pus coming out of it or if the person's face is swollen.

When to get prompt medical attention

If you suspect an abscess, get the person to a dentist as soon as possible.

For a suspected cavity, place a cotton ball soaked in oil of cloves on the tooth, and have the person hold it there. Then call the dentist right away.

How is a toothache treated?

For a cavity, the dentist:
- numbs the tooth
- removes the decayed area
- fills the resulting hole with one of several "filling" substances or with porcelain cement, plastic resin, or a gold onlay.

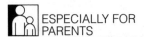

Starting your kids off right

The dental care you provide your children when they're young can have a positive effect on their health and appearance for decades to come. Here are a few tips to start your child off right.

Promote good habits
- Don't put your baby to sleep clutching a bottle of milk or fruit juice. If the child won't settle without a bottle, fill it with water.
- Begin teaching your child to brush regularly even before all baby teeth have come in.

Provide the right equipment
- Choose a toothbrush that fits your child's mouth. Make sure it can reach every tooth.
- Use only a soft-bristled toothbrush. Stiff bristles can damage the gums.
- Have your child use a fluoride toothpaste.

Other instructions
- Take your child to the dentist regularly. Choose a dentist your child likes.
- Talk to the dentist about dental sealants to protect against cavities when your child's permanent molars start to come in.

For a large cavity that would leave the tooth too weak to support a filling, the dentist may need to create a porcelain jacket or crown after taking a mold of the tooth.

For a severe abscess, the dentist may need to pull the infected tooth and prescribe antibiotics.

Performing root canal
If decay has spread to the tooth's pulp layer — even if it hasn't become an abscess yet — the person will probably need a root canal. In this procedure, the dentist removes the nerve and pulp from the roots of the tooth and fills the roots with an inert solid material. This leaves the shell of the original tooth in place. The shell may be more brittle than the original tooth, though, so the dentist may have to make a crown to support the tooth.

What else should you know?
The condition of an adult's teeth and the risk of future toothaches depend largely on how those teeth were treated in childhood. Parents can do much to prevent toothaches in their grown children by providing good dental care early in life. (See *Starting your kids off right*.)

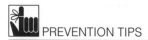
PREVENTION TIPS

Avoiding toothaches through good dental care

The best way to avoid toothaches is through sound dental care. Read on to learn how to take care of your teeth.

Basics of dental care
Taking care of your teeth can be as simple as following these three guidelines:
- Brush your teeth at least twice a day with a soft-bristled toothbrush and a fluoride toothpaste.
- Floss your teeth every day.
- Replace your toothbrush every 3 or 4 months, or whenever the bristles become bent. (The tips of the bristles do the cleaning.)

Brush or rinse after snacks
Rinse your mouth with water within 20 minutes after snacks if you can't brush. Try to avoid chewy, sticky snack foods. And remember — it's more harmful to eat sweets between meals than with meals. The worst thing you can do is drink sweetened drinks or suck on hard candy all day.

Floss daily
To remove harmful plaque, floss your teeth every day, preferably just before you brush your teeth at bedtime. Don't worry if your gums bleed the first few times you floss; it's most likely because the tissue has been weakened by plaque. If your gums keep bleeding after the first few times, talk to your dentist.

Use correct flossing technique
To floss properly, wrap about 18 inches (45 centimeters) of dental floss around your middle fingers. It doesn't matter whether you use waxed or unwaxed floss, string or tape. Try them all until you find the type you like best.

To floss your bottom teeth, stretch a short piece of floss between your index fingers, slide it between two teeth, and curl it around the base of one tooth. Slide the floss up and down against the side of the tooth to clean plaque away. Then floss the adjoining tooth. Repeat with a fresh section of floss for each bottom tooth. To floss your top teeth, stretch the floss between your thumb and index finger and repeat the process described above.

Make routine dental visits
See your dentist regularly, whether or not you get toothaches. Most people should have a professional cleaning twice a year and X-rays once a year.

An ounce of prevention
Even after a tooth problem arises, it can often be caught before it becomes a full-blown toothache. Seeing a dentist when tooth problems first begin can save you time, money, and pain. Of course, practicing good dental hygiene is the best way to prevent toothaches. (See *Avoiding toothaches through good dental care*.)

TOOTH INJURY OR TOOTH FALLING OUT

A sports injury, a car accident, or an assault can break, loosen, or knock out a tooth. If left untreated, these injuries could lead to a dead or missing tooth.

When a tooth gets knocked out, it means the ligament — the band of connective tissue that holds the tooth in place — has been severed. Fortunately, the tooth can usually be put back in as long as its root hasn't been damaged. But to preserve the tooth, you must take the right actions — fast.

What are the symptoms?

Besides the broken, loose, or knocked-out tooth, the person may have:
- mouth pain
- slight swelling of the mouth
- bleeding of the mouth.

Also look for other injuries that may have occurred at the same time. Such injuries are especially likely if the person fell, was assaulted, or was in a motor vehicle accident.

What should you do?

If a person's tooth gets broken or knocked out, check the mouth for bleeding. Remove any loose pieces of the broken tooth and retrieve any knocked-out tooth. Handle a knocked-out tooth by its crown (top), not its root. Take the person and the tooth to the dentist immediately. If a dentist isn't available, get the person to a hospital emergency department.

If the person's gums are bleeding, place a gauze pad, a clean handkerchief, or a tissue over the wound. Have the person hold the pad tightly in place.

Don't remove a loose tooth. Simply push it back into the socket and get the person to a dentist or a hospital emergency department at once.

Be sure not to put aspirin directly on the person's gums.

A knocked-out tooth can usually be put back in as long as its root hasn't been damaged. But to preserve the tooth, you must take the right actions— fast.

How to preserve a knocked-out tooth

A dentist may be able to replace a knocked-out tooth if its root doesn't suffer severe damage. Until the person gets to the dentist, preserve the tooth by placing it in a cup of cold whole milk, warm salt water, or a tooth-preserving solution. Be sure not to touch the root of the tooth while handling it.

Be prepared for emergencies
If you or your kids play on a sports team, talk to the coach about keeping a tooth-preserving solution on hand to use in dental emergencies. The coach can obtain it through a dentist or local drugstore.

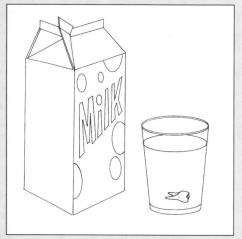

Preserve the tooth

If possible, carry the tooth in a cup of cold *whole* milk (not skim milk). Whole milk contains nutrients that can help keep the tooth alive. Or put the tooth in a tooth-preserving solution, available at many drugstores. If you don't have either, place the tooth in a container of salt water (add one teaspoon of salt to 1 quart of water). Or try to place the tooth back in its socket. (See *How to preserve a knocked-out tooth*.)

If you know the person won't get to the dentist within a few hours, rinse the knocked-out tooth to remove debris. If you rinse it over a sink, be sure to close the drain.

❌ Never put a knocked-out tooth back in a child's mouth because the child could swallow it. Worse yet, he or she could inhale it.

❌ Don't put the tooth in tap water because the water contains minerals that could harm the tooth.

❌ Be sure not to put the tooth in mouthwash or alcohol.

❌ Avoid putting the tooth in a dry paper towel or anything else that could scrape its surface.

Don't rub or scrape the tooth, and don't remove any pieces of flesh attached to it.

Avoid cleaning the tooth unless you're going to replace it in the socket.

Replace the tooth

If you don't have milk or other supplies to preserve the tooth of an adult, gently replace it in the socket after rinsing it. Make sure to position it correctly, using nearby teeth as a guide.

Push the tooth down or have the person gently bite down to make the loose tooth even with the adjacent ones. Get the person to a dentist as soon as possible.

> *If you don't have milk or other supplies to preserve the knocked-out tooth, gently replace it in the socket after rinsing it. Make sure to position it correctly.*

How is a tooth injury treated?

If possible, the dentist replaces the knocked-out tooth in the person's mouth. Usually, the person receives pain relievers to reduce pain and antibiotics to help prevent infection.

What else should you know?

After treatment, the person should place a cold compress on the face at the affected area for about 15 minutes each hour. If the doctor or dentist hasn't prescribed pain medication, taking acetaminophen (such as Tylenol) or ibuprofen (such as Advil) may relieve the pain.

TOXIC SHOCK SYNDROME

Toxic shock syndrome is a life-threatening form of shock. It starts suddenly and quickly becomes a severe illness that must be treated immediately.

Naming a new disease

Toxic shock syndrome got its name in the early 1980s, a few years after doctors started to see young women get severely ill or even die during their menstrual periods. Researchers found that many of the women had been using a new superabsorbent tampon when they developed it. (See *Tampons and toxic shock syndrome: A mysterious link.*)

Within a short time, the superabsorbent tampon was withdrawn from the market, and the incidence of toxic shock dropped.

Finding the bacterial culprit

Disappearance of the tampon didn't make the disease go away. But discovery of the tampon link led medical scientists to determine that toxic shock syndrome results from a strain of bacteria called *Staphylococcus aureus.*

People often have these bacteria on and in their bodies without suffering any harm. But sometimes, as in toxic shock syndrome, these germs become dangerous — even deadly — when they produce a toxin that can travel in the blood. When enough toxins build up in the blood, they may trigger a life-threatening condition called septic shock. (For more information, see "Shock," page 452.)

Who gets toxic shock syndrome?

Although about 15% of the victims are men, this disorder usually affects women — nearly all of them under age 30 and menstruating at the time the illness strikes. The typical victim has a history of steady tampon use and may not change her tampon very often.

However, toxic shock syndrome can strike anyone at any age, particularly the following people:
- those with abscesses
- those who have recently had surgery
- those with a bone infection called osteomyelitis.

What are the symptoms?

Toxic shock syndrome may cause:
- a sudden high fever (over 102° F [38.8° C])
- headache
- severe muscle aches
- sore throat
- swelling of the mucous membranes, which line the nose, mouth, and other orifices
- copious diarrhea
- nausea and vomiting
- a red rash that typically covers the palms and soles
- confusion
- light-headedness and dizziness (from low blood pressure)

Tampons and toxic shock syndrome: A mysterious link

Although we know tampons play a crucial role in toxic shock syndrome, we still don't know how or why they are related. Here are some possible explanations.

Tampons may aid bacteria
- Tampons may pull bacteria into the vagina when they're inserted.
- Tampons may absorb the bacterial toxin from the vagina.
- Tampons may create a vaginal environment that's favorable to *Staphylococcus aureus*.

Tampons may cause injury
Tampons may scrape the vaginal walls during insertion. This would make the vagina more vulnerable to bacterial invasion.

- fast pulse
- bluish arms and legs.

What should you do?

If you suspect a person has toxic shock syndrome, call for immediate medical help. Feel the person for a pulse and look, listen, and feel for breathing. Have her lie down, and cover her just enough to keep her from getting cold.

How is toxic shock syndrome treated?

To confirm that the woman has toxic shock syndrome, the doctor orders blood tests and takes a specimen of her vaginal fluids to see if they contain *Staphylococcus aureus*.

To treat it, the medical team administers an intravenous antibiotic that is known to work against the bacteria. They also give oxygen and other treatments, as needed, to help the person breathe.

To combat shock, the person receives large amounts of fluids through the intravenous line, plus medications to help raise the blood pressure. She also receives medicines to ease diarrhea, nausea, and vomiting.

What else should you know?

Although antibiotics can help prevent toxic shock syndrome from striking again, the recurrence rate may be as high as 30%. In fact, women who get it once are at increased risk for getting it again.

But you can take steps to prevent toxic shock syndrome or a recurrence by using common sense during your menstrual period. Here are some guidelines that may help you avoid a first, second, or third bout.

Use tampons safely

- Use tampons less often or stop using them altogether.
- Alternate tampons with sanitary pads.
- Use low-absorbency tampons if possible, or the lowest absorbency that works for you.
- When inserting tampons, be careful not to scrape the vaginal walls. To avoid injury, use a water-soluble vaginal lubricant like KY Jelly, if necessary.
- Change your tampon at least every 8 hours.
- If you've had toxic shock syndrome, don't use any tampons for several months.

To avoid getting toxic shock syndrome or a recurrence, use tampons less often or stop using them altogether. When inserting tampons, be careful not to scrape the vaginal walls.

UNCONSCIOUSNESS

People exist in what is called a state of consciousness. Unless sleeping, we are awake and alert. We know who and where we are. We know the time and date. We can speak logically with other people. And, unless paralyzed, we can move about at will.

But when a person experiences a reduced state of consciousness or unconsciousness, some or all of these things change.

Wrong picture?
When we think of an unconscious person, most of us picture what we typically see on television: someone who could pass for dead, eyes closed, completely lacking awareness, unresponsive to any stimulation.

Wide spectrum of states
A reduced state of consciousness is much more complex than total unresponsiveness. Reduced consciousness covers a spectrum of states, from slightly reduced (such as inability to recall the year or month) to extremely reduced (such as deep coma).

That's why health care professionals test and score three different types of responses — eye response, motor response, and verbal response — when evaluating a person's level of consciousness. A *deep coma*, which produces the lowest score, is the most profound state of unconsciousness; the person can't be aroused even by pain.

What are the symptoms?
A completely unconscious person can't be aroused even when you attempt to awaken him or her. The person remains unresponsive and unaware of surroundings.

Many conditions can reduce a person's level of consciousness without making him or her fully unconscious. For instance, a person may seem awake but disoriented and confused, unable to move purposefully. Likewise, a person may "black out" briefly and "come to" — yet still not be fully conscious.

Reduced consciousness covers a spectrum of states, from slightly reduced (such as inability to recall the year or month) to extremely reduced (such as deep coma).

What should you do?

■ If you come upon someone who seems completely unconscious, first make sure the person's airway is open.

■ Then ask the person if he or she is okay. If you get no response, ask again in a loud voice. If you still get no response, have someone call for medical help immediately.

■ Next, feel for a pulse and look, listen, and feel for breathing. If you don't feel a pulse or breathing, start CPR if you know how. (See *Performing CPR on an adult,* page 579, *Performing CPR on a child,* page 585, or *Performing CPR on an infant,* page 590.)

■ If the person *is* breathing and *does* have a pulse, loosen any tight clothing, especially around the neck.

■ Check for bleeding. If you see any, apply direct pressure to the bleeding part to try to control it. But don't waste time tending to minor cuts and scrapes.

■ Next, cover the person to prevent heat loss. Check for a medical identification bracelet or card that might reveal a medical condition. If the person "comes to," try to keep him or her awake and ask if he or she knows what happened.

> Never move a person unless his or her life is in danger. Any injury to the head, neck, or spine could get worse if the person is moved. If you must move the person, do so without bending the head and neck.
>
> Don't put a pillow under the person's head.
>
> Avoid giving the person anything to eat or drink.
>
> Be sure not to leave the person alone.

How is unconsciousness treated?

Rescue personnel take steps to keep the airway clear and help the person breathe, if necessary. They also monitor the heartbeat.

When the immediate danger has passed and the person is medically stable, the medical team runs diagnostic tests to see why the person passed out. They try to find out if the person has a disease that could affect consciousness. Tests may include a computed tomography scan (commonly called a CAT scan) and blood studies. The medical team also checks for internal and external bleeding and looks for signs that the person might have had a seizure.

If the person is breathing and has a pulse, loosen any tight clothing. Cover him or her to prevent heat loss.

What else should you know?

A person can lose consciousness from one of these conditions:

- a breathing problem
- shock
- drugs and other substances that depress brain function
- seizures
- stroke
- brain tumor
- brain infection
- brain injury
- complications of diabetes, poisoning, or an imbalance of the body's salt levels.

Urination difficulty

Normally, people expel urine effortlessly whenever they get the urge. But certain disorders can prevent a person from urinating freely at will. When this happens, some urine is retained. Retained urine is dangerous because it encourages the growth of bacteria in the bladder and nearby structures. (See "Painful urination," page 383.)

Understanding the causes

The most common reason for urination difficulty is an enlarged prostate gland, known as *benign prostatic hypertrophy*. As the prostate enlarges, it presses against the urethra, reducing the flow of urine. (See *How an enlarged prostate limits urine flow,* page 540.) Four of five men over age 50 have this condition.

Other causes of urination difficulty include:

- lower urinary tract infection
- irritation of the urethra by chemical irritants like bubble baths and feminine deodorants
- prostate infection
- prostate cancer (see *Prostate cancer: Recognizing the warning signs,* page 541)
- loss of nerve function to the bladder from spinal cord injury or disease

The most common reason for urination difficulty is an enlarged prostate gland. As the prostate enlarges, it presses against the urethra, reducing the flow of urine.

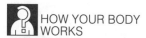

HOW YOUR BODY
WORKS

How an enlarged prostate limits urine flow

The prostate gland, found only in males, encircles the opening of the bladder and the starting point of the urethra. Its function is to add liquid to semen.

Squeezing an already small space

Normally, the prostate is about the size of a walnut, as you see in the picture on the left. When it enlarges, as it does in most older men, it may squeeze the urethra and restrict the flow of urine from the bladder, as you see in the picture on the right. When this happens, the bladder fills and the man feels the urge to urinate, but the urine has trouble escaping.

NORMAL PROSTATE

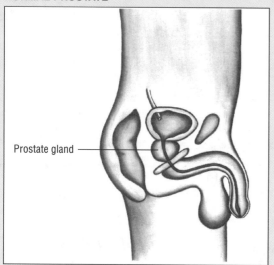

Prostate gland

ENLARGED PROSTATE

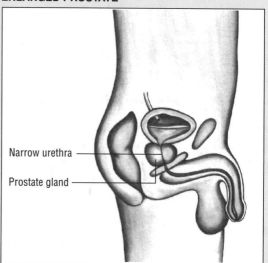

Narrow urethra

Prostate gland

- brain disorders
- metabolic disorders
- syphilis
- diabetes
- multiple sclerosis.

Another cause of urinary difficulty is when the kidneys fail to function. In this condition, called *acute kidney failure,* the person is unable to urinate because the body has stopped producing urine.

What are the symptoms?

The person feels the urge to urinate, but either has trouble starting the urine stream or produces little urine. Doctors call this problem *urinary hesitancy.*

With some underlying conditions, the person may also feel the urge to urinate more often than usual, called *urinary frequency.* For many people with difficulty urinating, the urine stream is weak and dribbles at the end.

Symptoms of a prostate infection

The man may have these additional symptoms:
- fever
- chills
- pain in the lower back
- pain between the rectum and testicles.

What should you do?

Complete inability to urinate is an emergency that requires immediate medical care. Call the doctor right away for someone who feels the urge to urinate but can't produce a normal urine stream.

How is urination difficulty treated?

Treatment depends on the underlying cause. For an older man, the doctor usually performs a rectal exam to check for an enlarged prostate.

Treating an enlarged prostate

This condition isn't dangerous and requires no specific treatment unless symptoms are troublesome. If symptoms *are* troublesome, the doctor may prescribe a medication called Proscar.

For severe symptoms, the man may need an operation to reduce or remove the prostate. These days, the operation performed most often is called a transurethral prostate resection.

Treating prostate infection

The doctor prescribes an antibiotic and may recommend sitting in a tub of warm water to soothe the affected area.

Treating other conditions

Prostate cancer usually calls for:
- cancer medications
- radiation

Prostate cancer: Recognizing the warning signs

Prostate cancer is the second leading cancer among men (lung cancer ranks first). Here are the warning signs to watch for.

Abnormal urine flow

- Weak or interrupted urine flow
- Inability to urinate or to control the urine flow
- Increasingly frequent urination, especially at night

Other unusual symptoms

- Blood-tinged urine
- Pain or a burning sensation when urinating
- Pain in the lower back, pelvis, or upper thighs

If you have any of these symptoms, see your doctor for a checkup.

Get checked out

To detect prostate cancer, the American Cancer Society recommends:
- a yearly rectal exam for men over age 40
- a yearly blood test to detect a tell-tale substance (prostate-specific antigen) in men over age 50
- an ultrasound test if either of the first two tests yields an abnormal result.

- surgery to remove the prostate
- some combination of the above three.

Acute kidney failure requires treatment in the hospital. The doctor usually prescribes a carefully monitored diet that's high in calories and low in protein, sodium, and potassium, plus vitamin supplements and restricted fluids.

What else should you know?

If you have difficulty urinating, avoid caffeine and alcohol, which tend to irritate the bladder. To help dilute your urine and flush bacteria from the urinary tract, increase your intake of fluids — especially water.

Also, stay away from bubble bath and bath salts. If you're a woman who has had several urinary tract infections, be sure to empty your bladder immediately before and after you have sex.

VAGINAL BLEEDING

Bleeding from the vagina is normal *only* during the menstrual period. It's abnormal when it occurs:
- between regular periods
- during pregnancy
- after menopause.

Even bleeding during the period can be abnormal if it's unusually heavy or lasts a long time. (See *Understanding how menstruation occurs,* page 544.)

Minor irritation or major threat?

Depending on the cause of the bleeding and the amount of blood lost, abnormal vaginal bleeding can range from a minor irritation to a life-threatening emergency.

Fortunately, it's rarely an emergency. More often, it comes from:
- a hormone imbalance
- an infection of the cervix or uterus
- polyps or noncancerous growths (such as fibroids) in the uterus, cervix, or vagina.

Regular pelvic exams and Pap tests can detect these and other problems before they cause serious illness.

Vaginal bleeding during pregnancy

Vaginal bleeding is perhaps most dangerous during pregnancy. The condition that's causing the bleeding may threaten the life of the mother, the baby, or both.

One such condition is *ectopic pregnancy*. In this disorder, the embryo attaches to a structure outside the uterus — typically, a tube that carries the egg to the uterus (fallopian tube). As the fetus grows, it stretches and may eventually rupture the tube. If this happens, the woman may experience:
- massive bleeding (called *hemorrhage*)
- shock

Vaginal bleeding is perhaps most dangerous during pregnancy. The condition that's causing the bleeding may threaten the life of the mother and her baby.

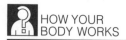

Understanding how menstruation occurs

Each month, if you're a fertile woman, one of your two ovaries releases a tiny egg. This process is called *ovulation*.

Tracing the egg's journey
The egg travels down a tube called the *fallopian tube* to the uterus, or womb. During this journey, which takes about 5 days, the egg may become fertilized by sperm that have traveled up into the fallopian tube after intercourse.

Making a baby
Before ovulation, the lining of the uterus, called the endometrium, thickens and fills with blood. If a fertilized egg reaches the uterus, attaches to the endometrium, and begins to develop into an embryo,

pregnancy begins. The blood-filled endometrium will develop into a placenta and nourish the growing fetus.

Shedding an unneeded layer
However, if an unfertilized egg reaches the uterus, the thickened, blood-filled endometrium isn't needed. So, about 14 days after ovulation, its top layer breaks down and flows out of the body. This flow, known as menstruation, consists of blood, mucus, and unneeded tissue. The flow lasts about 5 days.

Starting over
After menstruation stops, the endometrium begins to thicken again in preparation for another egg and the start of another cycle.

- inflammation of the abdominal wall lining (called *peritonitis*).

Placenta previa can also cause a pregnant woman to bleed. In this disorder, the placenta — the organ that delivers oxygen and other nutrients to the fetus — develops near or atop the opening of the cervix. Here, it has the potential to cause:
- massive vaginal bleeding
- shock
- anemia
- kidney damage
- possibly death.

Sometimes the placenta separates from the uterine wall — a condition called *abruptio placentae*. This can also cause vaginal bleeding and shock.

Vaginal bleeding after childbirth
Even after delivering her baby, a woman is at risk of vaginal bleeding. In this case, the bleeding, called *postpartum hemorrhage*, can lead to:
- shock

- kidney failure
- stoppage of the heart.

Any condition that causes trauma during childbirth can result in postpartum hemorrhage.

Vaginal bleeding after menopause

Although bleeding after menopause isn't an outright emergency as is bleeding during pregnancy, it can still be a serious concern. Such bleeding can indicate cancer, so regard it as a red flag that shouldn't be ignored.

More often, though, postmenopausal bleeding is linked to a hormone imbalance, an infection, or another relatively mild problem.

What are the symptoms?

Vaginal bleeding can appear as:
- slight brownish or red spotting
- oozing of fresh blood
- large clots
- a large amount of bright red blood.

Sometimes the bleeding is accompanied by varying degrees and types of pain, from crampy to excruciating.

Symptoms of placenta previa

A woman with this disorder develops painless, bright-red vaginal bleeding after the 20th week of pregnancy. The bleeding may stop and start without warning.

Symptoms of abruptio placentae

Abruptio placentae also typically arises after the 20th week of pregnancy. If the placenta separates only slightly, it may produce only minor vaginal bleeding and discomfort. But if it separates moderately or severely, it could cause vaginal hemorrhage and shock. Severe separation typically produces extreme, knifelike, or tearing uterine pain.

Postmenopausal bleeding

After menopause, vaginal bleeding may be painless. The bleeding may be spotty, steady, brown, or red. It may include pus or other discharge.

What should you do?

Get medical care immediately for any woman with heavy vaginal

Vaginal bleeding can appear as slight brownish or red spotting, oozing of fresh blood, large clots, or a large amount of bright red blood.

bleeding — especially if she feels weak, cold, or sweaty. And remember that for a pregnant woman, even minor bleeding can indicate a major problem.

If the bleeding is not heavy and the woman isn't pregnant or if she feels weak, cold, or sweaty, call the doctor. Have the woman rest, avoid strenuous exercise, and avoid using tampons until the doctor finds the cause of the bleeding.

Be prepared to give information

The doctor will need as much information about the woman's condition as possible, so be prepared to provide these details:

- how long it takes her to saturate a sanitary pad
- the number of sanitary pads she has used over a specified time (this will help the doctor estimate how much blood she has lost)
- which medicines she is taking, including birth control pills
- dosages of medicines.

How is vaginal bleeding treated?

Once the woman is medically stable, the doctor tries to pinpoint the cause of the bleeding. The woman will almost certainly undergo a pelvic exam and a Pap test, and may have blood drawn to measure her hormone levels and check for anemia.

To rule out cancer, the doctor may remove tissue from the lining of the uterus. An ultrasound test can help detect any tumors in the cervix or uterus. Cultures of vaginal and cervical fluids may be taken to help detect infection.

Treating a pregnant woman

If the woman is pregnant and the cause of vaginal bleeding turns out to be placenta previa, she may need no treatment. The advancing pregnancy may correct the condition. (As the uterus enlarges, it may raise the placenta away from the opening of the cervix.)

On the other hand, if a woman is bleeding heavily with either placenta previa or abruptio placentae, the pregnancy may have to be terminated to save her life.

To treat an ectopic pregnancy, the woman may undergo laser surgery to remove the affected area of the fallopian tube.

Treating other problems

Simple menstrual irregularity may not call for treatment. Some of the other conditions that cause vaginal bleeding can be controlled

Some of the conditions that cause vaginal bleeding can be controlled through birth control pills or other hormone therapy.

through birth control pills or other hormone therapy. For example:
■ a drug called Clomid can induce ovulation, if necessary
■ a procedure that kills tissue, such as application of extreme cold, can be used to remove cervical polyps
■ a procedure called a D & C (dilatation and curettage) can be used to remove polyps and a bleeding endometrium from the uterus.
A woman who has cancer or another large tumor may need to have her uterus removed in an operation called a hysterectomy. For cancer, she may also need radiation therapy, chemotherapy, or both.

What else should you know?

Excessive vaginal bleeding commonly leads to anemia. If you tend to bleed excessively during your menstrual period, be sure to ask your doctor whether you should take an iron supplement.

VISION LOSS

Because vision is so essential to our functioning, any degree of vision loss is frightening. What's more, without proper diagnosis and treatment, even a slight decrease in vision can progress to total blindness.

Sudden vision loss can range from slightly decreased vision to total blindness. Depending on the cause, the loss may be temporary or permanent.

Understanding the causes

Causes of sudden vision loss include:
■ a stroke
■ an eye disease called *acute closed-angle glaucoma*
■ blockage of the retinal artery. (See *A blinding blockage,* page 548.)

What are the symptoms?

The person who loses vision suddenly can't see visual images in one or both eyes. With stroke, retinal artery blockage, or acute closed-angle glaucoma, the vision loss affects only one eye. In this last con-

Sudden vision loss can range from slightly decreased vision to total blindness. Depending on the cause, the loss may be temporary or permanent.

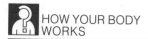

HOW YOUR BODY
WORKS

A blinding blockage

One cause of sudden vision loss is *central retinal artery occlusion.* In this disorder, the main artery of the retina — the part of the eye that receives and transmits visual images — becomes blocked.

Starving for blood

The retina can survive for a brief time because it still receives blood from other vessels. But it needs the full blood flow from the central retinal artery. If this flow isn't restored in 2 hours, the retina swells, its cells die, and blindness occurs.

From hardening to obstruction

A common cause of retinal artery blockage is hardening of the arteries (arteriosclerosis) or heart disease. A blood clot can break off from a hard-ened carotid artery or a diseased heart valve. After the clot breaks off, it travels into the retinal artery, blocking it.

Other causes of arterial blockage

The retinal artery may also become blocked from:
- too much pressure on the eye socket
- swelling around the eye
- poorly applied eye dressings
- lying prone with the feet elevated.

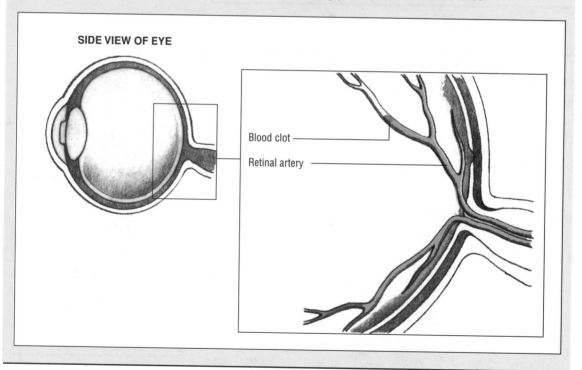

SIDE VIEW OF EYE

Blood clot

Retinal artery

dition, the person also may have additional symptoms, such as:

- severe eye pain
- pressure over the eye
- unusual light sensitivity
- halos seen around lights
- nausea and vomiting.

What should you do?

Sudden vision loss is a medical emergency. Call for medical help immediately or take the person to the nearest hospital emergency department.

How is sudden vision loss treated?

Treatment depends on the underlying cause.

Treating a blocked retinal artery

The doctor tries to widen the blocked artery so that more blood will flow to the retina. For instance, he or she may use light external eye massage over the closed eyelid.

Treating glaucoma

To treat acute closed-angle glaucoma, the doctor prescribes medications to reduce pressure within the eye and pain relievers to ease pain. Surgery may be necessary if the eye pressure doesn't decrease within a few hours.

What else should you know?

Sometimes sudden vision loss results from:

- injury to the eye
- concussion
- detachment of the retina (the eye's image-receiving structure) from the back of the eye
- a condition called *amaurosis fugax,* in which one eye goes blind for a few seconds or minutes, then regains sight
- bleeding into the vitreous humor, the eye's transparent, gelatin-like substance.

If a blocked retinal artery is causing the sudden vision loss, the doctor tries to widen the blocked artery to improve blood flow to the retina.

VOMITING BLOOD

Vomiting is never pleasant. But vomiting *blood* is more than just unpleasant — it can be life-threatening.

When you vomit blood, it usually means you're bleeding somewhere in your throat, esophagus, stomach, or the starting point of your small intestine (called the *duodenum*).

Old blood or new?

Sometimes, vomiting of blood is unmistakable, such as when the vomit is bright red or contains bright red streaks. This appearance means the blood is fresh, and may represent recent or rapid bleeding in the uppermost part of the digestive tract.

But sometimes the blood is less obvious — for instance, when the vomit is dark red, brown, or black (about the color and consistency of coffee grounds). This appearance means the blood has been in the stomach for a while and has had a chance to react with stomach juices.

No matter what the color, though, vomiting blood is a potentially dire problem if the person loses a lot of blood.

Understanding the causes

Severe vomiting of blood may result from the following life-threatening conditions:

■ acute inflammation of the stomach lining, caused by blood thinners, aspirin, nonsteroidal anti-inflammatory drugs like ibuprofen (Advil), steroids, or alcohol

■ damage to the esophagus, caused by swallowing a corrosive acid or alkali

■ rupture of enlarged, twisted veins in the esophagus or stomach, caused by chronic alcoholism, increased pressure in the abdominal veins, or some other condition

■ rupture of the esophagus, triggered by eating a large meal in people with a condition called Boerhaave's syndrome

■ inflammation of the lining of the esophagus, caused by chronic alcoholism or radiation therapy of the esophagus

■ a tear where the esophagus and stomach meet, caused by protracted vomiting (most common in alcoholics)

■ stomach ulcer, possibly compounded by alcoholism, trauma, illness, burns, or surgery

■ use of blood thinners.

Whether it appears bright red, dark red, brown, or black, vomited blood is a potentially dire problem if it leads to massive blood loss.

What are the symptoms?

Besides bright red or coffee-ground-like vomit, the person may have:

- diarrhea
- weakness
- thirst
- sweating
- light-headedness
- indigestion
- stomach pain or stomach injury
- difficulty eating or swallowing.

Other symptoms to watch for

Often, when blood comes up as vomit, some blood is also going down into the stool. When that happens, the stools may turn black and look like tar.

What should you do?

Unless you know the vomited blood came from a recent nosebleed, get emergency medical attention for the person immediately.

The person will probably be very anxious. Provide reassurance and try to keep the person calm. If you know the source of the bleeding, use direct pressure to try to stop the bleeding.

Watch for shock

Someone who is vomiting a lot of blood is at risk for shock caused by massive loss. Cool, clammy skin; light-headedness; and a rapid pulse mean that shock has already set in.

While waiting for help to arrive, keep the person lying down, preferably with the feet elevated; this will help keep as much oxygen-carrying blood as possible in the brain.

 Don't give the person anything to eat or drink.

How is vomiting blood treated?

Emergency rescuers replace lost body fluids to maintain the person's blood pressure. In the hospital, the medical team continues efforts to stabilize the person, such as by giving blood transfusions and oxygen and monitoring the blood's oxygen-carrying ability.

Finding the bleeding source

Once the person is medically stable, the medical team may pump the stomach contents. The doctor may insert a thin tube called an

> *If a person vomits blood, stay calm and reassuring. Watch for symptoms of shock, such as cool and clammy skin, light-headedness, and a rapid pulse.*

endoscope into the person's digestive system to pinpoint the bleeding site and determine how severe the bleeding is.

What else should you know?

Vomiting occurs in response to a message from the brain. Here's what happens:

- The muscles in the abdomen contract.
- Next, the ring of muscle between the stomach and the esophagus (called the *esophageal sphincter*) opens.
- Finally, the contents of the stomach, which normally would pass down through the digestive tract, are instead ejected upward and out of the mouth by reverse muscle contractions.

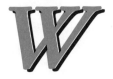

WHEEZING

Wheezing is a high-pitched breathing sound caused by air flowing rapidly through a narrowed airway. Sometimes, the wheezing can be heard only by a doctor or nurse who listens to the person breathe through a stethoscope.

On the other hand, you may hear obvious wheezing in a heavy smoker who has just climbed a flight of stairs. Or in another person, you may be able to hear wheezing if you put your ear on the chest or next to the person's mouth or by standing next to the person.

Understanding the causes
Usually, wheezing results from asthma, chronic bronchitis, or congestive heart disease. (See *What to do when your child wheezes,* page 554.)

Other reasons for wheezing include:
- a life-threatening allergic reaction (anaphylaxis)
- emphysema
- an inflamed airway
- croup, a childhood respiratory viral infection
- inflammation of the epiglottis (a flap that overhangs the voice box)
- lung cancer
- an inhaled object that's partially blocking the airway.

What are the symptoms?
Wheezing has a high-pitched, musical, squealing, creaking, or groaning quality. Even when the person coughs, the wheezing doesn't go away. (If the sound *does* go away with coughing, the person has a different problem that may still need medical care.)

Other symptoms to watch for
Symptoms that may accompany wheezing include:
- anxiety
- shortness of breath

Wheezing has a high-pitched, musical, squealing, creaking, or groaning quality. Even when the person coughs, the wheezing doesn't go away.

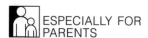

ESPECIALLY FOR PARENTS

What to do when your child wheezes

Children are especially susceptible to wheezing because it doesn't take much to block their small airways.

What causes wheezing in children?

Major reasons why a child wheezes include:

- spasm of the large airways, as from asthma
- swelling of the airway linings
- too much phlegm in the airways, as from cystic fibrosis
- choking on a foreign body.

Take action

Seek medical attention if your child starts to wheeze. However, if your child has been diagnosed with asthma, first have him or her take prescribed asthma medication by inhaler. If this doesn't halt the asthma attack, call the doctor.

- heaving of the chest
- tightening of the neck muscles.

What should you do?

 WHEN SECONDS COUNT

If the person is having difficulty breathing, call for immediate medical help. Assume the person is having such difficulty if you can answer *yes* to one or more of these questions:

- Is the person breathing abnormally — either too fast or too slow?
- Does the person's breathing seem too shallow or too deep?
- Is the person using the chest muscles in an effort to breathe?
- Does the person seems restless, confused, anxious, or afraid?

Provide information

If the person *isn't* having difficulty breathing, you don't have to call for emergency help. But the person does need prompt medical attention. Be prepared to tell the doctor:

- when and how the wheezing began
- if it started with a specific incident
- if it's ever happened before
- if anything makes it better or worse
- if it's accompanied by shortness of breath, pain, coughing, itching, sneezing, nausea, or other symptoms
- if the person recently had a broken hip or leg (this injury could lead to a serious condition that causes wheezing)
- if the person smokes or has allergies
- if the person has ever had a lung, heart, hormone, or immune problem.

How is wheezing treated?

The medical team administers oxygen, if necessary, or puts the person on a machine to aid breathing. They also:

- place the person in a position that eases breathing
- give respiratory treatments and medications to open the airways
- run blood tests to check the person's oxygen level.

What else should you know?

Although wheezing is common during an acute asthma attack, it may disappear if the attack gets worse. Consider its disappearance a dangerous sign. Why? During a worsening asthma attack, inability to wheeze means that the narrowed airways have completely closed up.

Emergency Response and Prevention Guide

HOW TO RESPOND IN AN EMERGENCY

Getting help with 911

The 911 system began in the 1970s to help people get emergency aid more quickly and easily by telephone. Today, this universal emergency number is available to more than 50% of the United States population and in most large cities.

Here's some advice that will help you to use the 911 system properly.

Take action fast

If you come upon someone who's had an emergency and you can't provide adequate assistance on your own, don't try to diagnose or solve the problem. Instead, call 911 as soon as possible. This number provides instant access to emergency services — medical, help, police, and fire — 24 hours a day.

If you're not near a standard phone, try to call from another person's car (cellular) phone. Don't call your doctor, friend, relatives, or neighbors first. This would only delay getting help for the victim.

Note: If the injured person is a child and you've been trained in CPR, begin it immediately and send someone else to call 911.

When to call

Call 911 for anyone who:
- is unconscious or seems to be losing consciousness
- is very confused
- has a severe headache or slurred speech
- has trouble breathing
- has persistent chest pain or pressure
- has persistent pain or pressure in the abdomen
- is vomiting or passing blood
- is having a seizure
- has suffered a serious head, neck, or back injury
- seems to have been poisoned
- can't be moved easily.

> *If you come upon someone who's had an emergency and you can't provide adequate assistance on your own, don't try to solve the problem. Instead, call 911 as soon as possible.*

Other times to call 911
Even if you don't see any victims, call 911 in these situations:
- fire or explosion
- downed electrical wires
- evidence of a gas leak
- rising flood water
- motor vehicle collision.

How to call
Just pick up a telephone and dial 911. A trained dispatcher will answer your call. You'll be asked what seems like a lot of questions. Listen carefully and cooperate fully. Your answers are necessary to help emergency personnel tailor their response to the situation.

Give the victim's location
Give the city or town, street name, and house number. Also provide names of nearby intersecting streets or other landmarks.

If the victim is in a rural area, don't give the post office box number because this won't help the rescue squad find the location. Instead, name the road or street, nearest intersection, and any landmarks.

Give the number of the phone you're using
The dispatcher will ask for your phone number so he or she can call you back if necessary. Asking for this information also helps discourage crank calls to 911.

Tell what happened
Describe the incident, such as a car accident, near-drowning, fire, or heart attack. Specify how many people need help and any special conditions that are involved, such as a dog in the house, a jammed elevator, or numerous flights of stairs.

Describe the victim's condition
Tell the dispatcher how old the victim is, whether the victim is conscious or not, and whether or not he or she is breathing (or is breathing with difficulty).

Also state what, if anything, is being done for the victim right now. For example, specify whether CPR is being given or if the victim's bleeding is being controlled.

Speak clearly and slowly

Don't be in a hurry to end the call. If someone else makes the call for you, have the person report back to you so you can be sure the call was made. Don't feel you must hang up right away in order for the ambulance to be sent promptly.

Stay on the line

The dispatcher will probably give you further instructions or ask for more information as needed. Don't hang up until the dispatcher tells you to.

Teach your family about 911

Make sure everyone in your home, including your children and the babysitter, know how to dial 911 or the emergency medical services number in your area. If you're not sure if 911 is available in your area, check the inside front cover of your local phone book for the number. Do this right now — not when you're faced with an emergency.

Post the emergency number on or near the phone, along with the poison control center number for your area. Also post your home address there; in the panic and excitement of an emergency, even the familiar can be forgotten. (And the babysitter may not recall your address right away.)

Finally, have family members rehearse the emergency call and what they will say.

Other important points

■ If you're alone and suspect you are having a heart attack or may need emergency medical treatment, call 911 immediately. You can't afford to spend time wondering whether you're truly having a heart attack. In the words of one paramedic, "It's not unusual for us to arrive to find the person dead with a bottle of antacid tablets in his hands."

■ Install a phone by your bed, especially if you live alone. Many heart attacks happen while the victim is resting.

■ If you have a programmable phone, don't set it up to automatically dial 911. Although it sounds like a great idea, many people dial this number accidently instead of another preprogrammed number. This wastes the dispatcher's time and may delay a real emergency call from getting through.

Who's who on the emergency response team

Until the late 1960s, most communities in the United States had few, if any, organized ways to quickly transport accident victims and other emergency victims to the hospital — much less to care for them on the way. Police, firefighters, and people trained to give first aid provided the only prehospital care available.

Modern emergency care network

Today, a carefully organized and trained array of rescue personnel provides most emergency care at the scene and on the way to the hospital, although fire and police remain part of the prehospital emergency care network. This network is called an *emergency medical service* (EMS) system.

Communication: Heart of the network

Communication is a vital component of emergency care at the emergency scene and on the way to the hospital. A large community may have a main communication center to coordinate all emergency calls, plus hospital-to-rescue-unit or hospital-to-hospital communications.

In most areas, the 911 emergency telephone system employs trained dispatchers who receive calls, gather pertinent information from the caller, and assess the information. Then the dispatchers summon the appropriate rescue service and maintain constant communication with rescue vehicles. The diagram on the opposite page shows how such a system might work in a typical urban area.

Field teams

Usually, special field teams within the EMS are organized to respond to the community's prehospital emergency care needs. Field teams may work for local hospitals, which administer the overall prehospital care programs and serve as communication centers for their rescue vehicles.

EMS field teams typically consist of:
- dispatchers
- emergency medical technicians (EMTs)
- nurses
- doctors

Today, a carefully organized and trained array of rescue personnel provides most emergency care at the scene and on the way to the hospital. This network is called an emergency medical service (EMS) system.

HOW AN EMERGENCY MEDICAL SERVICE SYSTEM WORKS

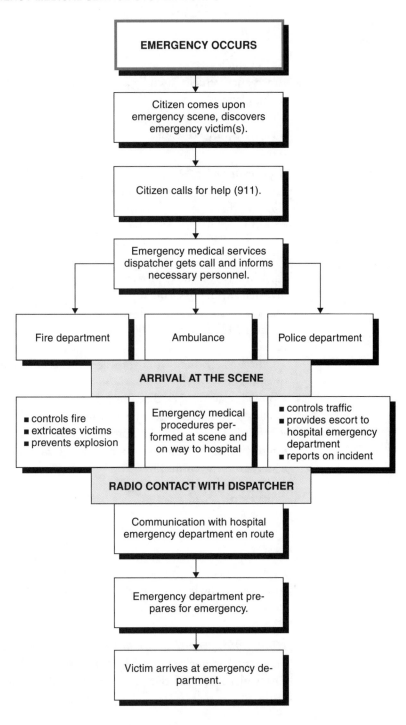

- fire departments
- police departments
- citizens.

EMS vehicles
Emergency vehicles used by an EMS system include:
- ambulances
- mobile rescue units
- air transport vehicles.

Two types of EMTs
Depending on the level of their training, EMS personnel are categorized as either emergency medical technicians (EMT-Basic, or EMT-B) or EMT paramedics (EMT-P).

What EMTs do
An EMT-B is trained to recognize life-threatening conditions and give first aid and basic life support, including CPR and rescue breathing. He or she may also assist with emergency childbirth. Training for an EMT-B averages 100 hours and includes lectures and skills reviews.

The EMT-B may work together with an EMT-P. An EMT-P is qualified to:
- provide advanced cardiac life support
- manage certain irregular heartbeats
- defibrillate ("shock") the heart to restore the victim's heartbeat
- insert tubes into the victim's airway or other opening
- start an intravenous line
- administer drugs.

EMT-P training is more advanced than EMT-B training — up to 2,000 hours.

Mobile rescue units
In an advanced life support (ALS) ambulance, the EMT-P communicates with the hospital, relaying assessment findings and receiving instructions from the doctor or nurse in the emergency department.

Emergency training for police and firefighters
Standards for emergency medical training for police and firefighters vary widely. Because they're often first at the scene of an accident,

most police and firefighters must have at least basic first aid training and some may also be certified in CPR. Some fire departments employ EMT-Ps as part of their own rescue teams.

How hospitals cope with emergency patients

States are divided into several EMS regions according to facilities, services, and staff. In each state, each hospital emergency department falls within certain a EMS region. This helps to ensure that high-quality medical and nursing emergency care are available. It also avoids needless duplication of emergency equipment and services.

How an emergency department is designed

The design of a hospital emergency department is based on:
- the community's emergency care needs
- size and capabilities of nearby emergency departments
- proximity of a trauma center
- size of the patient population.

Emergency department staff

The staff of a hospital emergency department typically includes doctors, nurses, and other personnel specifically trained to give emergency care. Many large departments have one nurse per shift who assigns treatment priorities to patients according to the severity of their injuries or condition ("triage"). This nurse may give preliminary care, such as wound care, before a patient is moved to a treatment area.

The *emergency doctor* has responsibility for medical care of patients in the emergency department. Not all hospitals are able to staff their emergency departments with doctors trained in emergency medicine. In hospitals lacking full-time coverage by doctors in the emergency department, area doctors may take turns being "on call" to manage emergencies.

Regional trauma centers

Within some EMS regions, regional trauma centers have been established to care for patients with serious multiple injuries.

In many large hospital emergency departments, a nurse assigns treatment priorities to patients according to the severity of their injuries or condition. This nurse may give preliminary care before a patient is moved to a treatment area.

What to do if someone has been poisoned

The chart that follows tells what action you should take for various kinds of poisonings. The number listed after each substance refers to the appropriate treatment listed below.

Important: This chart can't replace your call to a poison control center, doctor, or 911.

Suggested treatment

1. Small amounts of this substance aren't poisonous, so no treatment is necessary.

2. Make the person vomit. To do this, give ipecac syrup in the following dosages:

If the person is under age 1: 2 teaspoons followed by at least 2 to 3 glasses of water.

If the person is age 1 or older: 1 or 2 tablespoons followed by at least two to three glasses of water.

Don't make the person vomit if he or she is unconscious or having a seizure. Call the poison control center or 911.

3. Dilute the poison with water or milk. Don't make the person vomit. Call the poison control center or 911.

4. Dilute the poison with water or milk. Don't make the person vomit. The substance may burn the mouth and throat. Call the poison control center or 911.

5. Immediately rinse the skin thoroughly with running water. Continue for at least 15 minutes. Call the poison control center or 911.

6. Immediately rinse the eyes with running water. Continue for 15 to 20 minutes. Call the poison control center or 911.

7. Get the person to fresh air immediately; start artificial respiration if necessary. Call 911.

8. Call the poison control center or 911 before attempting any first-aid treatment.

A

acetaminophen, 2
acetone, 2
acids
    swallowed, 4
    eye contamination, 6
    skin contamination, 5
    inhaled if mixed with bleach, 7
aerosols
    eye contamination, 6
    inhaled, 7
after-shave lotions
    less than ($\frac{1}{2}$ ounce (15 milliliters), 1
    more than ($\frac{1}{2}$ ounce (15 milliliters), 2
airplane glue, 8
alcohol
    swallowed, 2
    eye contamination, 6
alkalies
    swallowed, 4
    eye contamination, 6
    skin contamination, 5
    inhaled, 7
ammonia
    swallowed, 4
    eye contamination, 6
    inhaled, 7
amphetamines, 2
aniline dyes
    swallowed, 4
    inhaled, 7
    skin contamination, 5
antacids, 1
antibiotics
    less than 2 to 3 times total daily dose, 1
    more than 3 times total daily dose, 2
antidepressants
    tricyclic, 2
    others, 2

antifreeze (ethylene glycol)
    swallowed, 2
    eye contamination, 6
antihistamines, 2
antiseptics, 2
ant trap
    Kepone type, 1
    others, 2
aquarium products, 1
arsenic, 2
aspirin, 2

B

baby oil, 1
ball-point pen ink, 1
barbiturates
    short-acting, 8
    long-acting, 2
batteries
    dry cell (flashlight), 1
    mercury (hearing aid), 2
    wet cell (automobile), 4
benzene
    swallowed, 8
    inhaled, 7
    skin contamination, 5
birth-control pills, 1
bleaches
    liquid swallowed, 1
    solid swallowed, 4
    eye contamination, 6
    inhaled when mixed with acids or alkalies, 7
boric acid, 2
bromides, 2
bubble bath, 1

C

camphor, 2
candles, 1
caps for cap pistols
    less than one roll, 1
    more than one roll, 2

APPROACHING AND MOVING AN INJURED PERSON

How to approach an accident victim

If you're the first person to come upon an accident victim, you can give aid and comfort at the scene, even if you're not trained in first aid. Follow the guidelines below.

Top priority: Get help

Make sure the emergency medical system (EMS) has been activated by calling 911 or the local emergency medical service as soon as possible. Either call 911 yourself or send someone else to call.

Stay with the victim

Next, try to aid the victim, within your abilities. Until the EMS team arrives, stay with the person. If his or her life isn't in imminent danger, providing constant reassurance is the best help you can give.

To move or not to move?

Don't try to pull an injured person out of a motor vehicle. Why? If the person's neck or back is broken and the spinal cord is damaged, moving him or her could cause permanent damage, paralysis, or even death. Or a broken bone may cut a blood vessel and cause massive bleeding.

Two exceptions

The only exceptions to the "Don't move the victim" rule are:
- when the victim's life in immediate jeopardy, such as from an imminent fire or explosion or from stoppage of the heartbeat or breathing
- when you don't have access to a phone and have no way to summon help.

In these cases, be sure to keep the victim's head and neck still when moving him or her. (See *Moving an injured person safely,* page 571.)

Begin resuscitation

If you have already called for emergency help and have determined that the victim is unconscious and isn't breathing, start CPR if you've been trained in it. If you're alone, don't wait to perform CPR on a child age 8 or younger; instead, give CPR for 2 minutes before calling for help. (See *Performing CPR on an adult,* page 579, *Performing CPR on a child,* page 585, or *Performing CPR on an infant,* page 590.)

Keep the airway clear

If the person's tongue falls to the back of the throat and blocks the airway, keep the head on a level surface and pull the lower jaw forward. This should clear the airway. Don't place pillows under the victim's head. This makes it more difficult to breathe and may cause further injury.

Stay at the scene

Continue CPR until the EMS team arrives. Then step back and allow them to do their job. Don't leave — they may need to question you to help them understand exactly what happened.

Try to stop any bleeding

If the victim has an open wound, try to control bleeding by pressing firmly and steadily on the wound. Don't use a tourniquet to stop the bleeding. If an object is protruding from a wound, don't try to remove it; doing so could cause life-threatening blood loss. (See "Bleeding," page 73.)

Stay calm

Try to keep the victim as calm and relaxed as possible. A person in pain may become agitated, verbally or physically abusive, or combative. Don't react defensively. Just keep reassuring the victim that help is on the way.

In a motor vehicle accident with multiple victims, both victims and bystanders may become dazed, disorganized, and confused. Try to help them stay focused until the rescue team arrives.

Obtain crucial information

Keep in mind that an accident victim may not be aware of his or her own injuries due to concern about others in the accident. Try to determine the victim's level of alertness and find out who he or she is. Ask simple questions, such as:

- "What's your name?"
- "Where are you?"

- "Do you know what day it is?"
- "What happened?"

If the victim loses consciousness before the rescue team arrives, be prepared to provide this information.

Moving an injured person safely

Before you read about *how* to move an injured person, remember that there are only two situations in which you *should* move an injured person:

- when you're certain there's an imminent threat to his or her life, such as from a fire or an explosion
- when you don't have access to a telephone or can't summon emergency assistance for some other reason.

At all other times, wait for an ambulance or other trained rescuers to arrive.

If you *must* move the person to safety, make sure you do so without causing further injury. Read on for guidelines.

How to carry the person

If the victim hasn't sustained a back or neck injury, you can use a two-person carry to move him or her out of danger quickly. This method immobilizes the person's upper body while allowing him or her to be carried more or less upright.

To perform this carry, the rescuers should stand facing each other, lock one pair of arms and hands together at wrist level, and grasp each other's shoulders with their free hands, as shown here, to fashion a sort of seat.

Move an injured person only if you're certain there's an imminent threat to his or her life or if you can't summon emergency assistance.

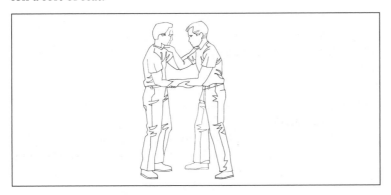

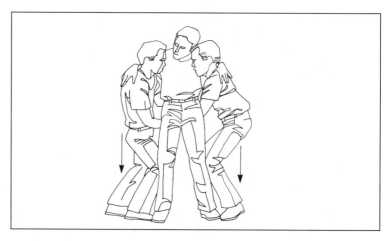

In unison with your helper, bend your knees and lower your body. Have the victim place his or her arms around your shoulders and your helper's shoulders, as shown above.

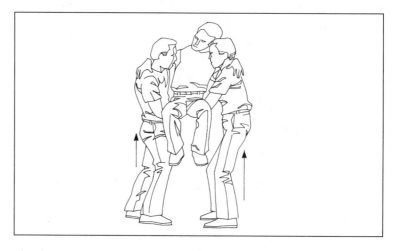

Slowly rise to a standing position along with your partner, as shown above.

Use proper body mechanics
When lifting, maintain a safe grip, using as much of your palms as you can. Keep your back straight, and tighten the muscles of your buttocks and abdomen. Keep your arms close to your body and keep your elbows flexed. Position your feet shoulder-width for balance, with one foot slightly in front of the other.

Keep the victim close to your body. Don't twist your back, but pivot with your feet. Lift and carry the victim slowly and smoothly and in unison with other helpers.

How to place the person on a stretcher

If other people are present to help you move the victim, use a stretcher. This is especially important if you suspect a neck or back injury. If a stretcher isn't available, use another firm, strong surface, such as an ironing board, a table leaf, or a door. Test the stretcher or other surface first to see if it's strong enough.

Immobilize the neck

Don't let the person's head bend forward or backward. And don't assume that a conscious person can keep the head level with the body without assistance.

If possible, support the head and neck with a collar made from such materials as fabric, folded newspapers, towels, or a blanket folded to a width of about 4 inches (10 centimeters).

Carefully slide the collar under the person's neck, taking care not to bend the head at the neck. Without obstructing the victim's breathing, fasten the collar and tie it loosely with long strips of fabric or other material.

Roll the person onto the stretcher

After you've immobilized the victim's neck, hold the neck and have volunteers help roll the person onto his or her side while someone else slides the stretcher or board as close to the person's side as possible. Then, gently roll the person's body onto the board, moving it as one unit, as shown below.

Important: When placing the person on the stretcher, be sure to keep the person's head, neck, and body aligned in a straight line at all times.

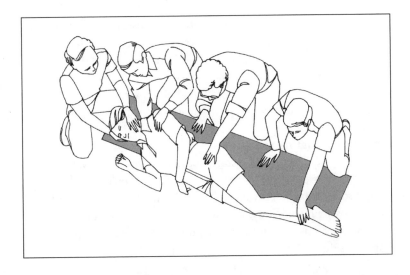

How to pull the person to safety

If you must pull a person to safety, use the victim's shirt or other article of clothing as a pulling device. Don't let the person's neck bend. Keep his or her head as close to the ground as possible and keep the body in a straight line. Avoid pulling the clothing so tightly that it obstructs breathing.

What to do if you can't reach the victim

If an injured person is literally out of your reach, you can still attempt a rescue or aid the person in other ways. Follow these guidelines.

Rescuing an electric shock victim

Let's say you're working at a building site and you hear a loud crash. As you follow the sound, you find a coworker lying on the ground, with a loose and apparently "live" wire from a temporary electrical pole lying next to him. What should you do?

Turn off the power

First, locate the power source (outside switch box, fuse box, or circuit breaker), and shut it off or disconnect it before you approach the victim.

Don't try to separate the victim from the electrical source until you've made sure it's turned off. Otherwise, you may receive a shock, even if you use a dry, nonconducting object, such as the dry wood of a broom handle, board, or chair. If you're unable to shut off the power source yourself, wait for trained help to arrive with the equipment needed to shut off the power or disconnect the wires.

Beware of a tingling sensation

If your feet and lower body start to tingle as you approach the victim, *stop*. This sensation means that the ground you're standing on is energized and the electrical energy is traveling up one foot, passing through your lower body, and leaving through your other foot. If this happens, raise one foot off the ground (to break the circuit) and hop to a safe place.

Don't try to separate the victim from the electrical source until you've made sure it's turned off. Otherwise, you may receive a shock.

Keep vehicle occupants safe

If you come upon a motor vehicle with power lines that have fallen onto it, tell the occupants to stay inside the vehicle until help arrives. Don't try to move a wire, the vehicle, or the occupants.

However, if you believe an explosion or a fire is about to occur, advise the occupants to try to jump out of the vehicle without making contact with either the vehicle or the wire.

Performing a water rescue

If you see someone who is struggling in open water or has fallen through ice, remember these four words, in this order: reach, throw, row, go. Here's an explanation.

Reach

If you can't reach the person with your arms, use a pole or a long stick and extend it to him or her. But make sure you have a firm footing before doing so. If bystanders are present, ask someone to hold your waist or your belt while you extend the reaching object.

Throw

Throw the victim any available object that will float, such as an empty picnic jug, a life jacket, a floating cushion, or a beach ball. If you're of average strength, assume you can throw something about 50 feet (15 meters).

If a rope is available, tie it to the floating object if possible. This will help you pull the victim to safety while he or she grasps the floating object. If your first throw misses the victim, having a rope tied to the floating object will enable you to try again.

Row

If you're too far from the person to throw him or her a floating object, paddle out to the person by using a rowboat, raft, canoe, or motorboat. Put on a life jacket first, if available.

When you reach the victim, pull him or her in over the rear end of the boat (stern), never over the side. This will prevent the boat from capsizing or turning over, which would make both of you go into the water.

Go

If all else fails and you're a capable swimmer trained in water lifesaving techniques, attempt a rescue by swimming to the victim. Be careful not to let the victim grab you; offer a shirt, sock, or other reaching item first.

What you should know about ice rescue

If the victim has broken through ice near the shore, try to extend a pole to the person or throw a line with something attached that floats. Then, pull him or her out onto the shore. Make sure you have a firm footing and won't be pulled into the water yourself.

If you can't reach the victim, don't walk to the edge of the hole in the ice. Instead, lie flat and have someone hold onto your legs as you extend your body to reach the victim. Or extend something for the person to grab, such as a ladder. This spreads your weight across the ice, lessening the risk of further ice breakage.

If you're afraid the ice won't support you, don't attempt a rescue. Instead, wait for emergency help to arrive.

Protecting yourself while aiding the victim

If you're giving assistance at the scene of a motor vehicle accident, don't forget to protect yourself from injury or an infection caused by a communicable disease. Read on to learn how to give yourself an extra margin of safety.

Check out the accident scene

Before approaching, quickly look over the accident scene to make sure it's safe to approach. Park your car at a safe distance.

Beware of explosions

To check for an explosion hazard, look to see if the vehicle is on fire. But keep in mind that even if it isn't already on fire, it may soon be. Look for leaking gasoline and, if you can see the engine's battery, check to see if sparks are present on exposed wires and terminals. If you see or smell gasoline, don't light or set safety flares.

Switch off the ignition of all vehicles involved in the accident. If a fire extinguisher is available, put out any fires.

Check for electric shock hazards

Are downed power lines on or near the victim? If so, don't touch the person. Instead, find the source of the power and turn it off before attempting a rescue.

Prevent further collisions

Observe where the car is on the highway. Is it in the middle of the road? Does oncoming or opposing traffic have to go around it? If possible, ask bystanders to help by directing traffic around the accident. Use a red reflecting signal, flashlight, or other device to warn oncoming traffic.

Avoid possible infection

Like many people, you may want to help a person in need but fear you may catch a disease if you're exposed to the person's blood or body fluids. Disease transmission is a legitimate concern, but it needn't keep you from giving aid. The following advice will help you protect yourself from communicable diseases, such as HIV and hepatitis.

Use protective equipment

Put on disposable latex gloves and other protective equipment whenever possible. If latex gloves aren't available, use the most waterproof material available or extra gauze dressings to form a barrier.

Unless you're wearing latex gloves or other reliable protection, don't touch the person's blood, body fluids, vomit, urine, feces, or an open wound.

Put on disposable latex gloves whenever possible. If gloves aren't available, use the most waterproof material available or extra gauze dressings to form a barrier.

Protect yourself during CPR

If you're trained in CPR, always carry a one-way breather mask, a face mask, or a shield that you can use as a barrier device to place over the victim's mouth during rescue breathing. Such barriers are light and compact and may even fit inside a handbag or small purse.

However, even if you don't have any protective equipment, be aware that the risk of contracting HIV infection or hepatitis while performing mouth-to-mouth resuscitation is very low.

Wash thoroughly if exposure occurs

If you've been exposed to the victim's blood or other body fluids or substances, wash the exposed area thoroughly with soap and running water as soon as possible.

Then seek medical treatment. If you haven't had a hepatitis vaccine, ask the doctor about HBV globulin. This vaccine can give short-term protection against hepatitis. However, it should be followed with the HBV vaccine.

If the accident occurred where you work, report the incident according to your workplace policy.

HOW TO PERFORM CPR

Saving lives with CPR

Cardiopulmonary resuscitation (CPR) is an emergency procedure that saves many lives every day throughout the world. Once you learn the techniques, you can perform CPR quickly in almost any situation, without assistance or equipment.

Why should you learn CPR?

Sudden death from a heart attack causes perhaps more deaths than any other medical emergency. Yet many victims might still be alive had a bystander performed immediate CPR.

The value of CPR isn't limited to heart attack victims. Effective CPR can also revive someone who has drowned, been electrocuted, or taken a drug overdose.

The two parts of CPR

CPR consists of two parts:

- *rescue (mouth-to-mouth) breathing,* which restores the person's breathing
- *chest compressions,* which, when done along with rescue breathing, get the person's blood moving until the heart can resume pumping blood throughout the body.

A person who has a pulse but isn't breathing needs mouth-to-mouth breathing but not chest compressions (because the presence of a pulse means the heart is beating). A person who doesn't have a pulse and isn't breathing needs both rescue breathing and chest compressions to force air into the lungs and get blood circulating throughout the body.

The AABCs of CPR

Remembering the letters A, A, B, and C will help you to follow the correct sequence when performing CPR. Here's what the letters stand for:

*A: A*ccess the emergency medical service system (call 911 or the telephone number for your local emergency medical service)

A: Open the *A*irway
B: Restore *B*reathing
C: Restore *C*irculation.

How to learn CPR
Although the instructions that follow will guide you through the steps of CPR, the best way to learn this lifesaving technique is by taking a course given by the local chapter of the American Red Cross or the American Heart Association. During the course, you'll practice on a mannequin and receive the individual instructions you need to master CPR.

CPR techniques vary somewhat with the victim's age. To learn how to perform CPR on an adult, read this page through page 585; on a child, pages 585 to 590; and on an infant, pages 590 to 593.

CPR techniques vary somewhat with the victim's age. The best way to learn CPR is by taking a course given by the local chapter of the American Red Cross or the American Heart Association.

Performing CPR on an adult

The sooner you begin CPR, the better the person's chance of survival. If no one else is available to help, follow this procedure to perform CPR on an adult.

Get ready
■ Gently shake the person's shoulders and shout "Are you OK?" This is to make sure you don't start CPR on a conscious person.
■ Quickly check the person for major injuries. Focus your inspection on the head and neck because you'll be manipulating these parts of the person's body.
■ Access the emergency medical service system. If possible, send a passerby to call 911 or the local emergency medical service.
■ Place the person on his or her back on a hard, flat surface, such as a floor or sidewalk. If you suspect a head or neck injury, try not to move the person at all. Otherwise, you could increase the risk of paralysis.

Open the airway

■ Kneel near the person's shoulders so you have easy access to the head and chest. Chances are that the muscles controlling the person's tongue will be relaxed, causing the tongue to block the airway. To restore breathing, you'll need to clear the airway.

If you don't suspect a neck injury

■ If you're certain the person hasn't injured the neck, open the airway by using the *head-tilt, chin-lift maneuver*. Place one hand on the person's forehead and place the fingers of your other hand on the bony portion of the lower jaw near the chin.

■ Gently push the person's forehead back and pull upward on the chin. Keep the mouth partly open, making sure the teeth are almost touching, as shown.

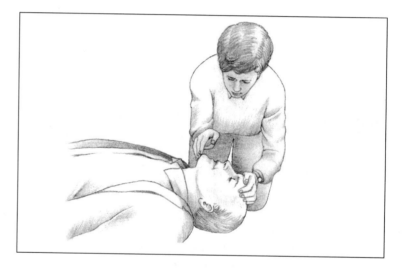

Avoid placing your fingertips on the soft tissue under the person's chin because you may accidentally block the airway you're trying to open.

If you do suspect a neck injury

If the person has suffered a neck injury, moving the neck could cause paralysis or death. So you must clear the airway using the *jaw-thrust maneuver*, which eliminates the need to move the neck. Follow these instructions:

■ Kneel at the person's head and position your elbows on the ground.

■ Curve your index fingers under the person's jaw and near the ears (see top next page). With a strong, steady motion, lift the jaw upward and outward. This action opens the airway without moving the person's neck.

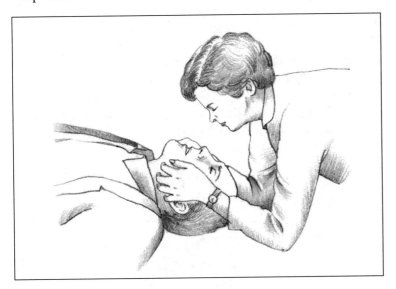

Restore breathing

■ While keeping the person's airway open, place your ear over the mouth and nose and look back toward the person's feet, as shown below. Listen for the sound of air moving and watch for chest movement. You may also feel air on your cheek.

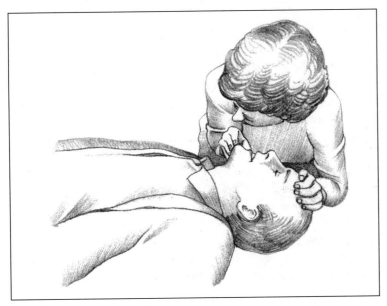

Start giving rescue breaths

■ If you don't detect breathing once you've opened the airway, begin rescue (mouth-to-mouth) breathing. Pinch the nostrils shut with the thumb and index finger of the hand you have on the person's forehead.

■ Take a deep breath and cover the person's mouth with yours, creating a tight seal, as shown below. Give two full breaths. After each breath you deliver, take a deep breath to allow enough time for the person's chest to relax. (This also helps prevent stomach bloating.) Each breath should last 1½ to 2 seconds.

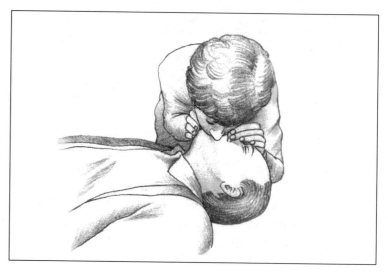

Using special disposable devices, such as a mask and face shield, can eliminate virtually all risk of catching AIDS and other diseases while giving CPR. Ask your CPR instructor how to obtain these devices.

Note: Although medical scientists don't believe AIDS is transmitted in saliva, some people may hesitate to give rescue breaths for fear of catching the disease, especially if they think the person might have AIDS. However, using special disposable devices, such as a mask and face shield, can eliminate virtually all risk of catching AIDS and other diseases while giving CPR. (See *Protection in a pocket mask,* page 437.) Ask your CPR instructor how to obtain these devices.

Check the person's response

■ To see if your breaths went in, watch for the person's chest to rise. If it doesn't, reposition the person's head and try again.

■ If the person's chest still doesn't rise after you've repositioned the head and given two more rescue breaths, suspect that a foreign object (such as dentures) is blocking the airway. To clear the airway, you must give abdominal thrusts (also called the Heimlich maneuver). For instructions on giving abdominal thrusts, see "Choking," page 142.

Restore circulation

■ Keep one hand on the person's forehead so the airway remains open.

Check for a pulse

■ With your other hand, check for a pulse by feeling for the artery in the neck, called the *carotid artery.* To do this, place your index and middle fingers in the groove between the windpipe and the muscle next to it on your side of the person's neck. Feel this artery for 5 to 10 seconds to detect a pulse.

■ If you can feel a pulse, *don't* start chest compressions. Instead, continue rescue breathing, giving 10 to 12 breaths per minute (or one every 5 seconds). Recheck the pulse every 2 to 3 minutes.

Get ready for chest compressions

■ If you don't detect a pulse and help hasn't arrived yet, you must start chest compressions. First, spread your knees apart for a wide base of support. Then, using the hand closer to the person's feet, locate the lower edge of the rib cage.

■ Move your fingertips along the edge to the notch at the end where the ribs meet the breastbone. Place your middle finger on that notch and your index finger next to it. Your index finger should be on the bottom half of the breastbone, just above the lowest point of the breastbone.

■ Put the heel of your other hand on the person's breastbone, next to your index finger, as shown.

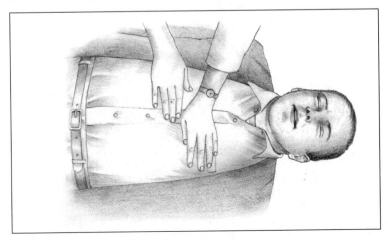

■ Take your fingers off the notch, and put that hand directly on top of your other hand, as shown.

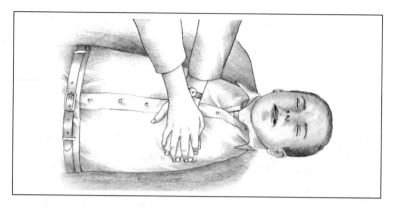

Make sure your fingers don't rest on the person's chest. If your hands are in the proper position, they will concentrate the force of the compressions on the breastbone. This reduces the risk of a broken rib, a punctured lung, or a ruptured liver.

Start giving chest compressions
■ With your elbows locked, arms straight, and shoulders directly over your hands, you're ready to start chest compressions. Using the weight of your upper body, press on the breastbone 1½ to 2 inches (4 to 5 centimeters). Make sure you deliver the pressure through the heels of your hands, as shown.

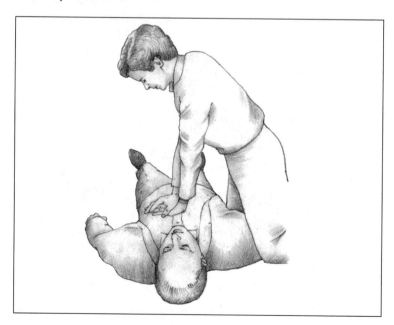

■ After each compression, release the pressure and let the person's chest return to its normal position. (This allows the heart to fill with blood.) To prevent injuries, make sure not to change your hand position during compressions.

■ Give 15 compressions at a rate of 80 to 100 compressions per minute. Count "ONE and TWO and THREE and..." up to 15. Press down on the number and release on the word "and."

Alternate compressions with rescue breaths

■ After 15 chest compressions, give two rescue breaths. Then find the proper hand position again and deliver 15 more compressions. Do four complete cycles of 15 compressions and two breaths.

■ Then, feel for a pulse in the neck (carotid) artery again. If you still don't detect a pulse, continue CPR in cycles of 15 compressions and two rescue breaths, beginning with breaths.

Check for a response

■ Every few minutes during CPR, check for breathing and a pulse.

■ If you detect a pulse but no breathing, give 10 to 12 rescue breaths per minute and check the pulse.

■ If you detect both a pulse and breathing, check the person's breathing and pulse closely.

Continue giving CPR

Don't stop giving CPR until one of the following occurs:

■ the person resumes breathing and a pulse returns

■ you're able to turn CPR over to a competent rescuer

■ you become exhausted.

Continue giving CPR until the person resumes breathing and a pulse returns, you're able to turn CPR over to a competent rescuer, or you become exhausted.

Performing CPR on a child

A child is most likely to need CPR because of a condition that has brought breathing to a halt. Perhaps the most common reason is choking on a small object like a toy or piece of food. Other conditions that can stop a child's breathing include:

■ motor-vehicle accidents

- drowning
- burns
- smoke inhalation
- falls
- poisoning
- suffocation.

When illness causes breathing to stop

Sometimes a child needs CPR to survive a crisis brought on by a respiratory infection that makes the throat swell and go into spasm. Such infections include the childhood illnesses croup and epiglottitis (infection of the flaplike lid that covers the voice box).

If you come upon a child who seems to have stopped breathing, follow this procedure to perform CPR.

Get ready

- Gently shake the child's shoulder and shout "Are you OK?" This is to make sure you don't start CPR on a conscious child.
- If the child is conscious but has difficulty breathing, help the child into a position that best eases breathing.
- Quickly examine the child for major injuries. Focus your inspection on the head and neck because you'll be manipulating these parts of the child's body.

Call for help

- Access the emergency medical service system. If possible, send a passerby to call 911 or the local emergency medical service.
- If you're alone and the child isn't breathing, perform CPR for 1 minute, as described below, before calling for help.

Position the child

- Place the child on the back on a firm, flat surface (usually the ground). If you must turn the child from a stomach-lying position, support the head and neck and turn the child as a single unit.
- If you suspect a head or neck injury, move the child as little as possible to reduce the risk of paralysis.

Open the airway

- Kneel beside the child's shoulder.

If you don't suspect a neck injury
- Place one hand on the child's forehead, and gently lift the chin with your other hand to open the airway.
- Avoid manipulating the soft neck tissue because you could block the airway you're trying to open. Also, never let the child's mouth close completely.

If you do suspect a neck injury
- Use the *jaw-thrust maneuver* to open the child's airway. (This action eliminates the need to move the neck.) To do this, kneel beside the child's head. With your elbows on the ground, rest your thumbs at the corners of the child's mouth, and place two or three fingers of each hand under the lower jaw. Lift the jaw upward.

Check for breathing
- While keeping the child's airway open, place your ear over the child's mouth and nose and look toward the feet. Listen for the sound of air moving and watch for chest movement. You may also feel air on your cheek.
- If you feel or hear breathing or see the chest rise, assume that the child is breathing. Keep the airway open and make sure the child keeps breathing.

Restore breathing
- If the child isn't breathing, maintain the open-airway position and begin rescue (mouth-to-mouth) breathing. Take a breath; then pinch the child's nostrils shut and cover the child's mouth with your mouth. Give two slow breaths (1 to 1½ seconds per breath), pausing between each.
- If your first attempt to give the child a breath doesn't work, reposition the child's head and try again. If that doesn't work, suspect that an object is blocking the airway.

Clear the airway
- A child's small airway can be easily blocked by the tongue. If this occurs, you may be able to clear the airway simply by lifting the child's chin while placing one hand on the forehead (as explained on the previous page under "Open the airway").
- If the airway is still blocked after you perform this maneuver, try to clear it by giving abdominal thrusts, as you would in an adult. (See *Aiding a choking infant or child,* page 145.) Remove any visible object with your fingers. However, don't blindly probe because you

A child's small airway can be easily blocked by the tongue. If this occurs, you may be able to clear the airway simply by lifting the child's chin while placing one hand on the forehead.

could push the object farther into the airway.

- Once you free an object that's blocking the child's airway, check for breathing and a pulse. If these are absent, proceed with chest compressions (described below).

Restore circulation

- Keep one hand on the child's forehead so the airway remains open. With your other hand, check for a pulse in the neck artery (called the *carotid artery*) on your side of the child's neck. To do this, place your index and middle fingers in the groove between the windpipe and the muscle next to it in the neck. Feel this artery for 5 to 10 seconds to detect a pulse.
- If you can feel a pulse, don't begin chest compressions. Instead, continue with rescue breathing, giving 20 breaths per minute (or one every 3 seconds). Recheck the pulse every 2 to 3 minutes.

Start chest compressions
- If you can't feel a pulse and help hasn't arrived yet, start chest compressions. First, spread your knees apart for a wide base of support. Then, using the hand closest to the child's feet, locate the lower border of the rib cage on the side nearest you.
- Hold your middle and index fingers together and move them up the rib cage to the notch where the ribs and sternum meet. Put your middle finger on the notch and your index finger next to it.

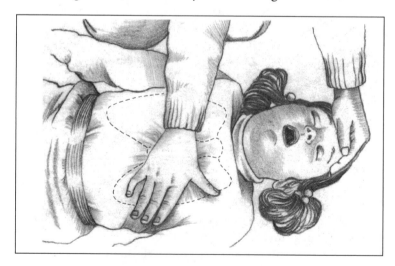

- Lift your hand and place the heel just above the spot where your index finger was. The heel of your hand should be lined up with the long axis of the breastbone, as shown above.

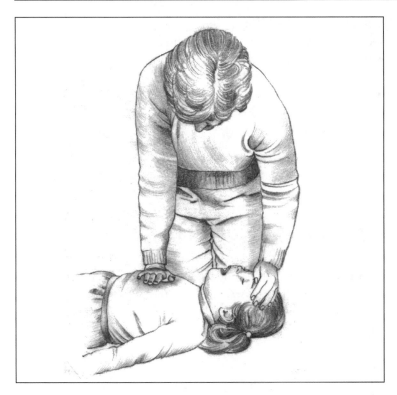

■ Using the heel of one hand only, apply enough pressure to compress the child's chest downward 1 to 1½ inches (2.5 to 4 centimeters). Press down five times in a row, at a rate of 100 compressions per minute.

Alternate compressions with rescue breaths

■ After every five compressions, breathe one breath into the child. Deliver one breath for every five compressions.
■ After 20 cycles (1 minute) of CPR, feel the pulse for 5 seconds to detect a pulse. If you can't detect a pulse, continue with chest compressions and rescue breathing.

Check for a response

■ If you can detect a pulse, check to see if the child is breathing on his or her own. If the child isn't breathing, give one breath every 3 seconds (20 breaths per minute), and continue to check the pulse. If the child begins to breathe on his or her own, keep the airway open and check both the breathing and pulse.

Continue giving CPR

Don't stop giving CPR until one of the following occurs:
- the child resumes breathing and a pulse returns
- you're able to turn CPR over to a competent rescuer
- you become exhausted.

Performing CPR on an infant

Like an adult or a child, an infant needs CPR when the heart stops beating and breathing ceases. However, the technique you use for an infant differs quite a bit from the one you use with an adult or a child. Follow these instructions.

Get ready

- Gently tap or shake the apparently unconscious infant's shoulder and shout "Are you OK?" This is to make sure you don't start CPR on a conscious infant.
- Quickly examine the infant for major injuries. Focus your inspection on the head and neck because you'll be manipulating these parts of the infant's body.

Call for help

- Access the emergency medical service system. If possible, send a passerby to call 911 or the local emergency medical service.
- If you're alone, perform CPR for 1 minute as described below. Then call for help. If necessary, you may move an uninjured infant close to a telephone so you can continue CPR while calling for help.

Clear the airway

- If the infant is choking or has something lodged in the airway, follow the instructions in *Aiding a choking infant or child,* page 145.

■ If you suspect a head or neck injury, move the infant as little as possible to reduce the risk of paralysis.

Try to restore breathing

■ If the infant becomes unconscious, open the airway by using the *head-tilt chin-lift maneuver.* Place one hand on the infant's forehead and gently lift the chin with your other hand to open the airway.
■ Avoid fingering the soft neck tissue beneath the chin because you may accidentally block the airway you're trying to open. Also, never let the infant's mouth close completely.
■ Deliver two rescue (mouth-to-mouth) breaths, as described below under "Provide ventilation."
■ If the infant doesn't begin breathing, reposition his or her head and try rescue breathing again. If this attempt fails, repeat the procedure you used to clear the airway.
■ After you've removed any object blocking the airway, check for breathing and a pulse. If needed, continue CPR.

Avoid fingering the soft neck tissue beneath the infant's chin because you may accidentally block the airway you're trying to open.

Provide ventilation

■ Take a breath, and tightly seal your mouth over the infant's nose and mouth, as shown.

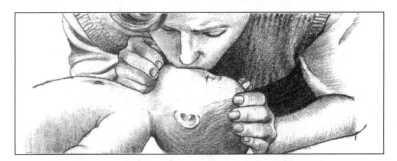

■ Deliver a *gentle* puff of air (because an infant's lungs hold less air than an adult's). If the infant's chest rises and falls, the amount of air you're delivering is probably adequate.
■ Continue rescue breathing, delivering one breath every 3 seconds (20 breaths per minute) if you can detect a pulse.

Restore circulation

■ Check the infant's pulse by feeling for the brachial artery. To find this artery, feel along the inside of the infant's upper arm between the elbow and the shoulder, as shown.

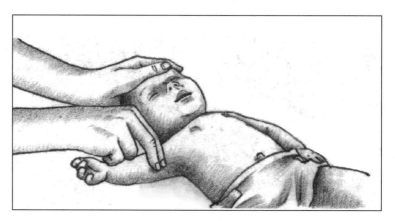

■ If you can feel a pulse, continue with rescue breathing but *don't* start chest compressions.

Start chest compressions

■ If you can't detect a pulse, you must start chest compressions. To locate the infant's heart, draw an imaginary horizontal line between the nipples. Place three fingers directly below — and perpendicular to — the nipple line.

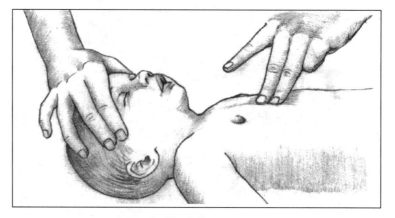

■ Then raise your index finger so that your middle and ring fingers lie one finger's width below the nipple line, as shown above. Use these two fingers only to press on the breastbone here half an inch to 1 inch (1.3 to 2.5 centimeters).

Alternate compressions with rescue breaths
■ After every five compressions, give one rescue breath. This ratio allows you to give about 100 compressions per minute and 20 breaths per minute to an infant.

Continue giving CPR
Don't stop giving CPR until one of the following occurs:
■ the infant resumes breathing and a pulse returns
■ you're able to turn CPR over to a competent rescuer
■ you become exhausted.

Clearing a blocked airway

A person with a blocked airway is in immediate danger of dying. The instructions below tell how to help yourself when you're choking and no one is there to help you, as well as how to cope with choking in a person who is obese, pregnant, or unconscious. To learn the standard technique for aiding an adult, a child, or an infant when none of these special circumstances apply, read "Choking," page 142.

Important: Anyone who starts to choke needs medical help, even if he or she has resumed breathing. Why? Because the trapped foreign body may have damaged tissues in the airway.

What to do if you're alone and you start choking
If your airway becomes blocked and no one is around to help you, give yourself an abdominal thrust. To do this, place the thumb side of your fist into your abdomen, slightly above your navel and below the ribs. Then grasp your fist with your other hand and press with a quick upward thrust.

Another method you may try
Another way to clear your airway is to lean with your abdomen against

If your airway becomes blocked when you are alone, place the thumb side of your fist into your abdomen, slightly above your navel. Grasp your fist with your other hand and press with a quick upward thrust.

the edge of a sink, table, or chair and then press against the object, as shown. Doing this applies sudden pressure to the same place you would when giving yourself an abdominal thrust.

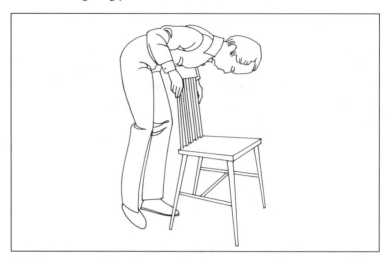

Clearing the airway of an obese person or a pregnant woman

The method for clearing the airway depends on whether or not the person is conscious.

If the person is conscious

■ Stand behind the person and place your arms under the armpits and around the chest, as shown below.

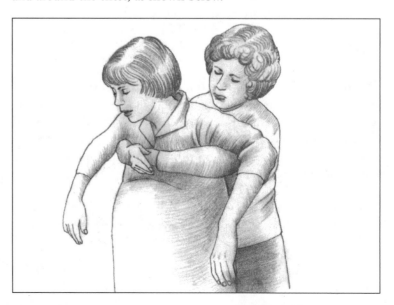

■ Place the thumb side of your clenched fist against the middle of the person's breastbone. Avoid the edges of the ribs and the bottom of the breastbone.

■ Grasp your fist with your other hand, and perform a chest thrust with enough force to expel the object from the person's airway. Continue until the person expels the object or becomes unconscious.

If the person loses consciousness
■ Carefully lower the person to the floor.

■ Kneel close to the person's side and place the heel of one hand just above the bottom of the breastbone. Line up the long axis of your hand with the long axis of the person's breastbone. Place the heel of your other hand on top of that, making sure your fingers don't touch the person's chest.

■ Deliver thrusts. Each thrust should be forceful enough to remove the object in the person's airway.

SPLINTING AND BANDAGING INJURIES

All about splints

Besides immobilizing a broken bone or dislocated joint, a splint supports and protects the injured part. A splint also can:
■ reduce pain
■ help prevent the person from going into shock
■ stop the injury from getting worse.

When you apply a splint, make sure it immobilizes and supports the joint or bone both above and below the injury site. That way, it will prevent movement at the nearest joint as well as at the injury site itself.

To learn about the different types of splints, read what follows.

Commercial splints
Several types of preformed or inflatable splints are available. The *air splint,* which inflates quickly, is easy to apply. It's used mainly for a broken arm or leg.

Make sure the splint immobilizes and supports the joint or bone both above and below the injury site. That way, it will prevent movement at the nearest joint as well as at the injury site itself.

The *SAM splint*™ can be wrapped around the injured part, folded in half to create two sides, or folded in a triangle.

Improvised splint

Of course, you can't count on having a commercial splint available when you need one. Instead, you may have to make a splint from materials at hand. You can make a splint from many common objects — for instance, a wooden board, cardboard, a broom, rolled newspapers or magazines, a rolled blanket, a stick, an oar, an umbrella, or a pillow.

Self-splint

With this splinting method, you attach the injured part to an uninjured part of the person's body. For example, you can tie an injured finger to the finger next to it, or you can tie the legs together.

Traction split

Used only on a broken thigh, this splint is normally found only on ambulances. It takes two trained people to apply it. You probably won't use it unless you're a trained paramedic, an emergency medical technician, or other health care worker.

Slings

Slings are used alone or with splints to support an injured arm, shoulder blade, or collarbone. If a commercial sling or bandage isn't available, you can use a belt, scarf, or necktie instead.

How to splint a broken bone or dislocated joint

To apply a splint safely, review the pointers below. For information on how to splint a specific part of the body, read the instructions given for that part, which follow "General guidelines."

General guidelines

■ Gently remove all clothing covering the part you think is injured.

■ Don't try to straighten a broken bone or dislocated joint or try to push any part of it through an open wound.

■ Cover any open wounds with a clean or sterile dressing before splinting.

■ Always try to get another person to assist you. One person supports, immobilizes, and stabilizes the injured part while the other applies the splint. Two-person splinting helps prevent further damage to the injured part.

Splint above and below the injured part

■ When splinting a bone, make sure the splint extends beyond both the joint above and the joint below the injured bone.

■ When splinting a joint, such as the knee or wrist, make sure the splint extends to the joints above and below that joint. For instance, when splinting an injured knee, tie the splint at both the hip and the ankle.

■ If possible, place the splinting materials on both sides of the injured part to prevent it from moving.

Pad the splint

■ Place padding (soft materials like blankets, cloths, or towels) between the splint and the skin of the injured part. This prevents excessive pressure on the injured part.

■ Also place padding under the person's knee, wrist, and other natural body hollows as well as around any deformities.

Check the person's circulation

■ Don't tie the splint too tightly or it could cut off the circulation or cause pain.

■ Loosen the ties if:
  — the person's fingers or toes become swollen or blue
  — the person can't move the fingers or toes
  — the splinted area becomes numb or starts tingling
  — you can't feel a pulse below the splint
  — the fingernail or toenail of the splinted limb doesn't return to its normal color within 2 seconds after you press on it.

Use elevation and ice

■ After splinting, raise the injured part to reduce swelling.

■ Apply an ice pack, if available, for 20 minutes — but only after you've checked the injured part for a pulse.

How to splint the collarbone

The collarbone may break from a blow to the shoulder or a fall on an outstretched hand. You may splint this injury by applying a sling or an elastic bandage.

Applying a sling

■ Put padding between the arm on the injured side and the side of the person's torso.

■ Place this arm in a triangular bandage or sling, with the person's hand raised 4 to 5 inches (10 to 12.7 centimeters). For instructions on making a sling from a triangular bandage, see *How to apply bandages,* page 606.

■ Secure the arm to the person's body with a triangular bandage that's been folded lengthwise.

■ Center the bandage on the outside of the arm.

■ Wrap the bandage across the chest and back.

■ Tie the bandage on the outside of the arm on the injured side, as shown below.

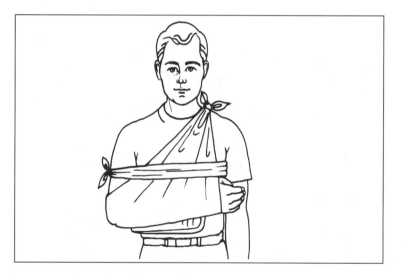

Using an elastic bandage

■ Starting under either arm, wrap an elastic bandage in a figure-of-eight pattern. First wrap it diagonally across the person's back.

■ Then wrap the bandage over the shoulder, under the arm, diagonally across the back, over the other shoulder, and under the other arm.

■ Repeat the figure-of-eight pattern several times.

■ Make sure the bandage isn't too tight. You should be able to slip a finger under the front of the bandage.

How to splint the shoulder blade

A broken shoulder blade is a relatively rare injury that may come from a direct blow to the shoulder. Follow these instructions to splint this injury.

■ Place the forearm (lower part) of the injured arm at a right angle to the person's chest.

■ Apply a sling around the neck, and tie it.

■ Bind the injured arm to the person's body by placing a bandage, towel, or cloth around the upper arm and chest and tying it under the other arm.

How to splint the upper arm

A broken upper arm bone typically causes swelling, deformity, and inability to use the arm below the break. Splint this injury as described below.

■ Place light padding in the armpit.

■ *Gently* place the injured arm at the person's side, with the forearm at a right angle across the chest.

■ Make a padded splint from newspapers, magazines, or other materials on hand.

■ Place the splint on the outside of the upper arm. Then tie it in place above and below the break.

■ Tie a sling around the person's neck to support the lower arm.

To splint the upper arm, gently place the arm at the person's side, with the forearm at a right angle across the chest.

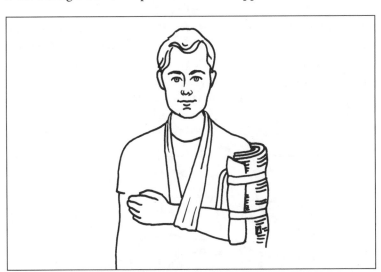

■ Place a towel, bed sheet, or other material around both the splint and the person's chest to bind the upper arm to the body. Then tie this material under the opposite arm.

How to splint the elbow

A broken elbow can cause damage to nearby tissues, nerves, and blood vessels. The injury may impede blood flow to the forearm, possibly causing a permanent disability. The person needs medical help at once.

Until help arrives, follow these instructions to make a splint.

If the elbow is straight

■ Don't bend the elbow to apply the sling.

■ Put padding in the person's armpit.

■ Place padded splints along one or both sides of the entire arm. If you can't find other splinting materials, center a pillow at the elbow and tie a bandage around it.

If the elbow is bent

■ Don't try to straighten it.

■ Place the forearm in a sling. (For instructions on making a sling, read page 598.) Tie the sling around the person's neck.

■ Place a towel or cloth around the upper arm, sling, and chest to bind the injured arm to the body. Then tie this material around the opposite arm.

How to splint the forearm or wrist

Improvise a splint as described below.

■ Gently place the person's lower arm at a right angle across the chest. Make sure the palm faces the chest and the thumb points upward.

■ Place a padded splint on each side of the lower arm. Or wrap padded, folded newspapers or magazines under and around both sides of the arm. The splinting material should extend from the elbow to well beyond the wrist.

■ Tie the splint in place above and below the break.

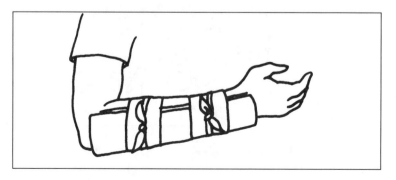

■ Next, tie a sling around the person's neck. Place the sling so the fingers are 3 to 4 inches (7.6 to 10 centimeters) higher than the elbow.

How to splint the hand

A broken hand usually results from a direct blow. Follow these instructions to make a splint.

■ Place padding in the person's palm and under the wrist.

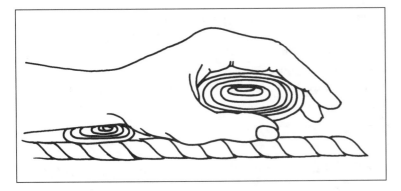

■ Place a padded splint — preferably a board — under the lower arm and hand.

■ Tie the splint in place.

■ Place the lower arm and elbow at a right angle to the person's chest. Then put the lower arm in a sling, and tie the sling around the neck.

How to splint a finger

Like other broken bones, a broken finger typically causes pain, swelling, and deformity. Follow these steps to splint this injury.

■ Place a narrow padded splint under the broken finger and under the palm.

■ Wrap a narrow strip of cloth around the splint and palm. Tie the cloth over the splint.

■ Next, wrap a second narrow strip of cloth around the finger and the splint above the fracture site. Tie the cloth over the splint.

■ Wrap a third cloth strip around the finger and the splint, below the fracture site. Then tie the strip over the splint.

■ Place the person's hand in a bandage sling. (See *How to apply bandages*, page 606.)

How to splint the thigh

The best way to splint the thigh is by using two board splints. If board splints aren't available, improvise with materials on hand. Here are instructions for both splinting methods.

Using board splints

■ Don't straighten the knee if it's bent, unless you must do so to move the person. If you must straighten the knee, pull it slowly and carefully.

■ Gather seven long cloth strips or bandages. Using a stick or a small board, push the strips or bandages under the person's body at a hollow, such as the small of the back or the ankle.

■ Slide each strip or bandage into place — at the ankle, below the knee, above the knee, at the thigh, pelvis, lower back, and just below the armpit.

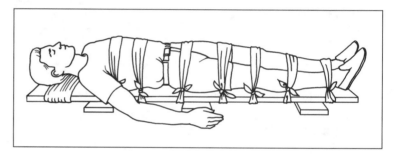

■ Place two padded board splints parallel to each other. The outer splint should reach from the person's armpit to below the heel; the inner splint, from the crotch to below the heel.

■ Tie the splints in place on the outer splint.

Making a splint if boards aren't available

■ Place a folded blanket or other padding between the person's legs.

■ Tie the injured leg to the other leg.

■ Then tie the legs together at a minimum of three places — around the thighs, above and below the knees, and around the ankles. *Don't* tie the splint directly over the fracture.

How to splint the kneecap

If the person's leg is bent, don't try to straighten it. Doing so could cause permanent damage. Instead, immobilize the knee in place, using padding to fill any space. Follow these instructions.

The best way to splint the thigh is by using two board splints. If boards aren't available, place a folded blanket between the person's legs. Tie the injured leg to the other leg. Then tie the legs together.

■ Place a padded board at least 4 inches (10 centimeters) wide under the injured leg. Make sure the board is long enough to reach from the person's buttocks to the heel.

■ Put extra padding under the knee and ankle.

■ Tie the splint at the ankle, just above and just below the knee, and at the thigh. *Don't* tie it directly over the kneecap.

How to splint the lower leg

If the injured leg isn't deformed, use an air splint, if available. Otherwise, use two board splints or improvise a splint from materials on hand. Here are instructions for using board splints or an improvised splint.

Using board splints

■ Pad both splints.

■ Place one splint on each side of the injured leg. (If a third board splint is available, place it under the leg.) The splints should extend from above the knee to below the heel.

■ Tie the splints together in several places — but *not* directly over the break.

Using other materials

■ Place a folded blanket or other padding material between the person's legs.

■ Tie both legs together.

How to splint the ankle or foot

Follow these instructions to make a splint.

■ Keep the person lying down.

■ Gently loosen or remove the shoe from the injured foot. If necessary, cut the shoe to prevent further injury to the ankle.

■ Place a pillow or rolled blanket around the injured leg, from the calf to beyond the heel. The pillow's edges should meet on top of the leg. For extra support, fold the ends of the pillow that reach beyond the heel.

■ Tie the pillow with three bandages. Tie the first bandage above the ankle, the second one around the ankle, and the third one below the ankle.

■ Place padding between the ankles. Make sure the padding extends above the knees.

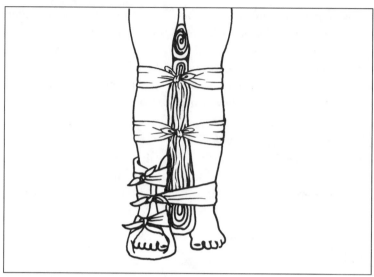

■ Tie one bandage around the knees, another below the knees, and another around both ankles, as shown.

How to splint the neck and spine

The spine, made up of bones called *vertebrae,* surrounds and protects the spinal cord. One or more vertebrae may be broken at any point along the spine — from the top of the neck, where the spine begins, to the tailbone, where it ends.

A broken vertebrae can injure the spinal cord by pressing against it or by becoming displaced and cutting the cord. No matter how a spinal cord injury occurs, it can lead to paralysis and death.

Check for symptoms of spinal cord damage

To help prevent a disabling injury and reduce the risk of further spinal cord damage, learn how to recognize symptoms of spinal cord damage. These include:
■ back or neck deformity
■ pain and tenderness at the injury site
■ cuts or bruises
■ numbness, tingling, or a burning sensation
■ paralysis.

One way to check for paralysis is to touch the person's feet and hands and ask him or her to wiggle the fingers or toes. If the person can't do these things, suspect paralysis. In an unconscious person, suspect paralysis if the feet or hands don't react when you stroke the soles or palms with a pointed object.

When in doubt, splint

If you're not sure whether the spinal cord is injured or whether the neck or spinal column may be broken, always assume that it is. First-aid for someone with a neck or back injury should be performed only by trained medical personnel.

If you can't get trained personnel to the injury scene, splint the neck and spine by following the instructions below. Have at least one other helper assist you. *Important:* Don't move the person until he or she has been completely immobilized from head to toe.

Immobilize the person's head

■ Keeping the person's head still, wrap a rolled towel, sweater, newspaper, or other padded object measuring about 4 inches (10 centimeters) wide around the person's neck. Keep his or her head as still as possible. *Be sure not to move the person's head because this could cause paralysis or death.*

■ Tie the padded object loosely in place around the person's head.

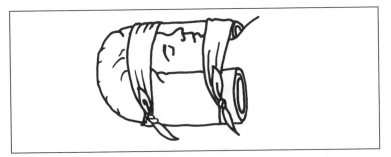

Make sure it's loose enough so it won't cut off the person's breathing.

■ Have a helper cradle the person's head in his or her arms to keep the head still while you splint the person's body.

Immobilize the person's spine

■ As the helper continues to keep the person's head still, place a wide board, door, or other rigid, padded support next to the person. The support should extend from beyond the head to the person's buttocks.

■ Obtain at least 10 bandages, gauze rollers, scarves, neckties, or other long, narrow objects; you'll use these tie the person to the support. Then slide these objects under the support.

■ If the person is breathing on his or her own, hold the head so it stays at the same angle to the body as it was when you found the person. Then have other helpers grasp the person's clothes and slide

If you're not sure whether a person's spinal cord is injured or whether the neck or spinal column may be broken, always assume that it is. Don't move the person's head because this could cause paralysis or death.

the support underneath him or her. Move gently, carefully, and slowly. Lift the person only high enough to slide the support underneath. Make sure to move the entire body, neck, and head together as a single unit. *Don't let the person's head move independent of the rest of the body.*

Secure the person to the splint

■ Tie bandages around the person's body at the sites shown in the illustration below. With the last bandage, tie the person's forehead to the support.

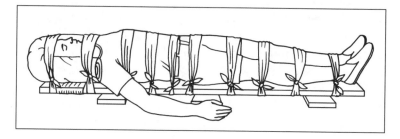

■ Finally, cover the person with a blanket.

How to apply bandages

A bandage has many uses in first-aid:
■ It keeps a dressing or splint in place.
■ It limits the movement of an injured body part.
■ It keeps pressure on a wound.
■ It provides support.

Materials you can use

Bandages are usually made of gauze (lightweight woven cotton) or elastic fabric. If these materials aren't available, you can improvise by using long, thin material, such as a necktie, handkerchief, scarf, or belt. Or you can tear strips of cloth from a bed sheet, towel, shirt sleeve, or pant leg.

A bandage doesn't have to be sterile. But whatever material you use should be as clean as possible.

General guidelines

When using any bandage, keep these pointers in mind.

Clean the skin

■ Before applying a bandage, make sure the injured part of the person's skin is clean and dry.

■ Don't apply a bandage directly to an open wound. First, cover the wound with a sterile dressing or other clean, absorbent material.

Wrap at the right place

■ Wrap the injury site starting at the area that's farthest from the person's head. Then wrap in an upward direction.

■ Always secure the bandage away from the person's body.

■ Never put a bandage around a person's neck.

Ensure comfort and safety

■ Don't tie the bandage too tightly or it could cut off circulation. Loosen it if:

    — the person can't move the fingers or toes.

    — the fingers or toes become swollen or blue.

    — the bandaged area becomes numb or starts tingling.

    — you can't feel a pulse below the bandaged part.

■ Never apply a wet gauze bandage because it will shrink when it dries and become too tight.

Applying a gauze bandage

Gauze bandages usually come in rolls 1 to 4 inches (2.5 to 10 centimeters) wide.

GAUZE BANDAGE

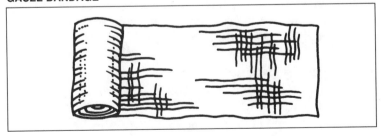

    Although the procedure that follows describes how to apply a gauze bandage to a person's hand, you can apply one to any part of the body the same way. The width of the bandage you use depends on:

■ the size, condition, and location of the wound

- the amount of blood and other body fluids present
- the bandaging material that's available.

Bandaging the hand

- With one hand, hold the loose end of the gauze roll just below the knuckles of the injured hand. With your other hand, pass the roll around the hand twice to secure the bandage.
- Angle the bandage to begin making a figure-eight turn. Then pass the roll under the wrist and back up toward the fingers to complete the figure-eight turn. Repeat until the wrist is covered.
- Finish wrapping by passing the roll around the person's wrist and circling up the forearm (lower arm) several times.

Secure the bandage

- Secure the end of the bandage with adhesive tape.
- If you can't find tape or another fastener, try this fastening technique: Slit the end of the bandage lengthwise about 8 inches (20 centimeters) and twist the two ends together several times. Wrap one of the ends around the bandage. Then tie the two ends together. Be sure not to tie the knot over the wound.

You can use recurrent bandaging to secure a dressing over an area that's hard to bandage. In this technique, you make circular turns and perpendicular turns to cover the desired area.

Using recurrent bandaging

You can use a method called *recurrent bandaging* to secure a dressing over an area that's hard to bandage, such as a finger, a toe, or the head. In this technique, you make the following turns:
- two circular turns
- additional turns perpendicular to the first ones to cover the desired area
- more circular turns to secure the bandage.
- more circular turns to secure the bandage.

   Although the procedure below describes how to bandage a finger, you can easily adapt it when bandaging any difficult area.

Use the right bandage size

- First, select roller gauze or an elastic bandage in the appropriate width. For a finger, you'll need a bandage that's 1 inch (2.5 centimeters) wide. For the head, use one that's 3 or 4 inches (7.6 to 10 centimeters) wide.

Make two circular turns

- Secure the bandage at the bottom of the finger with two circular turns.

■ With your index and middle fingers, hold the bandage at the bottom, where it's secured. Roll the bandage over the fingertip to the other side of the finger, as shown below.

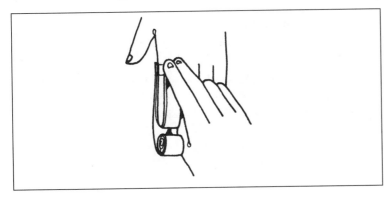

Wrap in layers

■ Now, using your thumb to hold the other side of the bandage, bring the bandage back and forth until the finger is covered with several layers of bandage.

■ To keep the bandage in place, start at the bottom and wrap in circles up the finger and back to the bottom, as shown below.

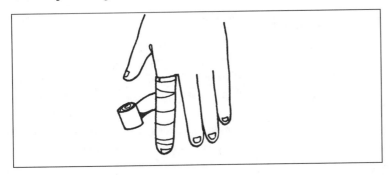

Finish securing the bandage

■ Apply a piece of tape about 6 inches (15 centimeters) long up one side of the finger, over the fingertip, and down the other side. Don't secure the dressing with a *circle* of tape, because this could act as a tourniquet and cut off the circulation.

Applying an elastic bandage

Elastic bandages are used to compress, or squeeze, the tissues around a sprain or a strain. This helps prevent swelling and provides support. Unlike gauze bandages, elastic bandages aren't meant for covering wounds.

The procedure that follows describes how to wrap an elastic bandage around a person's ankle. You can modify this technique if you need to wrap a knee, wrist, elbow, or hand.

Overlap the bandage

■ With one hand, hold the loose end of the elastic bandage on top of the foot between the instep and toes.

■ With the other hand, wrap the bandage twice around the foot, as shown, gradually moving toward the ankle. Make sure to overlap the bandage in a spiral, as shown below.

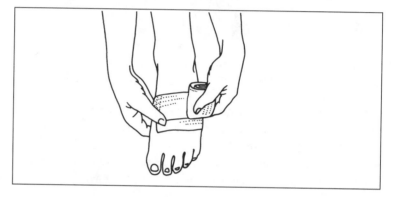

Make figure-eight turns

■ After wrapping the foot twice, support the heel with one hand.

■ Use your other hand to wrap the bandage in a figure-eight fashion, leaving the heel uncovered. To do this, wrap the bandage around the ankle in an upward direction, cross it over the foot, and pass it behind the ankle.

■ Next, wrap the bandage down toward the foot at an angle, cross it over the top of the foot, and pass it under the foot to complete the figure-eight turn. Do this step twice, as shown.

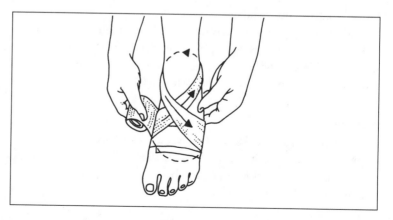

Circle the calf

■ Now, circle the bandage around the calf, moving toward the knee, as shown. Don't wrap downward. Overlap the bandage as you wrap.

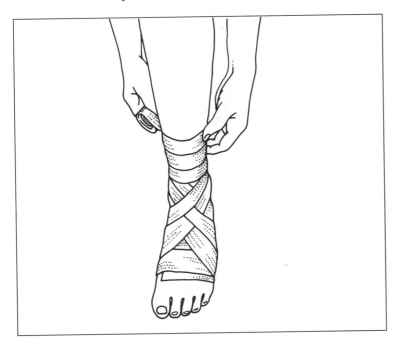

■ Stop wrapping just below the knee.

Secure the bandage

■ Secure the end of the bandage with a metal clip or adhesive tape.
■ If you can't find a metal clip or tape, try splitting the end of the bandage lengthwise about 8 inches (20 centimeters) and twisting the two ends together several times. Then wrap one of the ends around the bandage and tie the two ends together.

Using a triangular bandage

A triangular bandage can be used as a sling or as a tie that holds a splint or dressing in place. You can make a triangular bandage from any piece of cloth 36 to 40 inches (91.4 to 101.6 centimeters) square. If necessary, you can make one from a shirt or large handkerchief. To form two triangles, cut the cloth diagonally.

When fully opened, the bandage can be used as a sling to immobilize an injured arm. When folded into a tubular shape, it becomes a *cravat bandage*, commonly used to hold splints in place.

Making a sling

To apply a sling to support a person's arm or shoulder, follow these steps.

■ Place the center of the triangular bandage at the elbow of the affected arm. The longest side of the triangle should be parallel to the person's body, as shown.

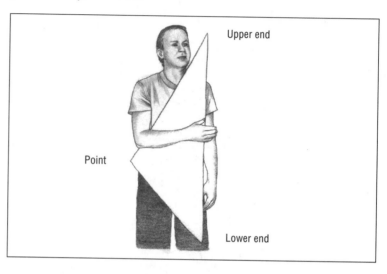

Upper end

Point

Lower end

■ Drape the upper end of the triangle over the uninjured shoulder. Help the person bend the elbow of the injured arm at a 90-degree angle, with the thumb pointing up.
■ Place the lower end of the triangle over the shoulder of this arm, enclosing the forearm in the sling.
■ Knot the two ends of the sling loosely around the person's neck. Always position the knot to the side — never at the back of the neck. To keep the knot in place and prevent skin irritation, place the sling outside the person's collar or insert a gauze pad under the knot.
■ If the knot is uncomfortable, pin each point to the opposite side. Make sure the edge of the sling extends to the first joint of the person's little finger. This holds the wrist in line with the arm to help prevent wrist damage. Now, use a safety pin to fasten the overlapping piece at the elbow to the sling fabric. This keeps the sling from falling off.

Bandaging a head wound

You can use a triangular bandage to dress an open wound on a person's forehead or in the back of the head. Follow these instructions.

■ Place the center of the triangle's base across the person's forehead, just above the eyes. Make sure the point of the bandage is at the back of the head, facing downward.

■ Bring both ends of the bandage above the person's ears and around to the back of the head.

■ At the back of the head, just below the natural bulge, cross the ends over each other snugly.

■ Then bring the ends back around to the center of the forehead and tie them in a knot, as shown. Make sure the knot lies over the wound.

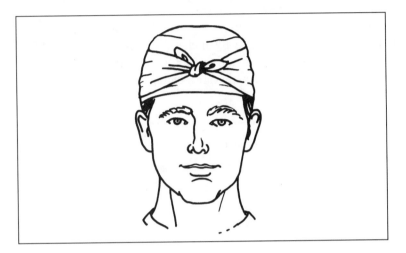

■ Finally, tuck the point of the bandage into the fold where the bandage crosses in the back.

*U*SING CRUTCHES AND CASTS

How to use crutches

The doctor prescribes crutches to prevent a person from putting weight on an injured leg or foot. Or if the person is allowed to bear some weight, the doctor may prescribe crutches to reduce the amount of weight placed on the injured leg.

To use crutches properly, first check to see if they're right for you. When you're certain the crutches are the correct size and properly padded, let the nurse show you how to use them. But remember, crutch-walking requires practice. Don't get discouraged if you have difficulty at first.

Are the crutches right for you?
■ Make sure the crutches have rubber tips to prevent slipping, as well as padded underarm and hand supports to prevent injury.
■ Check for proper size. When you're standing with the crutch tips 6 inches (15 centimeters) from the sides of your feet, the underarm pieces should be about 1 to 1 ½ inches (two finger-widths or 2.5 to 3.8 centimeters) below your armpits, as shown. If the underarm pieces touch your armpits, the crutches are too long. Ask the nurse to shorten them.

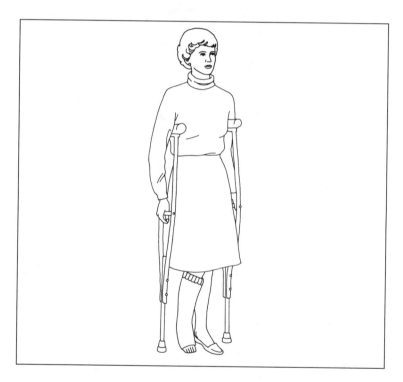

Remember — you should support your weight with the hand grips, not the crutch tops.
■ Check the placement of the hand grips. When you grasp them, your arms should be slightly bent — *never* straight.

Test your crutch technique

Support yourself by distributing your weight on your hands, wrists, and arms. If you feel tingling or numbness in the side of your chest below your armpits or in your upper arms, you're probably using the crutches incorrectly.

Crutch-walking with partial weight on your injured leg

The doctor may let you place some of your weight on the injured leg. The instructions below describe how to walk with crutches while putting some weight on your injured leg.

Stand correctly

■ Stand straight with your shoulders relaxed and your arms slightly bent. Lean your body slightly forward, distributing your weight between the crutches and your uninjured leg.
■ You can put some weight on your injured leg.

Move the crutches forward

■ Move the crutches forward about 12 inches (30.5 centimeters).
■ Move your injured leg up to meet them.
■ Put some weight on your injured leg as you move your uninjured leg ahead of the crutches.
■ Repeat these steps to keep walking.

Crutch-walking with no weight on your injured leg

Read what follows to learn how to walk with crutches if your doctor doesn't want you to put any weight on your injured leg.

Position your legs

■ Stand straight with all your weight on the uninjured leg. Relax your shoulders. Hold the foot of your injured leg off the floor, flexing your knee slightly.
■ Balancing all your weight on the crutches, position the foot of the uninjured leg so that it's even with the crutch tips, slightly in front of you. Use the uninjured leg and the crutches to support your weight as you lean forward slightly.

Shift your weight

■ Shift all your weight to the uninjured leg, and move the crutches forward together, swinging the injured leg along with them. Don't put any weight on your injured leg.

If you're allowed to put weight on the injured leg, walk by moving the crutches forward about 12 inches, then moving your injured leg up to meet the crutches.

- Now, shift all your weight back to the crutches by way of your hands and wrists, swing your uninjured leg forward and, again, place all your weight on this leg. Use the crutches to keep your balance.

Using crutches on stairs

Sooner or later, you'll have to get up and down stairs using your crutches. Assuming the banister is on your left and your *right* leg is injured, here's how to proceed.

Get into position

- Standing at the bottom of the stairs, shift both crutches to your right hand.
- Then grasp the banister firmly with your left hand.
- Using your right hand, carefully support your weight on the crutches.

Hop with the uninjured leg

- Next, push down on your crutches and hop onto the first step, using just your uninjured leg.
- Lift your injured leg as you go.
- Support your weight on your uninjured leg as you continue to grasp the banister tightly. Then swing the crutches up onto the first step. Now, hop onto the second step, using your uninjured leg. Repeat this procedure, but go slowly.

Reverse these maneuvers on the way down

To get down the stairs, reverse these maneuvers. But always advance the crutches and your injured leg first. Remember, your strong leg goes up first and comes down last.

Getting into and out of a chair

If you're on crutches, you'll need practice getting into and out of a chair. Follow these guidelines.

How to sit down

- Using your crutches, walk over to the chair. Turn around, and step backward carefully until the back of your uninjured leg touches the chair's front edge.
- Keeping your weight on your uninjured leg, transfer both crutches to the hand on the same side as your injured leg. Support most of

your weight on your crutches. Next, reach back with your other hand and grasp the chair arm.

■ Carefully sit down, making sure to keep your weight off your injured leg. Keep your crutches next to the chair.

How to get up

■ Move your uninjured leg backward until it touches the back of the chair's front edge. While you're still sitting, take both crutches and stand them upright.

■ Using the hand on the same side as your injured leg, hold onto the hand grips. With your other hand, hold onto the chair arm.

■ Slide forward, with your uninjured leg slightly under the chair. Push yourself up onto your uninjured leg.

■ Once you're standing, transfer one crutch to your uninjured side. Or push yourself up while grasping the handgrip of a crutch in each hand.

What to do if you fall

If you fall when using crutches, follow these steps to get back on your feet safely.

Look for support

■ Sit with your legs extended and your hands beside your hips.

■ Look around the room for a low, sturdy piece of furniture, such as a sofa (or chair).

■ Then, inch backward toward the sofa by alternately pushing your hands down on the floor and lifting up your buttocks. Slide the crutches along with you as you go.

Use your hands and crutches

■ When you reach the sofa, lean the crutches against it. Move the cushion to the side if the sofa is high. Then reach back and place both hands on the sofa seat.

■ Press down on the sofa seat with both hands, and lift your buttocks onto the sofa.

■ Grasp both crutches in one hand. As you steady yourself with the crutches, raise yourself to a standing position by pushing down on the sofa with your other hand. After that, transfer one of the crutches to your other hand.

How to care for a cast

Wearing a cast helps an injured muscle or bone heal properly after surgery. A person may wear a cast for 3 to 24 weeks, depending on the type and location of the injury.

If you must wear a cast, you'll need to give it careful attention to avoid problems, such as skin irritation and infection. Following the guidelines below will help you live more comfortably with your cast while it does its job.

Speed the drying time

Whether the cast is made of fiberglass, plaster, or another material, it must dry thoroughly and evenly to support your broken bone properly. Follow these tips to speed drying.

■ Keep the cast exposed to the air. Fiberglass and synthetic casts dry soon after application, but plaster casts take 24 to 48 hours to dry. Drying a plaster cast in less time will make it more comfortable sooner.

■ The doctor will probably instruct you to raise the casted part on pillows as the cast dries. Make sure the pillows you use have rubber or plastic covers under the pillowcase. Place a thin towel between the cast and the pillows to absorb moisture. Never place a wet cast directly on plastic.

Dry the cast evenly

■ To make sure the cast dries evenly, change its position on the pillows every 2 hours. Use your palms, not your fingertips, to move it. (If necessary, have someone else move the cast for you.)

■ Don't poke at the cast with your fingers while it's wet because you could create bumps inside the cast that cause skin irritation or sores. Also be sure not to dent the cast while it's still wet.

Keep the cast clean

■ After the cast dries, you can remove dirt and stains with a damp cloth and powdered kitchen cleaner. Use as little water as possible. When you've finished, always wipe off any moisture that remains.

Don't poke at the cast with your fingers while it's wet because you could create bumps inside the cast that cause skin irritation or sores.

Protect the cast

Avoid knocking the cast against a hard surface. To protect the foot of a leg cast from breakage, scrapes, and dirt, place a piece of carpet over the bottom of the cast. Slash or cut a V-shape at the back of the carpet so that it fits around the heel when you bring it up toward the ankle. Hold the carpet in place with a large sock or slipper sock. Extending the carpet a little beyond the toes also helps to prevent them from being bumped or stubbed.

Prevent snags

■ To keep an arm cast from snagging clothing and furniture, make a cast cover from an old nylon stocking. Cut the stocking's toe off, and cut a hole in the heel. Then pull the stocking over the cast to cover it. Extend your fingers through the cut-off toe end, and poke your thumb through the hole you cut in the heel.

■ Trim the other end of the stocking so it's about 1½ inches (3.8 centimeters) longer than the cast, and tuck the ends of the stocking under the cast's edges.

Care for your skin

■ Wash the skin along the edges of the cast every day, using a mild soap. Before you begin, protect the cast's edges with plastic wrap.

■ Use a washcloth wrung out in soapy water to clean the skin at the edges and as far as you can reach inside the cast. Avoid getting the cast wet.

■ Dry the skin thoroughly with a towel, and then massage the skin at and beneath the cast's edges with a towel or pad saturated with rubbing alcohol. This helps toughen the skin. To help prevent skin irritation, remove any loose plaster particles you can reach inside the cast.

Relieve itching safely

No matter how much the skin under the cast may itch, never try to relieve the itching by inserting a sharp or pointed object into the cast. This could damage your skin and lead to infection. Don't put powder or lotion in your cast, either, or stuff cotton or toilet tissue under its edges; this may interfere with blood circulation.

Itch-relief tip
Set a hand-held blow dryer on cool and aim it at the problem area, as shown.

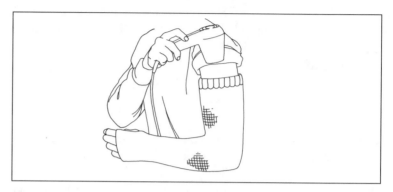

Keep the cast dry

If you have a plaster cast, you'll need to cover it with a plastic bag before you shower, swim, or go out in wet weather. You can use a garbage bag or a cast shower bag, available at a drugstore or medical supply store.

Important: Don't get a plaster cast wet. Moisture will weaken or even destroy it. If the cast gets a little wet, let it dry naturally; don't cover the cast until it's completely dry.

How to flush a cast

If you have a fiberglass or synthetic cast, check with the doctor to find out if you can bathe, shower, or swim. If you're permitted to swim, the doctor will probably tell you to flush the cast with cool tap water after swimming in a chlorinated pool or a lake. This removes any foreign matter trapped inside the cast.

How to dry a cast

To dry a fiberglass or synthetic cast, first wrap the cast in a towel. Then prop the cast on a pad of towels to absorb any remaining water. It will air-dry in 3 to 4 hours; to speed drying, use a hand-held blow dryer.

Use a sling as instructed

If you have an arm cast, the doctor may want you to wear a sling temporarily to support and rest your sore shoulder. Ask the doctor when and how often you can remove the sling.

Cast-signing precaution

It's all right to let family members and friends sign their names or draw pictures on the cast, as long as they don't paint over it. This could make the cast nonporous and damage the skin beneath it.

Troubleshooting your casted arm or leg

After you leave the hospital, you'll need to check for possible problems with your casted arm or leg, such as wound discharge and excessive swelling. Be sure to check your cast daily.

Watch for wound discharge

When a cast also covers a wound, you can expect some red or reddish-brown discharge during the first 48 hours after the cast is applied. This discharge may stain the cast or, if it leaks from the cast's ends, the bed linens.

If discharge occurs, use a felt-tipped pen to outline the stain on the cast. Jot down the date and time, too. Discharge may signal a problem that requires the doctor's attention.

Stay alert for danger signs

Notify the doctor if:
- discharge stains the cast or bed linens bright red.
- stains appear even though the cast wasn't applied over a wound (pressure from the cast may have caused a sore).
- a stain spreads.
- drainage changes color or odor (this may indicate infection).

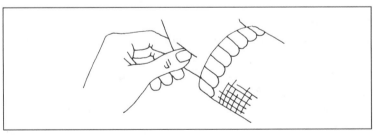

Test sensation and movement

- Several times a day, check for changes in sensation by touching the area above and below the cast, as shown above. Is the area numb? Do you feel tingling or pain?
- Wiggle the fingers or toes on the casted arm or leg. If you can't move your fingers or toes or if you have more pain than usual when you move them, call the doctor.

Call the doctor if discharge stains the cast or bed linens bright red, if stains appear even though the cast wasn't applied over a wound, or if a stain spreads.

Check circulation

■ Press a fingernail or large toenail on the casted limb, as shown, until the color fades. Then let go. If normal flesh color doesn't return quickly (within 2 seconds), contact the doctor at once. Repeat this check at least three times a day.

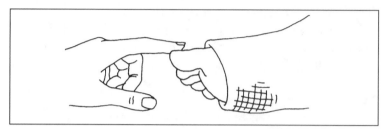

■ If your fingers or toes are cold, try covering them. If that doesn't warm them, contact the doctor.

Cope with arm or leg swelling

A little swelling of a casted limb is normal, but a lot isn't. To help prevent excessive swelling, follow these guidelines.

■ Keep the cast raised above the level of your heart as much as possible on two regular size pillows. Apply ice as directed by the doctor.

■ If your leg is in a cast, sit or lie down and raise the leg on pillows. If your arm is in a cast, prop up the arm so your hand and elbow are higher than your heart.

■ Check for severe swelling above and below the cast several times daily. To do this, compare the casted arm or leg with the uncasted arm or leg.

Relieve skin irritation

After the cast dries completely, rough edges may cause skin irritation. Smooth rough edges on a fiberglass cast with a nail file.

If the cast is plaster, "petal" rough edges using adhesive tape or moleskin. This prevents the material from catching on clothing or being peeled off accidentally. To petal your cast, follow these steps:

■ Cut several strips of tape or moleskin measuring 4 inches by 2 inches (10 by 5 centimeters). Trim the ends that lie outside the cast so they're rounded.

■ Place the first strip, rounded end down, on the outside of the cast.

■ Tuck the straight end just inside the cast edge. Smooth the tape or moleskin with your finger to remove any creases, which can also irritate your skin.

■ Apply the remaining strips. Overlap them, as needed, until you've covered all the cast's rough edges.

WHAT YOU SHOULD KNOW ABOUT FIRST-AID KITS

Supplies to keep in a first-aid kit

Keeping a properly stocked first-aid kit is one of the best ways to be prepared for medical emergencies. With such a kit, you can treat a wide range of health problems on the spot, eliminating the need for medical attention. And if the person does need professional health care, the kit can help you provide aid until help arrives.

Customize your kit

You can buy a ready-made first-aid kit in a drugstore. But if a family member has a chronic health problem, such as diabetes, asthma, or an allergy to bee stings, you may want to assemble your own kit. Ask the doctor what additional drugs or supplies to include in your kit.

Besides making up a first-aid kit for the home, consider making others to keep in your motor vehicle or with your boating or camping supplies and even to take to the workplace. (See *Stocking a first-aid kit for your car,* page 626.)

If you decide to make your own first-aid kit, refer to the general guidelines below when gathering supplies.

First-aid essentials

Most people without special health care needs can get by with just the following first-aid items:
- adhesive strip bandages
- coins (to call for help from a pay phone)
- latex gloves
- scissors
- triangle bandages.

Other first-aid supplies

The list below includes items you may want to add to your first-aid kit, especially if you or a family member has special needs.

General equipment
- Bandage scissors

You can buy a ready-made first-aid kit in a drugstore. But if a family member has a chronic health problem, such as diabetes, asthma, or an allergy to bee stings, you may want to assemble your own kit.

- Blanket
- Cotton-tipped swabs
- Extractor (to suction and remove snakebite venom)
- Folding pocket knife
- Latex disposable gloves
- Ice pack or ice bag
- Light sticks
- Mouth-to-mouth barrier device, face shield, or face mask with one-way valve
- Penlight with spare batteries
- Regular scissors
- Resealable plastic bags
- Safety pins
- Shears that can cut thick material or metal (such as EMT shears)
- Splint or a board to use as a splint
- Thermometer
- Tweezers

Bandages and dressings
- Adhesive strip bandages
- Adhesive tape (½-inch and 1-inch)
- Conforming, self-adhering bandages (1-inch and 2-inch)
- Duct tape (to hold splints in place)
- Elastic roller bandages (1-inch and 2-inch)
- Eye pads
- Gauze pads (in several sizes)
- Gauze roller bandages (1-inch and 2-inch)
- Hypoallergenic tape and waterproof tape (½-inch and 1-inch)
- Nonstick pads (2-inch by 3-inch and 3-inch by 4-inch)
- Triangular bandages

Medicines
- Acetaminophen (such as Tylenol, for pain relief)
- Activated charcoal (for some poisonings — only when medical authority directs)
- Alcohol prep pads (for cleaning skin around wounds)
- Antibiotic ointment (for burns, minor cuts, and abrasions)
- Antihistamine (for allergic reactions)
- Antiseptic towelettes (for cleaning hands and skin around wounds)
- Aspirin (for pain, swelling, and fever; don't give to children or teen-agers)
- Calamine lotion

- Glucose paste (to treat insulin reaction in a diabetic person)
- Ibuprofen (such as Advil or Motrin, for pain, swelling, or fever)
- Insect repellant
- Ipecac syrup (for poisoning — only when medical authority directs)
- Medicine for diarrhea, nausea, and vomiting
- Medicine for motion sickness
- Powdered electrolyte mix (for heat stress)
- Sting relief swabs (for insect bites and stings)
- Sunscreen with sun protection factor of 15 or higher

Use the right container

Keep your first-aid supplies together in a tool box, a fishing tackle box, or any plastic container with a tight-fitting lid. You can keep similar items, such as those needed to bandage a wound, together in sealable transparent plastic bags. This will help you locate the items more easily in the rush and excitement of an injury or an accident. Be sure to keep the kit out of the reach of children, just as you would anything that contains drugs.

Keep your first-aid supplies together in a plastic container with a tight-fitting lid. Be sure to keep the kit out of the reach of children.

Update the contents

Check the contents of your first-aid kit regularly — once a month, as well as after the kit has been used. Check the expiration date of perishable items, such as ointments; these lose their potency or degrade over time.

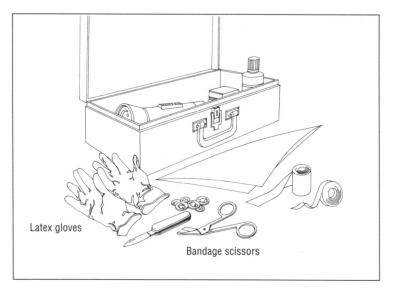

Latex gloves

Bandage scissors

Stocking a first-aid kit for your car

For most people, it's not enough to keep a first-aid kit in your home. You should also keep one anywhere you spend a lot of time. For many of us, this includes our motor vehicle.

Two kits are better than one

Better yet, keep a standard first-aid kit in the front of your motor vehicle and a second container of emergency supplies in the trunk. You'll want to change some of these supplies with the season. In the winter, for instance, keep extra gloves, a scarf, a snow shovel, a de-icing device, and a spare change of warm clothes handy. In the summer, keep chemical ice packs, additional bottled water, a sun hat, extra sunglasses, and salt packs.

Emergency supplies to gather

- Battery jumper cables
- Blanket
- Bottled water
- Can opener
- Electrical tape
- Extra fan belt and hoses for the car
- Fire extinguisher
- Gas can
- Maps
- Matches in waterproof container
- Nonperishable food
- Pocket knife
- Rope
- Shovel
- Tool kit
- Wire

Make regular checks

Be sure to check your first-aid kits periodically, especially before you take a long trip.

HOW TO PREVENT EMERGENCIES AT HOME

Home safety hints

To make sure your home is safe, you'll need to take steps to prevent injuries and other emergencies. Here are some general safety tips.

Keep essentials on hand
Keep a flashlight and a portable radio handy. These are helpful if the lights go out or an emergency occurs. Make sure to keep extra batteries.

Use one good lock
Install a single lock on each door. If you have an emergency and need to get out of your house quickly, opening a single lock is easier than struggling with several.

Get up slowly
To avoid getting dizzy from changes in blood circulation, rise slowly to a standing position when getting up from a chair or a bed. Also, be sure to turn your head slowly.

Keep in touch with others
If you live alone, ask a friend, neighbor, or family member to check on you each day.

Take your time
Don't rush. Most accidents happen because people try to do things too quickly. Take time to be safe.

Stay physically fit
Regular exercise, well-balanced meals, and plenty of rest are important to keeping healthy and safe. Before starting an exercise program, though, be sure to consult your doctor.

Don't rush. Most accidents happen because people try to do things too quickly.

Reducing fire hazards in your home

In North America, more than 2 million people suffer burns each year. Of these, 300,000 are burned seriously and over 6,000 die, making burns the continent's third leading cause of accidental death.

To make sure you and your loved ones don't contribute to these grim statistics, follow these tips.

Eliminate fire hazards

- Store matches out of the reach of children.
- Discard oil cans and oily rags properly.
- Turn pot handles toward the back of the stove when cooking food.
- Use appliances according to their instructions.

Use caution with heaters

- Don't fill kerosene heaters indoors.
- Keep kerosene heaters away from children. Or place a protective device around the heater or around a wood-burning stove.

Banish bad habits

- Never smoke in bed.
- Don't let newspapers or other paper products pile up.
- Don't overload electrical circuits.
- Never use spray cans near a flame.

Perform regular safety checks

- Make sure your home's electrical system is in good working condition.
- Routinely inspect your kitchen appliances.

Be prepared

- Keep a fire extinguisher in the kitchen and in the garage, especially an attached garage.
- Install at least one smoke detector on each floor of your house. Check smoke detectors for proper function several times a year — for instance, when daylight saving time begins and ends.
- Devise and practice a plan for fast evacuation in case of fire.

Safeguarding your home from electric shock

Electrical hazards in your home can cause potentially deadly injury. Use the guidelines below to identify and correct such hazards.

Don't mix electricity with water
■ Don't set a glass of water, a wet towel, or any other wet item on an electrical appliance or electrical equipment.
■ Wipe up accidental spills before they leak into electrical cords and other electrical equipment.

Watch what you touch
■ Don't use an electrical appliance when you're wet or when you're taking a bath or shower.
■ Never touch electrical appliances while touching faucets or cold water pipes in the kitchen. These pipes often provide the ground connection for all circuits in the house.

Keep electrical equipment safe
■ Check for cuts, cracks, or frayed insulation on electrical cords and appliances.
■ Keep electrical cords and appliances away from hot or wet surfaces and sharp corners.
■ If an appliance sparks, smokes, seems unusually hot, or gives you a slight shock, unplug it immediately.

Check plugs and outlets
■ Make sure the ground connections on electrical equipment are intact.
■ Electrical appliances should have three-pronged plugs. The prongs should be straight and firmly fixed.
■ Check to see if prongs on cord plugs fit the wall outlets properly.
■ Don't use adapters on plugs.
■ Inspect wall outlets to make sure they aren't loose or broken.

Beware of extension cords
■ Avoid using extension cords because they may bypass the ground circuit.
■ If you must use an extension cord, don't place it under carpeting or in areas where it will be walked on.

Check electrical cords and appliances for cuts, cracks, or frayed insulation. If an appliance sparks, smokes, seems unusually hot, or gives you a slight shock, unplug it immediately.

HOW TO KEEP YOUR CHILDREN SAFE

Protecting your baby

Understanding how your baby grows and develops will help you keep him or her safe.

Keep up with the changes
Your baby's needs and abilities change with surprising speed as he or she grows. Here are some examples:

■ From birth to age 4 months, babies spend most of their time in the crib. However, they can roll off a flat surface in an unguarded moment.

■ From age 4 to 7 months, babies explore the world outside the crib and can move about quickly, grasp objects, and put them in their mouths.

■ From age 8 to 12 months, babies learn how to climb on chairs and stairs and open cabinets, drawers, and containers.

The suggestions below can help you anticipate potential problems and guard your baby from accidents.

Prevent drowning
■ Keep one hand on the baby at all times while bathing him or her in a tub or bassinet. Never leave the baby alone during the bath; a baby easily can drown in a few inches of water.

■ Don't let your baby enter the bathroom unless you or another responsible person is present. He or she can drown in an open toilet or a cleaning bucket. For the same reason, never leave the baby alone in a wading pool.

Prevent falls
■ Never turn your back when your baby is on a table, in a bed, or in an infant seat.

■ Always use the restraining straps when your baby is in a high chair.

■ Keep the crib sides up.

■ If you're interrupted while caring for the baby, put him or her in the crib, under your arm, or on the floor.

■ Place gates at the top and bottom of stairways.

Reduce the risk of burns and fire hazards

■ Adjust the thermostat on your hot water heater to below 120° F (49° C).

■ Check the baby's bath water temperature with your hand or a thermometer before bathing the baby.

■ Put screens around radiators, floor furnaces, stoves, and kerosene heaters.

■ Don't smoke, and don't let babysitters or other caregivers smoke when caring for your baby.

■ Keep your baby away from flames, including candle flames.

■ Store matches and lighters out of the baby's reach.

■ Make sure all baby clothes and bed linens are flame retardant. Avoid products that have been treated with Tris, a toxic fire retardant that has been banned.

■ Install smoke detectors if you don't already have them. Keep a small fire extinguisher in the kitchen, out of a small child's reach.

Make sure all baby clothes and bed linens are flame retardant. Avoid products that have been treated with Tris, a toxic fire retardant that has been banned.

Avoid scalding accidents

■ Don't hold your baby when drinking a hot beverage.

■ Don't leave a hot beverage on a place mat or near a table edge where the baby could pull it down.

■ When cooking, turn pot or pan handles toward the back of the stove.

■ Don't warm baby food or formula in a microwave oven because it may heat unevenly.

Prevent sunburn and heat exposure

■ Make sure your baby wears a hat or stays in the shade when outdoors.

■ Apply a sunscreen on the baby only as advised by the doctor.

■ During hot weather, cover your child's car safety seat with a towel when parking your car in the hot sun.

Decrease smothering hazards

■ Make sure crib bars are no more than 2 ⅜ inches (6 centimeters) apart so the baby won't get caught between them.

■ Don't use a mesh playpen or a crib that has holes in the mesh.

■ Make sure the crib mattress fits snugly so the baby won't slip between the mattress and the sides of the crib.

■ Keep pins, coins, buttons, and plastic bags out of the baby's reach.

■ Make sure toy chests or trunks have safety hinges (which hold the

lid open). If they don't, remove the lid.
- Don't use a pillow in the crib.

Deter choking accidents

- Select crib toys that can't be swallowed or broken and don't have sharp points or edges.
- Place hanging toys or mobiles out of the baby's reach. Don't string them across the crib.
- Remove toys and other small objects from the crib or playpen before putting the baby down for a nap.
- Move the crib or playpen away from draperies or venetian blind cords.
- Never put a loop of ribbon or cord around your baby's neck — for instance, to hold a pacifier.
- Don't put necklaces, rings, or bracelets on the baby.
- Keep foods that might cause choking (such as nuts, popcorn, or raisins), out of the baby's reach.

Prevent electric shock

- Cover unused electrical outlets with safety caps or tape.
- Keep electrical cords out of the baby's reach so he or she can't chew or pull on them.
- Don't let your baby play with Christmas lights.

Prevent poisoning

- Keep toxic household products, such as cleansers, detergents, pesticides, bleach, liquor, and cosmetics, out of the baby's reach or in child-proofed cupboards, drawers, or storage areas.
- Never store poisonous household products in food jars, bottles, or soft drink cans. Someone may consume the contents or feed them to the baby.
- Keep medicines separate from household products and household products separate from food.
- Buy syrup of ipecac (not the fluid extract, which is toxic) at your pharmacy, and keep it available on your medicine shelf to treat poisoning. However, don't use ipecac unless told to do so by a doctor or a poison control center.

Remove lead from your home

- Paints made before February 1978 may contain lead. If a toy or crib is old and needs repainting, remove the old paint completely.

Use a chemical stripper; sanding spreads toxic particles. Repaint with lead-free household paint, such as a latex-based paint.

■ If your house is old and has chipped paint or plaster, repair it (again, without sanding) and cover it with wallpaper or new paint. If you find old chipped paint or plaster in places you can't repair, have it tested for lead by the health department. If it contains lead, cover the area with wallpaper or fabric, or place furniture in front of it.

Keep emergency numbers handy

■ Post telephone numbers of the doctor, fire department, ambulance, and poison control center near your telephone.

■ Teach older children how and when to dial 911, if available in your area.

What the babysitter needs to know

Besides instructing your babysitter when to put your child to bed, what TV shows and snacks are allowed, and whether or not to answer the door or the phone, make sure the sitter knows what to do in an emergency. Here are some suggestions.

Keep important phone numbers handy

■ Place stickers with emergency numbers on all phones in the house, and make sure the babysitter knows where they are.

■ If you have a pager, show the babysitter how to activate it. Practice using it with the babysitter.

Teach the babysitter about your home and family

■ Make sure the babysitter knows the location of all fire exits and fire extinguishers in your home and knows how to lock and unlock windows and doors.

■ Provide the babysitter with any pertinent medical information about your children.

Babysitter's emergency guidelines

You can use the handy form shown here to help the babysitter direct emergency personnel to your home in case they're needed. Once you fill in the information for the first three sections, you probably won't need to make changes unless you move. However, you may need to revise the information in the last section ("Where the parents are") each time you go out.

BABYSITTER'S EMERGENCY FORM

IN AN EMERGENCY, CALL 911

Non-emergency police telephone number: _____

Emergency rescue number if 911 unavailable: _____

Fire department number if 911 unavailable: _____

Ambulance number if 911 unavailable: _____

Poison control center: _____

Neighbor's phone number: _____

Doctor's phone number: _____

MY LOCATION

Name of resident: _____

Address of residence: _____

_____

Nearest cross street: _____

Directions from nearest cross street: _____

_____

_____

WHO'S HERE WITH ME

Names and ages of children at home: _____

_____

WHERE THE PARENTS ARE

Location (address): _____

_____

Name of resident or business: _____

Telephone number: _____

Pager: _____

Cellular or mobile phone: _____

Using child car safety seats

More children die in motor vehicle accidents than from any other preventable cause. Many of these children might still be alive if the proper safety equipment had been used.

A well-designed safety seat holds the child securely in the vehicle and helps absorb impact in a crash. For older children, lap and shoulder belts provide better protection than lap belts alone. (In fact, using lap belts alone can increase the risk of severe injury or death if an accident occurs). Here are some other tips that will help you keep your child safe in a car.

Select and install seats with care

■ Make sure the child safety seat you select has been crash-tested and meets federal safety standards.

■ Anchor the seat to the car with the car's manual lap belt exactly as specified by the manufacturer. The illustration below on the left shows how to secure a safety seat for an infant or child up to age 4. The illustration on the right shows how to secure a safety seat for an older child.

Many of the children who have died in motor vehicle accidents might still be alive if the proper safety equipment had been used.

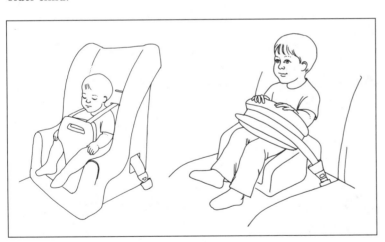

Use the right seat for your child

■ If your child weighs less than 20 pounds (9 kilograms), use an approved child safety seat that is semi-reclining and facing the rear.

■ If your child is age 4 or under and weighs 20 to 40 pounds (9 to 18 kilograms), use a child safety seat that faces forward.

■ If your child is age 4 or under and weighs over 40 pounds (18

kilograms), use a child safety seat intended for a child of that age and size.
- If your car has a passenger-side air bag, don't use a rear-facing infant safety seat in the front seat.
- Convertible safety seats — those that can be used by infants and young children weighing up to about 40 pounds — are usually secured by different belt arrangements. Be sure to use the one that's appropriate for your child.

Use built-in seat belts properly
- For an older child, the car's shoulder belt should cross from the child's shoulder across the chest to the hips. If the belt crosses the child's face and neck, tuck it behind the back — never under the arm. If the child is small, the shoulder belt will fit better if he or she sits closer to the center of the car rather than closer to the door. Adjust the lap belt until it's snug and rests over the child's hips.
- Don't use your vehicle's automatic (passive) safety belts to secure child safety seats. If your car doesn't have a manual lap belt in front, the child safety seat must be installed in the rear seat.

Other instructions
- If your vehicle has been involved in an accident, be sure to replace the child safety seat.
- Never use plastic feeder stands, car beds, pillows, or cushions that aren't certified for use in cars.
- Insist that everyone buckle up when riding in the car, no matter how short the trip.

Preventing accidental poisonings at home

Thanks to lead-free paints and childproof containers, fewer children die each year from accidental poisonings. However, poisoning still accounts for about 5% of accidental deaths in children younger than age 5.

Tireless explorers, young children learn about our world through taste. This means that anything within the child's reach may end up in his or her mouth.

How far can a child reach?

You've probably seen this warning hundreds of times: "Keep out of reach of children." That's easier said than done. Some children can reach as far as an adult can. What's more, children try to get into places that no adult would dream of going. For instance, to an adult a cupboard of common household products isn't exciting; to a child, it's a wonderland to be explored.

The "long arm" of the child

Despite their small size, young children can often find a way to get whatever they see. Because of a child's curiosity and zeal to explore, something placed in the back of a closet isn't necessarily out of his or her reach. Nor is a dangerous substance stored on a high shelf; if the child can see the container, he or she may try to reach it.

Dangerous imitation

Children are born imitators, aping what they see other people do — especially their parents. If they see a parent take medicine, they'll be eager to do the same.

And until they're taught otherwise, children don't know that medicines and other substances can hurt them. They have no fear and no notion of danger. To a child of 5, a box of rat poison looks like a box of cookies.

Of course, you can't watch your child every moment of the day. But you can make your home safe and teach your children the attitudes and behaviors that can keep them safe. Read on for details.

How to poison-proof your home

To keep your child safe, keep in mind the following fundamentals of poison-proofing:

■ Handle medicines properly.
■ Use household products safely and in the manner in which they were intended to be used.
■ Store household products and medicines in their original containers.
■ Keep hazardous substances out of the sight and reach of children.
■ Limit the number of dangerous substances in your home.
■ Keep dangerous substances in their original containers, and store them in assigned, locked locations.

SAFETY TIPS FOR OLDER ADULTS

Avoiding accidents when you're older

The physical and mental changes that come with aging put you at increased risk for accidents and injuries. These changes include:
- impaired vision, hearing, balance, and coordination
- slower reaction time
- reduced physical strength.

What's more, when an older person suffers an injury, it can be more serious because of brittle bones, reduced disease resistance, and slower healing. Here are some tips to help you avoid accidents in the home and outdoors.

Keep floors dry
- Wipe up floor spills immediately.
- Don't walk on a freshly washed or waxed floor until it's dry.

Get rid of skidding hazards
- Tack or tape down all carpet edges.
- Use nonskid tape or backings to secure throw rugs, or replace these with a more secure floor covering.
- Don't walk on bare floors when wearing only socks, slippers, or smooth-soled shoes.

Make stairs safe
- Make sure stairways in your home are well lit, have nonskid treads, and are equipped with handrails without sharp edges.
- Consider painting or marking the top and bottom steps with colored tape to make them easier to see.
- Take your time when climbing up and down stairs.

Make your bathroom a safe room
- Make sure bath mats have nonskid backings.
- Apply nonskid treads to the tub and shower floors.
- Install grab rails in the tub area and next to the toilet, if possible.

Reduce risks when reaching and carrying

■ Make sure your view isn't blocked when moving a heavy package. Get a firm grip on the package. Then slowly lift with your legs and knees bent and back straight, and walk slowly.

■ Get help to handle heavy or awkward objects.

■ Make sure you have a clear path through every room. Don't store things in a doorway, hall, or stair landing.

■ If you must climb, use a sturdy step stool or ladder instead of an unstable chair or box.

■ Avoid using your highest shelves, if possible.

Eliminate outdoor hazards

■ Remove snow, ice, and wet leaves from stairs, porches, and walks.

■ Keep stairs and walkways in good repair.

■ Install handrails at exterior stairways.

■ When walking on icy surfaces, wear rubbers with studded soles or use strap-on ice grippers. Don't wear shoes with smooth soles.

Use caution when walking

■ When walking in town, always use designated crosswalks — that's where drivers look for you. If there are no crosswalks, cross at corners.

■ Before crossing, look both ways, even if you have the right of way. Never assume that drivers obey safety rules.

■ When walking in the evening, wear light-colored clothing and carry a flashlight.

■ In bad weather, give yourself extra time and space. Cars and pedestrians can slip and slide easily in rain and snow.

Cross intersections properly

■ When crossing an intersection on foot, give yourself as much time as possible by starting across at the beginning of a new "walk" cycle on the traffic signal.

■ Don't start crossing in the middle of a "walk" cycle. The average traffic signal assumes a pedestrian walks at 4 feet (1 meter) per second — too fast for many people over age 60.

Stay safe on public transportation

■ Have your fare ready before you board a bus or train so you're not caught fishing for money as the vehicle starts moving.

■ Take your time getting on and off public transportation. Use a handrail to steady yourself.

> *In bad weather, give yourself extra time and space when walking outdoors. Cars and pedestrians can slip and slide easily in rain and snow.*

Safe driving guidelines

Motor vehicle accidents are the second leading cause of accidental death among people age 65 and over. As we age, our vision, energy level, and response time may diminish somewhat, and we may be more easily distracted. To adapt to these conditions, follow these safe driving tips.

Be prepared

■ Plan your travel and errands in advance. Know exactly where you're going and how to get there.

■ Always fasten your seat belt. Its proper use reduces your risk of suffering a serious injury or death if you're in a collision.

Obey traffic laws

■ Watch for and obey traffic signs and traffic lights. They're there to warn you and help you anticipate road and traffic conditions.

■ Always signal before turning to let other drivers know your intentions.

Stay alert or limit your driving

■ If you feel drowsy, pull off at the nearest well-lit rest stop and nap for a few minutes with your doors locked and the motor off. Or leave your car and take a short walk.

■ If you find it harder to drive as you age, do yourself and others a favor by limiting the roads you drive on and the distances and times you drive. For instance, drive fewer miles and stick to familiar roads and streets, if possible. Avoid driving at night, during rush hour, and in winter weather.

Other tips

■ Use your car's rear-view and side-view mirrors to observe other cars on the road. That way, you'll have less need to turn your head and strain your neck to see behind or beside you.

■ Yield the right-of-way. Be safe, not stubborn, and yield to other cars whenever necessary. Insisting on your rights may lead to an accident.

HOW TO STAY SAFE ON THE JOB

Protecting yourself in the workplace

If you work in a factory or other industrial site, you may be at risk for exposure to toxic chemicals, dusts, and fumes. Most workplace chemicals are inhaled; some are absorbed through the skin. Contact with these substances can cause occupational diseases of the skin and lungs, including cancers.

To protect yourself against these workplace hazards, be sure to wear the appropriate protective equipment, such as gloves, goggles, aprons, masks, and special clothing. If your employer provides these items, be sure to take advantage of them. Here are some other tips.

Keep your clothes and skin clean
- Launder protective clothing daily.
- Don't take the clothing home to wash it.
- Use only approved cleaning procedures.
- Wash all exposed skin — hands, arms, and face — with soap and water frequently during the work day, especially before eating, smoking, using toilet facilities, and leaving work.

Learn what to do in emergencies
- By law, certain employers must provide eye fountains and showers for immediate removal of spilled chemicals. Learn where the eye fountains and showers are, and use them when necessary.
- Use an air or gas mask or a respirator, if necessary. Your employer should keep these items and other safety equipment available for employees who work under dangerous conditions.

By law, certain employers must provide eye fountains and showers for immediate removal of spilled chemicals. Learn where the eye fountains and showers are, and use them when necessary.

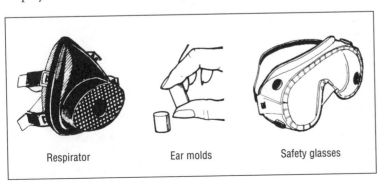

Respirator   Ear molds   Safety glasses

■ In the event of a hazardous chemical spill, leave the room at once. Don't try to clean up the spill yourself. Decontamination of spills is the job of specially trained personnel with adequate safety equipment.

Stay alert for symptoms

Any discomfort or body change can be a sign that you've been poisoned. Be alert for:

■ skin rashes, eruptions, or swelling
■ coughs
■ tightness in the chest
■ difficulty breathing
■ difficulty swallowing
■ a cold that won't go away
■ repeated respiratory infections
■ headaches
■ dizziness or light-headedness
■ eye irritations
■ fatigue
■ nausea
■ loss of appetite
■ numbness in any body part.

If you have any of these symptoms, report to your supervisor and seek medical assistance immediately.

INDEX

A

Abdomen
  injuries to. *See* Abdominal injuries.
  pain in. *See* Abdominal pain.
Abdominal aortic aneurysm, symptoms of, 6, 7, 53. *See also* Abdominal pain.
Abdominal breathing as relaxation technique, 392
Abdominal gunshot wound. *See also* Gunshot wounds.
  damage resulting from, 267i
  symptoms of, 265-266
  treatment of, 267-268
Abdominal injuries, 1-4
  causes of, 1
  delayed symptoms of, 4
  prevention tips for, 3
  symptoms of, 1-3
  treatment for, 3-4
  types of, 1
  what to do for, 3
Abdominal organs, location of, 5i
Abdominal pain, 4-9
  causes of, 5, 5i
  parents' tips for, 8
  symptoms of, 5-7
  treatment of, 9
  what to do for, 7-9
Abdominal stab wound, 487. *See also* Stabbing.
  symptoms of, 487
Abdominal thrusts. *See also* Respiratory arrest.
  how to perform, 434-435
  positioning hands for, 143, 144i
Abrasions, 439-440
  aftercare for, 440
  infection risk for, 439
  symptoms of, 439
  treatment of, 440
  what to do for, 439-440

Abruptio placentae, 544. *See also* Vaginal bleeding.
  symptoms of, 545
  treatment of, 546
Absence seizure, symptoms of, 448. *See also* Seizures.
Absorption of poisons, 411i. *See also* Poisoning.
Abused child, help for, 13. *See also* Child abuse.
Abuse of child. *See* Child abuse.
Abuse of older person. *See* Older person, abuse of.
Abuse of spouse. *See* Spouse abuse.
Abusive man, profile of, 17
Acceleration-deceleration injury, 150. *See also* Concussion.
Accidental amputation. *See* Amputation.
Accident scene, checking out, for safety, 576-577
Accident victim. *See* Injured person.
Achilles tendinitis, 344, 345i. *See also* Leg injuries.
  causes of, 344
  symptoms of, 346
Acquired immunodeficiency syndrome
  human bite and, 62
  mouth-to-mouth resuscitation and, 437-438, 437i
Acute pyelonephritis, 383. *See also* Painful urination.
Adenofibroma, symptoms of, 96. *See also* Breast lump.
Adrenalin, how to inject, 25
AIDS. *See* Acquired immunodeficiency syndrome.
Air bags, advantages of, 129
Air splint, 595. *See also* Splints.

Airway
  blocked, as cause of respiratory arrest, 432. *See also* Respiratory arrest.
  removing foreign object from, 144-145. *See also* Choking.
Akinetic seizure, symptoms of, 447. *See also* Seizures.
Alcohol abuse, effect of, on body, 21. *See also* Alcohol intoxication.
Alcohol intoxication, 20-23
  symptoms of, 20, 22
  treatment of, 22-23
  what to do for, 22
Alcoholism, self-help groups for, 23. *See also* Alcohol intoxication.
Alkali burns, 106. *See also* Chemical burns.
Allergic reaction
  to a drug, 27-30
  to food, 30-33
  to an insect bite or sting, 23-27
Allergy-related swelling, 518i. *See also* Swelling.
Altitude sickness, 33-35
  symptoms of, 34-35
  treatment of, 35
  types of, 33
  what to do for, 35
Amnesia, types of, 351, 352. *See also* Memory lapse.
Amphetamine overdose, 204t. *See also* Drug overdose.
Amputation, 36-40
  symptoms of, 36
  treatment of, 40
  types of, 36
  what to do for, 36-39
Anal fissure, 431. *See also* Rectal pain.
Anaphylactic reaction. *See* Anaphylaxis.

i indicates illustration; t indicates table.

i indicates illustration; t indicates table.

i indicates illustration; t indicates table.

i indicates illustration; t indicates table.

i indicates illustration; t indicates table.

i indicates illustration; t indicates table.

i indicates illustration; t indicates table.

i indicates illustration; t indicates table.